Multicultural Play Therapy

T0383659

Multicultural Play Therapy fills a wide gap in the play therapy literature. Each chapter helps expand play therapists' cultural awareness, humility, and competence so they can work more effectively with children of diverse cultures, races, and belief systems.

The unique perspectives presented here provide play therapists and advanced students with concrete information on how to broach issues of culture in play therapy sessions, parent consultations, and in the play therapy field at large. The book includes chapters on multiple populations and addresses the myriad cultural background issues that emerge in play therapy, and the contributors include authors from multiple races, ethnicities, cultural worldviews, and orientations.

Dee C. Ray, PhD, LPC-S, NCC, RPT-S, certified CCPT-T/S, and CPRT-T/S is Distinguished Teaching Professor and Elaine Millikan Mathes Professor in Early Childhood Education in the Department of Counseling and Higher Education at the University of North Texas, where she is also the director of the Center for Play Therapy.

Yumiko Ogawa, PhD, LPC, ACS, RPT-S, BC-TMH, certified CCPT-S, and CPRT-S is Associate Professor in the Department of Counselor Education at New Jersey City University. She provides play therapy trainings in the U.S. and throughout Asia and is one of the founders of the Play Therapy in Asia Summit.

Yi-Ju Cheng, PhD, LPC, NCC, RPT, certified CCPT-S, and CPRT-S is an assistant professor at Rider University. Her clinical and research interests center on play therapy and diversity in counseling. She is a trainer for the international certification program for Child-Centered Play Therapy and Child-Parent Relationship Therapy.

Multicultural Play Therapy

Making the Most of Cultural
Opportunities with Children

Edited by
Dee C. Ray, Yumiko Ogawa and
Yi-Ju Cheng

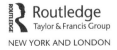

NEW YORK AND LONDON

Cover image: © Getty Images

First published 2022
by Routledge
605 Third Avenue, New York, NY 10158

and by Routledge
4 Park Square, Milton Park, Abingdon, Oxon OX14 4RN

Routledge is an imprint of the Taylor & Francis Group, an informa business

Library of Congress Cataloging-in-Publication Data
Names: Ray, Dee C., editor. | Ogawa, Yumiko, editor. | Cheng, Yi-Ju, editor.
Title: Multicultural play therapy : making the most of cultural opportunities with children / Dee C. Ray, Department of Counseling and Higher Education, University of North Texas, Yumiko Ogawa, Department of Counselor Education, New Jersey City University, Yi-Ju Cheng, Department of Graduate Education, Leadership, and Counseling, Rider University Department.
Description: New York : Routledge, 2022. | Includes bibliographical references and index. |
Identifiers: LCCN 2021050201 (print) | LCCN 2021050202 (ebook) | ISBN 9781032038544 (hardback) | ISBN 9781032038537 (paperback) | ISBN 9781003190073 (ebook)
Subjects: LCSH: Play therapy. | Play therapy--Cross-cultural studies.
Classification: LCC RJ505.P6 M85 2022 (print) | LCC RJ505.P6 (ebook) |
DDC 618.92/891653--dc23/eng/20211119
LC record available at https://lccn.loc.gov/2021050201
LC ebook record available at https://lccn.loc.gov/2021050202

ISBN: 978-1-032-03854-4 (hbk)
ISBN: 978-1-032-03853-7 (pbk)
ISBN: 978-1-003-19007-3 (ebk)

DOI: 10.4324/9781003190073

Typeset in Bembo
by Taylor & Francis Books

To the patient, accepting, and loving children and students who have taught me so much about cultural humility through the years. And to Yumi and Yi who are my greatest examples of cultural humility, opportunity, and comfort.

– Dee C. Ray.

To my family, friends, professors, mentors, colleagues, clients, and students, you all are my greatest teachers who have taught me humility and acceptance.

– Yumiko Ogawa.

To my family, who always encourage me to experience and learn from the world. To my professors, friends, colleagues, students, and clients who have nurtured my growth. Also, to Dee and Yumi, whom I have the honor to learn from and work with.

– Yi-Ju Cheng

Contents

Illustrations

Figures

Tables

Contributors

Elizabeth V. Aguilar, MS, LPC-Associate, NCC is a doctoral student at the University of North Texas specializing in play therapy. Elizabeth's experience and research interests are focused on Latinx and Spanish-speaking populations, trauma, and multicultural related issues.

Peggy Ceballos, PhD, NCC, CCPT-S, CPRT-S is Associate Professor in the Counseling Program at the University of North Texas. Dr. Ceballos specializes in multicultural and social justice issues in play therapy and school counseling.

Yi-Ju Cheng (she/her), PhD, LPC (TX & NJ), NCC, RPT, Certified CCPT-S, Certified CPRT-S is an Assistant Professor at Rider University and her clinical and research interests center on play therapy and diversity issues in counseling. She serves as a trainer for the international certification program for Child-Centered Play Therapy and Child-Parent Relationship Therapy.

Regine K. Chung, MS, LPC Associate, CAS is a doctoral student in the Department of Counseling and Higher Education, and assistant director at the Center for Play Therapy, University of North Texas. She actively promotes the awareness of cultural and diversity issues in the play therapy field through research and scholarship while developing as a counseling supervisor and educator.

Geri Glover, PhD, LPCC, NCC, RPT-S has worked with children and families for over 30 years in education, day treatment programs, private practice, mental health clinics, and is currently Professor and Chair of the Counseling Department at New Mexico Highlands University. She completed her early research in Filial Therapy with Native Americans residing on the Flathead Reservation in northern Montana in honor of her Salish ancestry and has worked for and with a number of tribal nations throughout her career.

Tamara Iliff, MS, LPC, NCC, RPT is a doctoral counseling student at the University of North Texas, where she specializes in play therapy and psychoeducational assessment of children. Tamara currently serves as the Assistant Director of Assessment Services at the Child and Family Resource Clinic, where she provides supervision and training for doctoral students in psychoeducational assessment of children.

Kimberly M. Jayne (she/they), PhD, LPC, NCC, RPT-S, Certified CCPT-S, Certified CPRT-S is an Associate Professor in Counselor Education at Portland State University, a practicing play therapist and supervisor, researcher, and author of numerous book chapters and research articles on play therapy and child development.

Yung-Wei Dennis Lin, PhD is an Associate Professor at New Jersey City University, and is currently the Research Committee Chair at the Association for Play Therapy.

Natalya Ann Lindo, PhD, LPC, Certified CCPT-S, Certified CPRT-S is an Associate Professor and Department Chair at the University of North Texas with more than 15 years of experience as a researcher and clinician with specialized training in working with children and families, diverse and at-risk populations. Dr. Lindo's primary research areas are school-based play therapy, child-parent relationship therapy, teacher-child relationship building, and career development across the lifespan.

Ahou Vaziri Line, LPC, CSC, NCC is currently working as a mental health counselor in a private practice where she serves children, adolescents, and adults. Ahou is also a doctoral student at the University of North Texas where she specializes in play therapy and has research interests in clinical considerations for immigrants and work with parents.

Yumiko Ogawa, LPC, ACS, RPT-S, BC-TMH, CCPT-S, CPRT-S is Associate Professor in the Department of Counselor Education at New Jersey City University. Dr. Ogawa has been providing play therapy trainings in the U.S. and Asian countries, and she is one of the founders of the Play Therapy in Asia Summit.

Kristie K. Opiola (she/hers), PhD, LCMHC, RPT, CCLS is an Assistant Professor in the Department of Counseling and Counselor Education and Assistant Director of the Multicultural Play Therapy Center at UNC Charlotte.

Katherine E. Purswell, PhD, LPC-S, RPT, CCPT-T/S is Assistant Professor and Director of the Institute for Play Therapy at Texas State University. She has experience working with children in play therapy in a variety of settings and has published articles and book chapters on the subject.

Dee C. Ray, PhD, LPC-S, NCC, RPT-S, Certified CCPT-T/S, Certified CPRT-T/S is Distinguished Teaching Professor and Elaine Millikan

Mathes Professor in Early Childhood Education in the Counseling Program and Director of the Center for Play Therapy at the University of North Texas.

Mónica Rodríguez Delgado, MA, LPC, NCC, Certified CCPT-S, Certified CPRT-S is a doctoral student at the University of North Texas where she specializes in play therapy. During her tenure at UNT, Mónica has worked with Spanish-speaking populations across multiple environments including schools, clinics, agencies, and in communities after disasters.

April Schottelkorb, PhD, LCPC, RPT-S, Certified CCPT/CPRT-Supervisor is a former school counselor and counselor educator who currently works in private practice at Big Sky Pediatric Counseling and Consulting in Kalispell, MT, with specializations in CCPT, CPRT, and play therapy supervision.

Hayley Lurie Stulmaker, PhD, LPC-S, NCC, RPT-S, Certified CCPT-T is the Owner and Counselor at HLS Counseling, PLLC. She is currently a private practitioner, specializing in play therapy. She has also worked in school and community agency settings with a wide variety of clients, taught at the university level, and has over ten years of experience in play therapy.

Alyssa M. Swan, PhD, LCPC, RPT, NCC is an Assistant Professor in the Counseling and Integrated Programs Department at Adler University in Chicago, IL.

Karrie L. Swan, LMHC, LPC, CCPT-T/S, CPRT-T/S is an Associate Professor at Missouri State University as well as consultant and clinician with Marimn Health, the Coeur d'Alene Tribal Hospital.

LaKaavia Taylor, PhD, LPC, NCC, RPT is a Clinical Assistant Professor in the University of North Texas Counseling Program, with clinical expertise in counseling children, adolescents, and families. She has delivered presentations at numerous national and state professional conferences, published research on play therapy, and contributed to *A Therapist's Guide to Child Development: Extraordinarily Normal Years*.

Sarah Tucker, PhD, LPC (TX), NCC, RPT, Certified CCPT-S is a Clinical Assistant Professor of Counseling at the University of Louisiana Monroe and a private practice owner/clinician. She specializes in Child-Centered Play Therapy and Child-Parent Relationship Therapy, and supervises counselors seeking CCPT certification.

Krystal K. Turner, MA, LPC-Associate, NCC hails from NC, where she received both her Bachelor's and Master's degrees from the University of North Carolina at Charlotte and is currently completing her PhD in Counseling and Play Therapy at the University of North Texas. Krystal's education and career have largely been focused on play therapy and trauma with a multicultural lens, with hopes to continue serving as an advocate in the African American community through teaching, research, and clinical work.

Cody T. (Lankford) Wehmeier, MS, LPC (TX), NCC, Certified CCPT-S, Certified CPRT-S is currently a doctoral candidate within the UNT Counseling Doctoral Program, where he has focused on child-centered play therapy and relational depth in counseling and counselor training. He additionally works full-time as a counselor and play therapist in private practice, specializing in power and control seeking children, filial therapy, and LGBTQ+ experiences.

Terence Tsien Li Yee, PhD is an Assistant Professor at Villanova University who is passionate about the intersection between play therapy, cultural competency, and anti-racism.

Introduction

The origins of this book began in small conversations in small offices over many years. Our conversations have been professionally focused on sharing the most effective ways to address cultural inclusivity in our counseling and classrooms, and they have been personal in sharing our vulnerability regarding our challenges, pride, excitement, hurt, and anger stimulated through our intercultural interactions. Although our roles for this volume are co-authors and co-editors, the three of us have relationships that span student-teacher, counselor-supervisor, mentee-mentor, and eventually colleague-to-colleague and friend-to-friend. Conversations encompassing cultural diversity and its impact on play therapy are typical for our personal interactions, taking place in a trusted and safe relationship. It is through this long-standing relationship that we embarked on this idea that we wanted to share the framework and types of conversations that keep us encouraged and enthusiastic about cultural inclusivity.

As the three of us are play therapists, we are characteristically concerned about cultural inclusivity, or lack thereof, and its impact on children. Over the last 20 years, we have all worked with children and families of diverse identities and from varied backgrounds. We have spent countless hours in discussions on play therapist attitudes and skills that best serve diverse children, as well as modifications to structures and materials in the playroom to provide safety and sense of belonging for child expression and exploration of cultural identity. We have participated in our own personal exploration of bias, contribution to systemic oppression, and ways to raise our self- and other-awareness of cultural embeddedness. We have sought training and knowledge on varied cultures, and taught others to increase cultural competence. Although we have actively sought to grow in our cultural awareness, attitudes, and skills through formal opportunities, we acknowledge that we have learned the most through our clients, the children we serve. A child in the playroom who expresses their pride, confusion, or hurt related to cultural identity is the best teacher of how critically important it is for play therapists to embark on a journey of cultural awareness, humility, and competency. We offer this book as a support for this journey.

DOI: 10.4324/9781003190073-1

Multicultural Orientation Framework

We conceptualize this book from the multicultural orientation (MCO) framework presented in Owen et al. (2011) and further examined in Davis et al. (2018). MCO embraces a way of being with clients in which the therapist is "guided primarily by therapists' philosophy or values about the salience of cultural factors (e.g., racial/ethnic identity, client's cultural background) in the lives of therapists as well as clients" (Owen et al., 2011, p. 274). The MCO consists of three pillars including cultural humility, cultural opportunities, and cultural comfort. *Cultural humility* is the organizing principle of the MCO (Davis et al., 2018) in which the therapist holds an attitude of humility and focus on the other person in therapeutic interactions and is manifested in overall way of being. It is through an attitude of cultural humility that a therapist engages in *cultural opportunities* whereby a therapist recognizes opportunities and actively enters into exploration of a client's cultural identity and experiences. When operating from cultural humility and actively engaging in cultural opportunities, the therapist is ideally able to enter into relationships and conversations with a greater sense of ease and less reactivity around clients' cultural identities, noted as *cultural comfort* (Davis et al., 2018). The MCO theoretically results in deeper therapeutic relationships with clients overall. We are particularly encouraged by MCO research that supports the relationship between MCO constructs and positive therapy outcomes related to client reports of the therapeutic relationship and progress toward therapy goals (Davis et al., 2018).

Our choice to embrace the MCO is grounded in the philosophical consistency between the MCO and child-centered play therapy (CCPT). CCPT is a humanistically oriented play therapy in which the relationship between therapist and child is considered the primary agent of change (Axline, 1947; Landreth, 2012). Play therapy developed from the observation that play is the developmental language of children, the language by which they express their feelings, wishes, experiences, and thoughts. In play therapy, children use toys and materials to express what they struggle to express through verbalization. The humanistic philosophy of CCPT guides the therapy approach with the belief in the innate forward-moving nature of children to grow toward self- and other-enhancing ways of being when provided with a safe, accepting environment. The safe, accepting environment is facilitated by the play therapist who provides attitudinal conditions of genuineness, empathic understanding, and unconditional positive regard (Ray, 2011). When children feel safe, understood, and highly regarded, they will naturally move toward feelings, behaviors, and thoughts that enhance themselves and others. They will typically use play to work through their struggles, express their experiences and perceptions, and build relationships. CCPT therapists trust children to direct their play where it needs to go, and therefore value permissiveness within the play therapy relationship (Landreth, 2012). CCPT therapists are called upon to engage in their own work toward authenticity, ability to fully empathize with the child, and movement toward deep relationships. CCPT is an evidence-based intervention with decades of research to support its effectiveness (Lin & Bratton, 2015; Ray et al., 2015).

Our commitment to effective multicultural practices and identification as CCPT therapists led us to a theoretical exploration of intersecting constructs between MCO and CCPT. Both CCPT and MCO are grounded in a focus on the relationship between client and therapist. In CCPT, relationship is the therapy (Landreth, 2012), and in MCO, the therapist's orientation is designed to deepen the relationship between client and therapist (Davis et al., 2018). As CCPT therapists, we are particularly motivated to explore relationship variables in order to create fuller, more meaningful relationships with children. MCO provides an avenue for creating such relationships. When a child is seen holistically through the lens of multiculturalism, we believe that we are engaging in deeper levels of relational connection, the goal of the CCPT therapist. The attitudes of the therapist as humble, authentic, motivated to engage in cultural opportunities with ease, and valuing those interactions are constructs that crossover between CCPT and MCO. The MCO emphasis on cultural inclusivity as an ongoing process is also consistent with CCPT advocacy for play therapists to engage in life-long pursuit toward genuineness, authenticity, and self-regard. The purpose of these pursuits in CCPT is the recognition that when play therapists engage in continued self- and other-awareness, they are more fully capable of providing acceptance and regard for clients (Ray, 2011). As a CCPT therapist pursues awareness and knowledge regarding self and relationships with others, this journey certainly requires exploration of cultural aspects of self and others. Additionally, this journey requires accountability for play therapists' contribution and advocacy toward an environment that facilitates optimal development for children, inside and outside of the playroom.

Furthermore, CCPT is an approach rooted in humanistic philosophy that promotes the positive potential of the person. The humanistic approach to therapy values the self-direction of the client which underlies advocacy for freedom and autonomy in therapeutic encounters. Play therapies based in humanistic philosophy typically value the therapeutic relationship over techniques and structured activities initiated by the therapist. Because CCPT is one approach to humanistic play therapy, we embrace the broader reference to humanistic play therapy throughout this book. The reader will find that authors often interchangeably refer to the specific approach of CCPT while at other times speaking more broadly to humanistic play therapy.

Due to the integration of CCPT humanistic philosophy and MCO in our conceptualization, we chose to frame and structure the book toward these ideals. We seek to explore the connection between play therapy and MCO through a deeper look at cultural humility (Chapter 1) and cultural opportunities and comfort (Chapter 2). Chapter 3 broadens the conceptualization of seizing cultural opportunities through emphasis on advocating for social justice in the larger field of play therapy. These chapters are followed by explorations of ways in which we can attend to understanding the needs of specific populations and seize cultural opportunities to deepen our relationships.

Group Populations

The MCO framework allowed us to explore multicultural inclusivity in play therapy from a process perspective. Through an emphasis on the process, including the personal work for which play therapists are responsible, we hoped to provide support for play therapists to develop the capacity to embrace and effectively serve in cross-cultural relationships (Grauf-Grounds et al., 2020). However, through this volume, we also sought to provide content training on multiculturalism; specifically, ways in which play therapists can engage in cultural opportunities with distinct populations. Content-oriented chapters can be problematic because they tend to focus on between-group differences (Grauf-Grounds et al., 2020) or they can negate within-group differences and perpetuate stereotyping. However, the content chapters are deeply embedded in the constructs of the MCO, resulting in a process orientation that leads to richer exploration of specific populations.

In addition, as we discuss in Chapter 1, we embrace accompaniment of cultural humility and cultural competence rather than seeing them as mutually exclusive (Greene-Moton & Minkler, 2020). I (YO) remember a conversation with a Black therapist friend when I started learning about cultural humility. My excitement about this concept and the limited knowledge on it back then emphasized too much of the other-oriented perspective and the stance of learning from the client. My therapist friend said, "But Yumi, we are tired of teaching others about our culture…" I stopped breathing for a moment but I really appreciated her honest feedback because it made me think more about the balance, balancing a way of being and doing. The content-oriented chapters in this volume facilitate the "doing," encouraging the work we do outside of therapy to enhance our knowledge and skills, nourishing our curiosity about a client's life in all of its aspects. This is the homework. On the other hand, the process-oriented chapters discuss how to be with a client given enhanced knowledge of a client's cultural background while holding the courage to put aside what we know "about" a client's culture and concentrate on creating moments of connection through seeking to know the person of the client and how they experience their intersecting cultural identities.

Specifically, in Chapter 4 on LGBTQIA populations, the authors explore the integration of the gender affirmative model with the humanistic approaches to play therapy to provide a myriad of cultural opportunities that honor children's autonomy. Chapter 5 on religious populations focuses on ways that religion affects the lives of children and their families and how play therapists can recognize and incorporate such impacts in the process of therapy. The authors of Chapter 6 on populations with disabilities present how child-centered play therapy is uniquely positioned to support children with disabilities and how play therapists can work with families and systems to advocate for the population. Chapters 7 through 11 look deeply into different ethnic groups including Indigenous, Black, Latinx, Asian, and Middle Eastern populations. The authors highlight the mental health of children of these racial/ethnic groups and share specific considerations and implications in play therapy when cultural opportunities emerge. The authors of Chapter 12 discuss the developmental journey of White play therapists to become allies through raising awareness and responding to cultural opportunities in the playroom. In Chapter 13, the author emphasizes the psychosocial concerns of childhood poverty, as well as the intersectional connections between poverty and cultural identities, and provides concrete ideas for integrating socioeconomic considerations into work with children in play therapy.

Special Topics in Multicultural Play Therapy

The final section of this volume presents principal topics that serve to extend a culturally inclusive movement in play therapy. In Chapter 14, the author provides a comprehensive discussion of play therapy supervision, including the intersecting identities of supervisor, supervisees, and child clients and how they impact the play therapy process. In Chapter 15, the authors present outcomes from a recent research study on developing consensus for the definition, structure, and materials of a multicultural playroom. Chapter 16 summarizes the findings from both quantitative and qualitative research regarding the impact of humanistic play therapy approaches on racially/ethnically diverse children and families. In the appendix of the book, we offer reflective questions matched to book chapters for the purpose of encouraging self-reflection while building cultural competencies. Overall, the chapters share a certain level of structure; at the same time, each chapter also demonstrates its distinct features and writing styles which reflect the specific content covered and the cultures of chapter authors.

The Authors

We are particularly honored to have worked with the chapter authors for this volume. The authors represent a diverse group of scholars who are also practicing play therapists. The contributors to this book actively practice play therapy, advocate for multiculturally inclusive practices in and outside of play therapy, and are representative of diverse identities. Each population-focused chapter is authored by scholars who personally identify with the population about which they are writing. We noted early in the writing process that authors approached their chapters from an attitude of cultural humility and commitment to encouraging play therapists to embrace cultural opportunities. Even though many of our authors have endured racism, sexism, and homophobia, as well as xenophobic, ableistic, and religious oppression, among other prejudicial aggressive acts, they emerged with a strong commitment to helping play therapists better serve their clients of intersectional identities. Throughout the chapters, they vulnerably share their stories of their personal work and the work of their clients. The personal and professional knowledge they share are incredibly poignant for our day-to-day work in play therapy.

Due to the multicultural framework and the commitment to the humanistic approach to play therapy that grounds this book, we are pleased to include positionality statements for each author. As is traditional in most textbooks, we provide a professional description of each author. Yet, within each chapter, authors were influenced by their experiences, identities, and understandings. We believed that the contributed chapters were so helpful and so moving that we anticipated readers would want to know the "truth" of the authors. In each chapter, the reader will find positionality statements in which authors vulnerably and humbly share their perspectives and framework from which they personally see the world. The three of us share our positionality statements at the end of this introduction in order to disclose our realities within the context of multiculturalism.

Conclusion

We present this book as a potential source of support for play therapists who are engaged in their own cultural journeys. We know that we have made many mistakes with clients through low levels of awareness or discomfort in seizing opportunities. We do not pretend to have the answers. In our safe spaces, we talk with each other and other colleagues about our shortfalls and ways to become more culturally sensitive to children and their families. We seek to grow in our skills of cultural inclusivity and advocacy. We offer forgiveness, grace, and acceptance to others and ourselves as we navigate the complexity of culture with the intention of growing from each and every relationship in play therapy. In this book, we hope to provide encouragement to all play therapists on this journey.

Positionality Statements

Dee

I am typically seen by others as a middle-aged, educated, White woman. In order of personal salience, I identify with being White, woman, mother, Christian, southerner (in U.S. terms), middle-aged, wife, and middle-class. I realize I listed many identities but I often find it difficult to tease them apart as the ones I listed are intimately integrated into how I see myself and each identity holds cultural implications for me. At any given time, I will identify more closely with one identity over the other. The identity of being White is an identity that I have only come to claim as salient to me in the last decade. Being raised in the generation where "not seeing color" was considered progressive and the way to end racism, I was slow to embrace being White as an identity. As I have worked to raise my awareness and knowledge, I have found that acknowledging and claiming my "whiteness" is essential to my relationships with others and keeps me more attuned to how I am being perceived by others. It is an aspect of my identity that I consistently have to keep at the forefront of my awareness, an acknowledgment of my privilege. I have identified as a strong feminist and Christian since a young age, both which have propelled my advocacy efforts for women and girls. Although I am now educated and considered in middle-class, my early childhood was influenced by a strong identity with the working class, as both my grandparents who I spent considerable time with while growing up were factory workers in rural Georgia. The feminist, Christian, Southern, and maternal aspects of my identity drive my need for advocacy in helping others. Yet, I often need to step back to reflect on my identification as a "White savior," and my need to step in to take control rather than staying in the background as a foundational support for others. I have learned the most about my personal limitations in my work as a counselor educator through interactions with my students and clients. I have had the great honor over 24 years to work with people of diverse identities and cultures. It is in conversations where students/clients share vulnerability, where I am confronted, where I am challenged that I have grown in my cultural awareness, humility, and competence in doing better. This book has been a labor of love that I embarked on with two people who have taught me so much about cultural humility and opportunities by simply being who they are, and being in safe spaces with them for almost 20 years.

Yumi

"Being a minority" was not a part of my perceived identity until I moved to the U.S. more than 20 years ago. I first attributed it to the fact that the country that I grew up in (Japan) is a very monocultural country. Yet, later, I realized it was also because of my ignorance and unawareness because there are in many aspects diversities in my own country. Once I faced the undeniable fact that I am a minority in the United States, my journey to embark on racial identity development started. I can remember many instances that reflected my place in identity development at different points in my life; however, there was one salient moment.

During my graduate program which was my very first formal educational experience in the U.S., I became extremely self-conscious about my accented English and started receiving accent reduction speech therapy. In one session, a speech therapist was trying to help me make a perfect shape of a tongue by pressing my tongue with a tongue presser so that I could pronounce a certain word accurately. My tongue was not flexible enough to make such shape that it never made in my life, and I gagged.

Then, a stream of tears came out from my eyes. My speech therapist thought it was because of gagging but I knew it was because of the sudden and intense wave of frustration, helplessness, and sadness. Walking back from the speech therapy session to home, I talked to myself. "I will never speak English like a native speaker, my friends still accept me despite of my accented English. I can try to speak better but why am I working so hard hoping to be someone that I can't be?" I chose not to go back to speech therapy after this session; however, something shifted in me as a play therapist since this incident. I became less anxious when a child noticed cultural differences between us; "You speak funny." "Are you from China?" "Your hair is so black!" I became more able to respond to those cultural opportunities from a place of understanding, empathy, and attunement; with greater cultural comfort.

Through my cultural identity development, I profoundly experienced that famous "curious paradox" that Carl Rogers wisely but simply put: "the curious paradox is that when I accept myself just as I am, then I can change" (Rogers, 1961, p. 17). I deeply appreciate all children that I worked with for giving me a courage to be becoming. The process of becoming continues and I am eager to move forward in this process because there is nothing more rewarding when I feel connected with children from an authentic place. A long time ago, when I introduced myself to a child client saying, "Hello, my name is Yumi," her face brightened up and she said, "It sounds like 'You' and 'Me'!" I look forward to having more authentic "you and me" time as a play therapist.

Yi

I (Yi) am from Taiwan. I fit under the category of Asian, but I am not Asian American. I also identify myself with being a middle-class, able-bodied, heterosexual woman, and a mother. Before coming to the U.S. to pursue an education in counseling and play therapy, I had the privilege of not having to think about my race and how it impacts my life and societal status. As someone who comes from an international and Asian cultural background, culture shock and homesickness were not the only two things I experienced in the U.S. Some of the personal and professional encounters I have experienced were characterized by microaggressions, discrimination, doubt, and exclusion, while many others featured support, care, acceptance, and recognition. These cultural opportunities have not only cultivated but also challenged my understanding and acceptance of myself and my cultural humility for others.

I don't speak "perfect" English, and I will always have an accent. This is hard to share but my accent and the way I look, for some reason, have caused me to experience distrust and even rejection by my clients. I have been asked by some parents where I am from, how long I have been in the U.S., and whether the cultural differences may impact the therapy process for their child. Sometimes, they have requested a different therapist even before we start therapy. Their concerns were understandable, but having this understanding did not make it less hurtful or discouraging for me. I remember asking the clinic director (it was Dee during that time): "When is this going to end?" Sharing these experiences reminded me of how powerless and small I felt, and in this very moment, I also realized maybe these are the same feelings that many children often experience in their daily life.

Touchingly, my same accent, skin color, and ethnicity have become points of connection between myself and many of my play therapy clients. I worked with a Black boy who simply stood and stared at me during our first play therapy session. All of a sudden, he said, "I am from China too, and I know Kung Fu!" Delving more deeply into my interactions with this child will certainly yield a fruitful discussion. However, what I most earnestly want to share at this time is that the boy recognized that we are different and wanted to connect with me. He made the connection by presenting how "he and I were alike," based on his perceptual world of information and understanding. The desire to convey connection and acceptance was the most powerful thing that the child and I were able to offer to each other in our relationship. I hold moments like this close to my heart because they have become a part of who I am today.

I know I will never be able to truly, fully know or understand all cultures, and maybe it is not my optimal goal to do so. I do hope, though, I will be able to attend to each child and our relationship from a place of humility, genuine curiosity, and vulnerability. The question I have for myself as continuing to work with children is: How can I connect with my child client as who they are, through their unique worldview, and with who I am? All children need a safe relationship in which their whole self, including their cultural self, can be recognized, cared for, and regarded, and I believe play therapy can be a place for such experience to unfold (it needs to be).

References

Axline, V. (1947). *Play therapy*. Ballantine.

Davis, D. E., DeBlaere, C., Owen, J., Hook, J. N., Rivera, D. P., Choe, E., Van Tongeren, D. R., Worthington, E. L., Jr., & Placeres, V. (2018). The multicultural orientation framework: A narrative review. *Psychotherapy*, 55(1), 89–100. doi:10.1037/pst0000160.supp (Supplemental).

Grauf-Grounds, C., Sellers, T., Edwards, S., Cheon, H.S., MacDonald, D., Whitney, S., & Rivera, P. (2020). *A practice beyond cultural humility: How clinicians can work more effectively in a diverse world*. Routledge.

Greene-Moton, E., & Minkler, M. (2020). Cultural competence or cultural humility: Moving beyond the debate. *Health Promotion Practice*, 21, 142–145. doi:10.1177/1524839919884912.

Landreth, G. (2012). *Play therapy: The art of the relationship*. Routledge.

Lin, Y.-W., & Bratton, S. C. (2015). A meta-analytic review of child-centered play therapy approaches. *Journal of Counseling & Development*, 93(1), 45–58. doi:10.1002/j.1556-6676.2015.00180.x.

Owen, J. J., Tao, K., Leach, M. M., & Rodolfa, E. (2011). Clients' perceptions of their psychotherapists' multicultural orientation. *Psychotherapy*, 48(3), 274–282. doi:10.1037/a0022065.

Ray, D. (2011). *Advanced play therapy: Essential conditions, knowledge, and skills for child practice*. Routledge.

Ray, D. C., Armstrong, S. A., Balkin, R. S., & Jayne, K. M. (2015). Child-centered play therapy in the schools: Review and meta-analysis. *Psychology in the Schools*, 52 (2), 107–123. doi:10.1002/pits.21798.

Rogers, C. R. (1961). *On becoming a person*. Houghton Mifflin.

Part 1

The Multicultural Orientation in Play Therapy

1 Cultural Humility and the Play Therapist

Dee C. Ray, Yumiko Ogawa and Yi-Ju Cheng

As we talked about writing this book, we started with our experiences as play therapists and in play therapy. All three of us are practicing play therapists, play therapist supervisors, and play therapy educators. We talked about our experiences with children who were similar to and different from us culturally. We talked about supervisees and their experiences with us and with their child clients. We talked about our students and our experiences in understanding, teaching, and modeling cultural self- and other-awareness. We all had experiences of missed opportunities, misunderstandings, and defensiveness. However, we also all had experiences of true encounters with children, students, supervisees in which we authentically and vulnerably made contact with another person, seeing all of the person. All of the person is comprised of hopes, dreams, beliefs, struggles, pain, joy, relationships, and so much more; and all of the person is comprised of multiple identities intersecting in complex ways and developed in cultural contexts. To really know a person, to really know a child, the play therapist seeks to understand all of the child, embraces the child's worldview, and holds the utmost respect for that worldview. As discussions about the book progressed, we acknowledged our sincere desire to know children culturally and the reality that we are always limited in fully knowing another person. This is a humbling place to be. Yet, embracing this humility seemed to be the chord that struck all three of us. We cannot ever fully know the cultural experiences and perceptions of another but we *seek* to know with great curiosity, care, and empathy for the person. Hence, we have attempted to write this chapter and edit this book from this place of humility.

Let us start with the word "culture." What is it? There are so many academic texts, popular books, and research studies conceptualizing culture that it can be dizzying to take it all in. We find that conceptualizing culture in its complexity may be more helpful than providing a singular definition. In synthesizing over 300 definitions across disciplines, Faulkner et al. (2006) defined culture as consisting of seven themes: structure/pattern (patterns or regularities among a group/norms for behavior), function (what culture does or accomplishes/outcomes), process (an active creation by group of people/ongoing actions), product (symbolic or material products produced

DOI: 10.4324/9781003190073-3

by groups), refinement (moral development/intellectual attainment), power/ideology (focus on power as central characteristic of culture), and group-membership (shared understanding of world/shared communication system). The multiple and diverse definitions of culture are likely a main reason that any discussion regarding culture can become confusing and lead to misunderstandings. Faulkner et al. caution against attempting to provide one definition due to the variations in perspectives. For our purposes, we hope play therapists will see that culture can be a group defined by a specific similarity such as skin color, orientation, nationality, gender, culture can be ongoing process in which a group may be continually progressing in communication or productivity, or culture can be defined as power-holding/dominant groups in comparison with non-dominant groups. A child may see their culture as belonging to a group who looks like them, while the child's parent may see that the child's culture is defined as being in a powerless/oppressed position, while the play therapist may see the child's culture as the ongoing development of childhood. When these three perspectives come together, the key is for the play therapist to have high awareness of the various perspectives and activate empathic understanding for each worldview. Coming back to our focus on cultural humility, the play therapist does not assume that the meaning of culture is the same for everyone.

In one example of cultural intersection, I (DR, a White play therapist) supervised a case in a school setting in which a Black child was being seen by an Asian play therapist who consulted regularly with a White teacher. As the child was leaving the playroom, he accidentally fell and suffered a serious injury to his face. The play therapist took the child to the school nurse who administered aid and then called the mother for the child to be taken to the doctor. I reviewed the incident carefully with the play therapist and it was clear that the therapist could not have prevented such an unexpected accident. In the meantime, the teacher had made quite a few assumptions about the play therapist, seemingly based on the therapist's race, including that the play therapist must have been unassertive and unable to handle the child which led to the accident. The teacher shared this view with the mother, a Black woman. The mother was not only upset about receiving this information, but was also humiliated at the doctor's office when it was assumed that she might have abused or neglected her child and had to defend herself to keep protective services from being called. The mother was understandably upset and immediately wanted play therapy services terminated. In this situation, as a White supervisor, I simply wanted to figure out how to problem-solve and did not initially consider all the cultural implications of the persons involved (example of the privilege I unknowingly operate from at times). So, I ensured that the play therapist had acted competently and that the child's injury had been treated. It was only when I received calls from school administration about the mother's complaints that I began to consider and explore all the cultural intersections taking place. Although, being White, I was familiar with previous experiences related to the teacher's bias, the humiliation experienced by the mother in taking her child to the doctor was not something that had even come into my awareness. And, of course, there were implications for the play therapist who had done her job well and yet her competency was being questioned due to what appeared to be racial bias. I was humbled in empathizing with the mother's experience and worldview and the therapist's experience of the situation. It was humbling because it was a moment of in-your-face awareness of my privilege and how comfortable it is for me to see children as children, and not all the cultural intersections and meanings of those intersections that surround them. It was humbling because I felt an intense amount of White guilt in that I never had the experience of taking my child to the doctor and being worried that I might be reported to protective services – and more guilt relative to the teacher, a White woman like me, who acted with such prejudice and destructiveness. I was angry, sad, and guilty all at the same time. And yet, ultimately, this situation was about how to put the child first; a Black child who obviously felt connected to and positively regarded by his Asian play therapist. In order to put the child first, it was essential for me to put aside all my feelings and tap into the worldview of all the adults to work out a way for the child to continue with his therapist in play therapy. I needed to engage in the humility that I did not know what was best and my role was to bring together the perspectives of all involved.

What is Cultural Humility?

We hope to provide real-life play therapy examples of cultural humility in action but we also want to contextualize those examples in literature. The term cultural humility was coined by Tervalon and Murray-Garcia (1998) in the context of training medical professionals to work more effectively with culturally diverse patients. Hook et al. (2017) defines cultural humility as, "an awareness of one's limitations to understanding a client's cultural background and experience... an interpersonal stance that is other oriented rather than self-focused in regard to the cultural background and experience of the client" (p. 9). Through cultural humility, the play therapist honors the reality that there are a multiplicity of truths and experiences based on a person's identities, background, and experiences. Hook et al. go further to discuss aspects of intrapersonal and interpersonal dynamics that make up cultural humility.

Intrapersonal dynamics include the therapist's awareness of personal cultural identities and background and the impact of those identities and background on the ability to honestly evaluate personal reactions to clients. For example, if my five-year-old client begins to curse in session, do I have immediate thoughts that such cursing is wrong for a young child and must be the result of his low socioeconomic status? If this is my automatic thought, what do I do with it? Intrapersonal cultural humility calls for honest introspection regarding my biases toward people and communities who are impoverished and my rigidity in accepting the child as is rather than seeing him as just one of his "group." What is the extent of my bias? How did I get to this bias? How do I work within myself to challenge this bias? Furthermore, the culturally humble play therapist is open to feedback and integrates feedback into self-evaluation. Feedback may come in the form of children, parents, supervisors, or supervisees.

Interpersonal dynamics involve my openness and curiosity toward others in therapeutic interactions, my willingness to engage in beliefs and values that are different from my own (Hook et al., 2017). Do I allow my biases to get in the way of truly knowing others, engaging in conversations that are difficult, or accepting others' experiences? In order to practice the interpersonal element of cultural humility, I attempt to operate from a place of curiosity and respect when working with others. I want to know how the child sees the world, how the parent sees the world, and further how the child's teacher or grandparent sees the world. My curiosity drives my willingness to engage in uncomfortable conversations that bring us closer together. In Chapter 2, we will talk more about how to move toward cultural comfort when operating from interpersonal cultural humility. Going back to the five-year-old who curses, holding interpersonal cultural humility means that I want to know more about what motivates this child from this child's complex background to express himself through cursing. Instead of setting a limit which I may have done operating from implicit bias (i.e. lacking intrapersonal cultural awareness), if I am operating from high intrapersonal and interpersonal cultural humility, I will likely recognize my automatic thought as out of my control, forgive myself for harboring unacknowledged biases, commit to working on this bias outside of session, and move into engaging with the child with curiosity with a possible response of "You are using all kinds of words to show how you feel." Such a response allows the child to continue to engage in expression to lead to therapist's greater understanding of the child's world. Of course, all of these dynamics take place in seconds flat in order to be present with the child but these are practices that help play therapists move toward greater depths of cultural humility.

Cultural Humility and the Philosophy of Play Therapy

As editors of this book, we believe one reason we were so drawn to the concept of cultural humility as part of the guiding framework for this book is that humility is a cornerstone of child-centered play therapy (CCPT), a humanistic developmentally appropriate intervention for children. One of our favorite quotes from Dr. Garry Landreth (2012) is that it is the play therapist's job to "discover that which I don't know that I don't know I don't know" (p. 81). A fun but accurate quote. The play therapist's role is characterized by intense curiosity to fully know the child with no a priori assumptions coming into the relationship. The play therapist enters the relationship with the child with no preconceived notions about who the child is or the child's worldview. The therapist recognizes that the best way to understand a child's behaviors and emotions is to empathically discover the way in which a child sees his or her world (Ray & Landreth, 2019).

Originating from Rogers' (1951) person-centered approach to therapy, CCPT holds that children enter the world with a self-actualizing tendency toward maturity, freedom, and self- and other-enhancing behaviors. Yet, as children develop and interact with others, they develop concepts of self, made up of perceptions from such interactions with their immediate and outside worlds. Interactions may or may not be congruent with the child's self-concept. This part of the theory is especially salient to cultural understanding from a CCPT perspective. A child whose needs are met through immediate family members, who develops a strong attachment bond, and who lives in non-threatening circumstances is expected to experience self as congruent with interactions and assumed to be well-adjusted. However, a child who is of a non-dominant race may grow up in those same family circumstances yet receive negative messages about the way they look, experience daily microaggressions, and be forced to navigate unmanageable obstacles due to systemic oppression. For this child, the greater culture has introjected values that are likely to be internalized by the child, even under favorable familial conditions, leading to incongruence between the child's experience of self within the family and the child's experience of self outside of family. In person-centered language, these introjected values are internalized by the child and may become conditions of worth (Rogers, 1951). For example, a Mexican-American child who experiences acceptance and worth from her immediate family may struggle when she watches children who look similar to her being detained in poor environments, being told that she cannot speak Spanish outside of her home, and experiencing daily reminders that her Mexican-American looks and culture do not measure up to expectations of the dominant culture. The world sends messages that she may internalize as conditions of worth (e.g. I am only of worth if I speak English, I am only of worth if my skin is light). We can also further this example to attempt to understand how complexities increase when a child is receiving messages that they are not of value from both family and society. Such experiences of incongruence are likely to lead to emotions and behavior that are developmentally beyond the ability of the child to understand or express in words.

In play therapy, the child is able to use the language of play to express through the symbols of toys/materials how they see themselves, how they see those with whom they are in intimate relationships, and how they experience the outside world. The play therapist trusts that the child is innately designed to move toward enhancement if provided with a carefully designed therapeutic relationship in which the child experiences the therapist's congruence (i.e. authenticity), unconditional positive regard, and the communication of empathic understanding (Ray, 2011). The CCPT experience has the potential to provide an optimal environment for the child's expression of intersectional identities and cultures. With cultural humility, the play therapist follows the lead of the child to enter the child's internal framework, working to fully grasp all identities and experiences of the child. And with cultural humility, the play therapist engages with the child to facilitate full expression of the child's perception of culture or cultural experiences. The play therapist does not shy away from the difficult and complex expression of culture but remains present and attuned to the child to provide safety and relational support for the journey of exploration. It is through the experience of feeling entirely understood and accepted as a person of worth and belonging that a child is able to explore and express self and world in the developmentally appropriate language of play.

In cultural context, the therapist attitudinal conditions of genuineness, unconditional positive regard, and empathic understanding are therapeutic factors that lead to meaningful cultural encounters and healing. Genuineness, also referred to as congruence, requires therapist self-awareness, acceptance of such awareness, and appropriate expression of awareness to the client (Ray, 2011). Cultural humility intersects the CCPT concept of genuineness in that both focus on the therapist's commitment to ongoing self-awareness, including awareness of beliefs, values, biases, and privileges. Furthermore, these areas of awareness are accepted by the therapist and accurately symbolized as part of the self-structure. For particular areas of bias or privilege, the acceptance of their existence within the self-structure allows for the therapist to openly and honestly work through harmful implicit and explicit predispositions that interfere with the therapeutic encounter, rather than denying or distorting beliefs that lead to relational disconnection.

The therapist's experience and communication of unconditional positive regard for the client sends the message that the child is accepted without any requirement to change or be different from who they are (Axline, 1947; Ray, 2011). The connection between cultural humility and the therapist's ability to experience unconditional positive regard for the client rests in the therapist's desire to accept and honor all identities and cultural beliefs/expressions of the child. The therapist's effectiveness in experiencing and communicating unconditional positive regard is the antidote to the conditionality that has been internalized by the child (Bozarth, 1998). For children who have been sent messages with conditions of worth, particularly children of color, the play therapist offers a therapeutic environment in which all parts of the child are valued and where there are no conditions of worth. The child is free to be exactly who they are. This freedom is a powerful force for children who struggle with cultural identity and feelings of belongingness.

The third therapist attitudinal condition is empathic understanding and it is within this concept that we find the greatest bond to cultural humility. Rogers (1975) said it best himself when he defined empathic understanding as

> entering the private perceptual world of the other and becoming thoroughly at home in it. It involves being sensitive, moment to moment, to the changing felt meanings which flow in this other person, to the fear or rage or tenderness or confusion or whatever, that he/she is experiencing.
>
> (p. 4)

Through empathic understanding, the therapist sets aside their own world and elevates the world of the child as cultural humility requires. The therapist never assumes that they completely know and understand the child's world but actively seeks to see the world from the child's eyes necessitating the therapist act of setting aside their own worldview.

These therapist attitudinal conditions are operationalized through the therapist's way of being and actions in the playroom. In CCPT, the therapist follows the child's lead in play and conversation, seeking to understand the child and the child's world without interference based on the therapist's worldview. The therapist's desire to follow the child's lead potentially results in minimizing power differences. Through reflections of content, feeling, relationship, and themes, the therapist sends the message that the therapist is present, attuned, and accepting of the whole child and the child's worldview. The therapist sends messages of encouragement and belief in the child's capability through self-esteem building responses, returning responsibility to the child, and facilitating creativity. Finally, the therapist provides ample opportunity for the child to explore self-regulation and self-initiated outcomes through limit-setting (Ray, 2011). An ideal CCPT session is a manifestation of a therapist's willingness to engage in cultural humility.

The connections between congruence, unconditional positive regard, empathic understanding, and cultural humility are meaningful and at first glance may seem uncomplicated in their delivery. However, in play therapy, when the identities and culture of the client meet the identities and culture of the play therapist, there are challenges to the play therapist to remain self-aware, authentic, and fully present in the child's world.

Nia's Story

I (DR) saw Nia, a five-year-old Black girl who was referred for a high level of aggression exhibited in school. At Nia's school, the population was majority Latinx, with the second largest demographic being White, and a small minority of Black students (approximately 10%). From the first session, Nia identified the spider as her toy of focus (a large black spider) and demonstrated fear of the spider. When she finally picked up the spider to begin playing with it, she placed the spider under the white sand of the sandbox. She verbalized that the spider needed to be covered with white so that people would like him. If people saw the black on the spider, they would think he was bad and scary. Over the next couple of sessions, Nia continued to play and verbalize that people were scared of the big black spider but really it was the spider that was scared of them. She further expressed that they did not really know the spider which is why they were scared of him. It was clear that at five years of age, Nia had internalized messages of how the dominant culture viewed her as a Black girl, including that her skin color was scary to others. She further expressed how lonely and misunderstood she felt which led to the "spider" being aggressive toward others. As the play therapist, I was aware that I was having strong feelings as a White woman watching this play and hearing her story. My first reaction was wanting to tell her, "You don't have to be White to be worthy and understood," "Your Blackness is beautiful," "You're worthy just the way you are," "You can love your Blackness." "You should love yourself the way that I love you." I realized all of these reactions were born from my own worldview, my White guilt, my need to act as a White savior, and a need for her to feel worthy so that I could experience relief from my own uncomfortable feelings. Fortunately, this disconnection from the moment lasted for a few seconds, and then I was able to come back to being present with Nia. In entering her world, I was able to respond with empathic understanding and hopefully with some cultural humility by putting her world first, "You think if he's White, they'll like him better." "If he's Black, you think they'll be scared." "It's confusing about whether he should be Black or White." "He really just wants people to know he's nice and not scary." Her response to my responses was to continue her expression of confusion and then she moved into finding ways to nurture the spider herself so that he would be taken care of. In reading this story, one might ask my rationale for not trying to build her up with positive affirmations, or question whether my reflective responses could be taken as agreement with her. My response to these types of questions is that Nia already experienced racial discrimination and its effects on her self-concept. She had already internalized conditions of worth based on her race. If my response was that it does not have to be that way and you can feel better about yourself, not only would that have probably been an inauthentic reaction to soothe my own cultural discomfort, it would have sent the message that what she has already experienced in her few short years is somehow not true or that it is not something that is okay to share. Rather, I wanted to offer her the environment to fully express all the reality of discrimination and its resulting confusion so that she had the opportunity to work through what the world is like for her and how she is going to navigate in the world as a young Black girl. Through accepting the reality of her world and her need to express her confusion, I sought to be a supportive partner who journeyed with her as she worked through the reality that she was going to have to nurture herself in order to cope with discrimination and oppression. I sought to send her the message that she is not alone in this confusing world and I would be with her through it, but not attempt to inauthentically rescue her from it.

In reflecting on this interaction further, each co-author of this chapter had a unique perspective on relational dynamics and cultural messages. I (YO) responded to the potential of highlighting power differences between therapist and child if the play therapist had responded with a "it doesn't have to be this way and you can feel good about yourself" type of response, as if the play therapist has the authority to determine what a child should feel and not feel. Because the play therapist is an adult, children naturally see that power is not distributed equally and this sense can be amplified by the difference in race between child and play therapist. Instead, the play therapist seeks to diminish power differences through providing the attitudinal conditions and accepting the child's reality. I (YC) noted the power difference beyond the playroom in that if a White play therapist who has substantial societal power based on race sought to minimize or invalidate the child's experiences due to their own discomfort, guilt, or desire to rescue, this would be confirmation of the child's lived experiences of being unseen or misunderstood.

Laura's Story

I (YO) met Laura, a third-grade Latinx female, at an elementary school where I provide school-based play therapy. Laura's school is located in an urban area and the majority of the student population is Latinx (approximately 95%) and about 90% of the students are from economically disadvantaged households. Laura's teacher referred her for play therapy because of her inattentiveness, lack of motivation and confidence. Laura was polite, articulate, and seemingly more mature than typical third graders. She liked drawing, in particular drawings of animals, and preferred talking to playing with toys for the first couple of sessions. During the second session, she asked me where I was from, if I was living with my "mom and dad" and if I had a brother or a sister. While I reflected her curiosity about my background, I briefly answered her question because I sensed that this was a part of her exploratory "play" and her way of expressing her desire to create contact with me. When I told her that my parents were back in my country and I did not have a family member in the United States, her eyes lit up and she said, "Me, too!" Then she started sharing that she came to the United States with her grandmother three years ago, and her parents and her younger brother were staying in her home country in Central America. She said she was missing all the animals that she had at her house in her home country: dogs, a cat, chickens, and a horse. In the next moment, her emotional tone changed and she shared in a somber voice how much she was missing her parents and her brother, and that she was told by her parents that they would send her to the United States with her grandma so that she could have a better life. She wondered if they might like her younger brother better than her because they did not send him to the United States, and said she still preferred living in Central America with her family. While she was sharing her painful thoughts and feelings, her eyes welled up with tears.

My knee-jerk reaction was wanting to console her by giving a pseudo pep talk such as, " I bet your mom and dad really love you, too," or giving her some other ways to think about her situation based on the knowledge I had learned about the sociopolitical situation in Central America like, "I heard gang members in Central America are really bad and perhaps it is safer for girls to live in the U.S." Those responses felt effective for a moment, effective particularly to reduce my pain, discomfort, and anxiety. The pain was stemming from witnessing her sadness. The discomfort and anxiety emanated from how she appeared to feel connected with me because I also lived away from my parents. I knew, however, that my situation was a much more privileged one than hers and I felt a sense of guilt about it.

Moreover, those responses are not theoretically grounded within CCPT and would not embody the therapist attitudinal conditions of genuineness, unconditional positive regard, and empathic understanding. I was trying to "do something" for her and myself, rather than being with her. The main task of a CCPT therapist is to offer a healing relationship, not the expert knowledge and application of techniques. It is important to be aware in the power of staying with a client's actual process and experience and the importance of letting go of knowledge. Wilkinson (2010) stated, "whatever experience and knowledge person-centered therapists bring to the practice, their job is to immerse themselves in the client's experience and to respond to that and only that" (p. 197).

Of course, thorough grounding in the theoretical orientation and acquisition of knowledge about a child's cultural background and additional skill sets are essential to work effectively with them, and they are what constitute competence. Yet, when play therapists enter the therapeutic relationship with children, they need to be courageous enough not to clutch to that knowledge and skills, but rather to let go of them and be open to the child's worldview, and imbue ourselves in it. That is, in fact, the "other-oriented" stance that cultural humility is based upon.

My training and experience allowed me to engage in such mental gymnastics to process multiple reactions and feelings in a split second and make decisions to deliver therapeutic responses. I tamed the original urges and instead chose to see the world from her eyes. "You miss your family so much and wish you were with them…" She also mentioned that she had not shared her feeling of missing her family with anyone, particularly with her grandma because she did not want to make her sad. After a couple of sessions of her sharing her longing for her family, she started playing with the kitchen toys, and she started sharing her future dream of opening her own bakery when she grew up.

Cultural Humility and Common Cultural Terms

Now might be a good time to discuss definitions a little more in relationship to the concept of cultural humility. Literature on culture and multicultural therapy have presented a myriad of terms that are ubiquitously yet unevenly used. And just as culture itself changes over time, communication and description of cultural terms progress. One of the terms with which most therapists are familiar is "cultural competence." Cultural competence is one of the earliest terms used to provide standards to mental health professionals for increased awareness and engagement in multicultural practices. The difficulty with cultural competence is the grammatical structure of the term and how it has been interpreted over the years. The word "competence" is a noun (i.e. person, place, or thing), and as such implies that you either have the thing or you do not. Based on the term competence, professional mental health organizations have now spent decades defining what makes up competence by creating "competencies," also a noun. Therefore, cultural competence standards are typically filled with competencies of which the therapist possesses or does not possess (e.g. National Association of Social Workers, 2003; Ratts et al., 2015). Writers and researchers in the cultural arena have pointed out the fallacy in the expectation that cultural competence is a place that a therapist arrives at or a thing that is possessed by the therapist (Grauf-Grounds et al., 2020; Hook et al., 2017). Instead, a therapist aspires toward being more culturally aware, culturally humble, and culturally engaging, knowing there is no end state to the process. The play therapist will never arrive at competence because if competence is achieved then there is no place for greater learning which is an essential component of cultural humility. There is always more to learn. In Sue et al.'s (2019) seminal text on counseling the culturally diverse, they emphasized the aspirational nature and lifelong process of cultural competence during which the therapist engages in actions or conditions that promote the development of clients and client systems. Greene-Moton and Minkler (2020) suggest that cultural humility and cultural competence do not have to be a forced choice but are terms that are complementary to the process of inclusivity, as cultural humility is a way of being while cultural competence is a way of doing. The integration of cultural humility with cultural competence is a pathway to self-reflection and reflective practice resulting in serving clients more effectively and challenging systems of oppressions that impact clients.

Additional terms that have emerged over the years include culturally responsive, culturally adaptive, and culturally sensitive. These terms are typically used interchangeably and indicate that a mental health professional is operating from awareness and responding to the needs of a particular client population or culture. I (DR) have personally used the term culturally responsive most frequently and up until the writing of this book felt that it was a way to be inclusive in my language when talking about culture and play therapy. When embarking on the multicultural playroom research project (see Chapter 15), as a research team, we were writing our research proposal and I automatically used the culturally responsive term. One of the research team members graciously stopped me to express her hesitation with the term. I could not imagine that there would be an issue with this term so I was curious as to her thinking, moving into an awareness of a need for increased cultural humility on my part. Because I was intrigued by her viewpoint, I wrote a quote from her, "Responsive indicates that I am reacting when someone different walks through the door," rather than our goal of creating an inclusive environment for all clients (K. Turner, personal communication, February 22, 2021). This statement really hit me as an accurate interpretation of the word and my use of the term. I have since moved to using terms such as culturally inclusive or multiculturally inclusive. I aspire to not just react to the children and families coming through my door but to be open, ready, and inviting to all who come through my door. I believe this is the difference between the responsive/adaptive/sensitive terms and cultural humility. As play therapists have learned over the last decades, language is integrally related to the expression of and communication between cultures. The ability of play therapists to adapt to language use is crucial to the expression of unconditional positive regard for clients in their cultural contexts.

Research on Cultural Humility and Therapy

To date, research exploring cultural humility and various aspects of the mental health profession is still developing, yet a few studies have supported the role of cultural humility in treatment outcomes perceived by clients. For example, clients who perceived their counselors as more culturally humble reported stronger working alliances (Hook et al., 2013). An association was found between clients' perceptions of their counselors' cultural humility and microaggressions experienced in counseling sessions (Hook et al, 2016), and that cultural humility and microaggressions were negatively related to counseling outcomes (Davis et al., 2016). Also, Owen and colleagues (2014) found that when clients with higher religious commitment see their counselors as culturally humble, greater counseling outcome was reported. In addition, scholars have started paying attention to the manifestation of cultural humility in clinical supervision (e.g. Cook et al., 2020). Although research conceptualizing and investigating cultural humility has not been explored in the field of play therapy, these findings support the integration of cultural humility as an essential aspect of working clients in therapy process.

Ways for Play Therapists to Embrace Cultural Humility

As mentioned, cultural humility is an aspirational process in which the play therapist seeks to raise self and other-awareness in the context of culture and intersecting identities for the purpose of understanding and elevating the child's worldview. For play therapists, cultural humility is essential not only with child clients but with parents, teachers, and all other systemic partners in the child's life. The practice of cultural humility with multiple clients and systemic partners is a substantial process for the play therapist and may be aided by preparation for engaging in this work toward humility.

Self-Evaluation

The first exercise we recommend toward cultural humility is raising awareness through self-evaluation. Hook et al. (2013) developed a client-rated measure of therapist cultural humility which included rating items such as therapist is respectful, considerate, open to exploring, genuinely interested in learning more, open-minded, open to seeing things from client's perspective, asks questions when uncertain, assumes they know a lot already, makes assumptions about clients, is a know-it-all, acts superior, and thought they understood more than they actually did. For play therapists, an honest self-evaluation of these types of questions related to play sessions and parent consultations may help raise self-awareness. Additionally, the scale could be provided to parents to measure the parent's perception of the play therapist's cultural humility. The scale is readily available in Hook et al. (2013; 2017). This could also be used as a supervision tool by which supervisors could engage in observations and discussions with supervisees on issues related to these items.

Earliest Memory of Race

Consistent with a play therapy approach to expression and growth, we recommend engaging in expressive arts activities to raise awareness and explore identities for therapist and client. One such activity is the "Earliest Memory of Race Drawing." For this activity, each person is provided with a large piece of art paper and markers/crayons/colored pencils. The person is asked to close their eyes as the facilitator leads a brief relaxation exercise of breathing and presence. The facilitator then asks the person to visualize the first time they became aware of race. The script is:

> As your eyes remain closed, I'd like for you to remember the first time you became aware of race. What was the first time you became aware of your own race, someone else's race, or race in general? Now take a minute to picture yourself in that moment. How old were you? What do you look like? How are you dressed? Where are you? Who is around you? What is happening? How are you feeling in the moment? What are you doing? What are you thinking? What is happening with others? How are they feeling? What are they doing? When you're ready, I'd like for you to open your eyes and draw your vision.

The facilitator will provide ample time for the drawing. When the person finishes the drawing, the facilitator asks the person to share their drawing, including their story of the event, their feelings, and thoughts. Once the person has shared with the facilitator or fellow group member, the facilitator asks the person to share their feelings about participating in the drawing and what it meant for them. This particular activity is helpful in small, cohesive groups in which participants can share openly and safely with each other. The goal of this activity is two-fold in that it serves to raise self-awareness of the play therapist regarding origins of beliefs about race. And secondly, this drawing activity is specifically helpful for play therapists because it is intended to remind them that awareness and resulting beliefs about culture start at very early ages, the same ages as the clients they serve; thereby raising their awareness that culture is a living dynamic for their current clients.

Play Therapist/Client Culture Collide

The use of sandtray to explore cultural identities and their connection to play therapy offers a visceral experience to raise awareness. The "Play Therapist/ Client Culture Collide" activity begins with dividing the sandtray into two sections. In one section, the play therapist is asked to create a scene in which the play therapist shares all their salient cultural identities. The play therapist may need to be prompted to share identities related to gender, race, ethnicity, sexual orientation, socioeconomic status, religion, ability, and any other salient identity for the therapist. In the second section, the play therapist is asked to do the same scene for their child client. In the processing of the tray, the play therapist is asked to share their feelings as they look at their scenes and reflect upon similarities and differences between the two sides. Another extension of this activity is to divide the sandtray into three sections and the play therapist is asked to add an identity scene for the parent, as well as therapist and child.

World Without Power and Privilege

The sandtray activity discussed above can also be modified and used to explore the play therapist's awareness of the power and privilege related to their cultural identities. The "World without Power and Privilege" activity begins with asking the play therapist to divide the tray into two sections. The facilitator asks the play therapist to spend some time reflecting on the cultural identities that are salient to them and create a scene that represents their world consisting of their feelings, thoughts, and experiences related to these identities in the first section. Then the play therapist is asked to close their eyes and imagine that they now live in a world without power and privilege. The play therapist is guided to reflect on how their life and lived experiences might have been changed as a result of no power and privilege existing in this new world. The facilitator gives the play therapist 30 seconds to one minute to immerse themselves in this world of imagination followed by asking the play therapist to present this scene in the second section. To process, the facilitator helps the play therapist to reflect on their experiences creating these two scenes, what they notice about these two scenes, and what they learn about themselves and meanings of the power and privilege they hold in the society. Lastly, the facilitator invites the play therapist to ponder how the cultural identities that bring them power and privilege interact with the therapeutic process, the relationship building, and the understanding and conceptualization of clients in play therapy. This activity can also be done using drawing or collage.

There are several additional resources available to play therapists to engage in activities that focus on awareness and greater cultural humility. We recommend *Cultural Humility: Engaging Diverse Identities in Therapy* (Hook et al., 2017), *The Racial Healing Handbook* (Singh, 2019), University of Oregon Division of Equity and Inclusion Cultural Humility Toolkit (https://inclusion.uoregon.edu/cultural-humility-toolkit), and *Connecting Across Cultures: The Helper's Toolkit* (Hays, 2013).

Conclusion

In this chapter, we sought to introduce the concept of cultural humility as essential to the play therapy process and highlight the intersecting philosophies behind cultural humility and child-centered play therapy. The decision to place the chapter on cultural humility as the first chapter of this volume was intentional, as we firmly believe that an attitude of cultural humility is necessary for the practice of cultural inclusion, as well as general effective practice in play therapy. The ability of the play therapist to be "other-oriented" and place self as second when moving into the world of a child are qualities of humanistic and culturally humble play therapists. The humanistic culturally humble play therapist knows that they are limited in their abilities to fully know all the cultural intersections of a child's world but continuously strives toward self-awareness of bias, privilege, and oppression in order to guide practice and develop deeper relationships with children. Cultural humility is the very cornerstone of relational connection in play therapy.

References

Axline, V. (1947). *Play therapy*. Ballantine.

Bozarth, J. (1998). *Person-centered therapy: A revolutionary paradigm*. PCCS Books.

Cook, R. M., Jones, C. T., & Welfare, L. E. (2020). Supervisor cultural humility predicts intentional nondisclosure by post-master's counselors. *Counselor Education & Supervision*, 59, 160–167. doi:10.1002/ceas.12173.

Davis, D. E., DeBlaere, C., Brubaker, K., Owen, J., Jordan, T. A., Hook, J. N., & Van Tongeren, D. R. (2016). Microaggressions and perceptions of cultural humility in counseling. *Journal of Counseling & Development*, 94(4), 483–493. https://doi.org/10.1002/jcad.12107.

Faulkner, S., Baldwin, J., Lindsley, S., & Hecht, M. (2006). Layers of meaning: An analysis of definitions of culture. In J. Baldwin, S. Faulkner, M. Hecht, & S. Lindsley (Eds.), *Redefining culture: Perspectives across the disciplines* (pp. xxx). Lawrence Erlbaum Associates.

Grauf-Grounds, C., Sellers, T., Edwards, S., Cheon, H.S., MacDonald, D., Whitney, S., & Rivera, P. (2020). *A practice beyond cultural humility: How clinicians can work more effectively in a diverse world.* Routledge.

Greene-Moton, E., & Minkler, M. (2020). Cultural competence or cultural humility: Moving beyond the debate. *Health Promotion Practice*, 21, 142–145. doi:10.1177/1524839919884912.

Hays, P. (2013). *Connecting across cultures: The helper's toolkit.* Sage.

Hook, J. N., Davis, D., Owen, J., & DeBlaere, C. (2017). *Cultural humility: Engaging in diverse identities in therapy.* American Psychological Association.

Hook, J. N., Davis, D. E., Owen, J., Worthington, E. L., Jr., & Utsey, S. O. (2013). Cultural humility: Measuring openness to culturally diverse clients. *Journal of Counseling Psychology*, 60(3), 353–366. doi:10.1037/a0032595.

Hook, J. N., Farrell, J. E., Davis, D. E., DeBlaere, C., Van Tongeren, D. R., & Utsey, S. O. (2016). Cultural humility and racial microaggressions in counseling. *Journal of Counseling Psychology*, 63(3), 269–277. doi:10.1037/cou0000114.

Landreth, G. (2012). *Play therapy: The art of the relationship.* Routledge.

National Association of Social Workers (2003). *Standards and indicators for cultural competence in social work practice.* Retrieved from www.socialworkers.org/LinkClick.aspx?fileticket=PonPTDEBrn4%3D&portalid=0.

Owen, J., Jordan, T. A., Turner, D., Davis, D. E., Hook, J. H., & Leach, M. M. (2014). Therapists' multicultural orientation: Client perceptions of cultural humility, spiritual/religious commitment, and therapy outcomes. *Journal of Psychology & Theology*, 42(1), 91–98.

Ratts, M. J., Singh, A. A., Nassar-McMillan, S., Butler, S. K., & McCullough, J. R. (2015). *Multicultural and social justice counseling competencies.* Retrieved from www.counseling.org/docs/default-source/competencies/multicultural-and-social-justice-counseling-competencies.pdf?sfvrsn=20.

Ray, D. (2011). *Advanced play therapy: Essential conditions, knowledge, and skills for child practice.* Routledge.

Ray, D., & Landreth, G. (2019). Child-centered play therapy. *Play Therapy Magazine*, 14, 18–19.

Rogers, C. (1951). *Client-centered therapy: Its current practice, implications, and theory.* Houghton-Mifflin.

Rogers, C. (1957). The necessary and sufficient conditions for therapeutic personality change. *Journal of Consulting Psychology*, 21, 95–103.

Rogers, C. (1975). Empathic: An unappreciated way of being. *The Counseling Psychologist*, 5, 2–10.

Singh, A. (2019). *The racial healing handbook: Practical activities to help you challenge privilege, confront systemic racism & engage in collective healing.* New Harbinger.

Sue, D. W., Sue, D., Neville, H., & Smith, L. (2019) *Counseling the culturally diverse: Theory and practice* (8th ed.). Wiley.

Tervalon, M., & Murray-Garcia, J. (1998). Cultural humility versus cultural competence: A critical distinction in defining physician training outcomes in multicultural education. *Journal of Healthcare for the Poor and Underserved*, 9(2), 117–125.

2 Cultural Opportunities and Comfort in Play Therapy

Yumiko Ogawa, Yi-Ju Cheng and Dee C. Ray

During the past decade, exploration of cultural humility as a concept and practice has pervaded the mental health literature and it has been promoted through numerous trainings, workshops, and presentations. Accordingly, studies of cultural humility in clinical practice have proliferated (Hook et al., 2017). This rapid recognition of cultural humility is partially a response to current incidences of systemic inequalities and structural racism. In the meantime, cultural humility has also been criticized for not offering a practical advantage over multicultural competence (Danso, 2018) and promoting a superficial tolerance to cultural difference rather than the stated goal of cultural humility as cultivating an intentional, lifelong commitment of cultural self-analysis, learning, and growth (Ross, 2010).

However, it is often forgotten that cultural humility is only one of three pillars that make up the multicultural orientation (MCO) framework. The two other components of MCO that serve as equal foundational principles are cultural opportunities and cultural comfort (Hook et al., 2017; Owen et al., 2016). Cultural opportunities and cultural comfort offer a practical framework from which to enact the principles of the MCO. In this chapter, we will take a deeper look into those two components and how they can be applied in play therapy practice.

Cultural Opportunities

Cultural opportunities are the moments during a counseling session when there is an opening to directly attend to clients' cultural identities (Owen, 2013). Cultural opportunities are markers that occur in therapy because of the clients' cultural beliefs, values, or other aspects of the client's cultural identity, all of which may be explored (Owen, 2013; Owen et al., 2016) as a way to deepen the therapeutic relationship. Seizing cultural opportunities is the expression of cultural humility within the MCO framework (Hook et al., 2017). Play therapists seek to consistently engage in opportunities to explore the child's and the family's salient cultural identities.

Cultural opportunities emerge in play therapy in various formats. Children's lived cultural experience may be embedded in their symbolic play or

DOI: 10.4324/9781003190073-4

it may be played out in pretend play. Other times, cultural opportunities are presented verbally as concrete information that children express and, often, originates from the systems in which they live. For example, a Black child client creates an animal kingdom with animal dolls during a play therapy session. He chooses a black horse as the main character of his narrative and creates a story in which the black horse was a kind and caring horse but other animals were scared of him and underestimated him because of his color; because he was black. Another Black child may play out a scene in a playroom where he, his family, and neighbors are having a party by "blasting" music and dancing. He asks the play therapist to be one of the guests of the party. Then, he pretends that he and the play therapist heard a police car, have to turn the light off, and stay quiet, otherwise they will be taken to a jail or shot. Another playroom example may be a Caucasian child who goes to a school with 90% Latinx population says in a concerning tone, "Our president is saying that we should build a wall…" All of these examples are real-life examples from our play therapy practices. Cultural opportunities emerge often in play therapy, providing the play therapist with ample opportunities to facilitate cultural exploration.

In addition, cultural content may emerge during play therapy in a relational context between the child and the therapist. For instance, in one session a child client asked me (YO) why I came all the way from China to Texas to play with her. In another case, my car key accidentally fell from my pocket during a play therapy session. As soon as the child client saw it, he said, "So you have Mercedes? BMW? Lexus? What kind of fancy car do you have?" He lived in an economically disadvantaged neighborhood and the family had to take public transportation because they did not own a car.

In play therapy, cultural opportunities may emerge as a unified theme as demonstrated through three markers of theme identification: repetition, intensity, and context (Ray, 2011). Themes are typically identified when children engage in repetitive play scenes or verbalizations, approach their play with a different intensity than is typical for them, and the therapist is knowledgeable of the fit between the child's play and the child's background experiences. Culture itself can be an independent theme or imbued in other themes. In the aforementioned example, the child who created the animal kingdom was dealing with the theme of his cultural identity, which also contained the more specific themes of helplessness and powerlessness. Alternately, unlike a theme, cultural opportunities may emerge as one-time events, or more sporadically and ephemerally.

Responses to cultural opportunities in play therapy vary based on multiple factors such as a child client's developmental stage and also a therapist's theoretical orientation. We propose that it is crucial for all play therapists to be aware of and capture cultural opportunities in play therapy by responding to them therapeutically, even in those instances when they are presented briefly or subtly. Owen et al. (2016) found that therapy outcomes were negatively associated with clients' ratings of therapists' missing cultural opportunities. Children may not be cognizant of a moment when a play therapist missed a cultural opportunity in a session; however, they may viscerally experience the missed moment as dissonance or disconnection. Cultural opportunities are typically described within the context of adult counseling. Hence, it may be challenging for play therapists to picture ways in which cultural opportunities are addressed in session with children. In the next section, we will introduce examples of cultural opportunities and play therapists' responses to such moments.

Examples of Cultural Opportunities in Play Therapy

Aaron

Aaron, a seven-year-old White boy, puts animals in the sand. Suddenly, he walks toward the corner of the shelves and reaches out his arm to get the cardboard blocks underneath. He takes a bunch of them and starts building something in the sandbox.

I (YC) reflect, "It looks like you just had an idea, and you are building something in there."

Aaron replies, "I am building a wall."

I say, "Oh, you want me to know that you are building a wall."

"Yes! We have to build a wall so that Mexicans can't come to our country," Aaron says, putting the blocks next to each other across the big sandbox on the floor. I feel stunned and do not know what to say, and then he moves on with his play.

We would like to ask the reader to pause here and examine your reactions and comfort level at this moment? Does your mind just go blank, or are there a million thoughts and feelings coming through? How would you respond if you were the play therapist? How sure are you about how you would respond? For me, I was overwhelmed by my immediate emotional reaction. "How can he say that? That is racist!" As judgmental thoughts emerged, I doubted myself and failed to focus on the child's experience, instead focusing on my own internal processes. Even today, I still wonder what I could have said and what might have been different afterward.

One question that students often ask in the play therapy course is, "What should we say if the child client makes racist comments?" Is it the play therapist's role (ethically) to address racism and prejudice shown by a child in the playroom to promote antiracism? If we do not educate the child client about racism and the effects of racism when the moment happens in the playroom, what does it imply about our ability to address multicultural issues and our sense of social justice as play therapists? We encourage play therapists to continue reflecting on and having discussions with each other on these topics because there are no simple yes or no answers. Although reaching a consensus on these issues may be difficult or even impossible, play therapists are encouraged to continue to practice being aware of and staying within cultural opportunities with a sense of cultural humility to further our understanding of the child and ourselves, as well as deepen therapeutic relationships with children.

Just because a child is the one who makes a racist comment, the comment is no less disturbing or hurtful. However, the play therapist's responsibility is to recognize how children develop and make meaning of their experiences in order to respond therapeutically to situations with perceived discomfort or offensiveness. Play therapists can honor and allow cultural opportunities to unfold while maintaining a child-oriented interpersonal stance when they understand that children's racial identities and attitudes form through complex processes in which their cognitive and social development, social interactions, and contextual factors simultaneously interact (e.g. Quintana, 1998; Rogers et al., 2021; Spencer, 2008). As Quintana and McKown (2008) discussed, children's understandings of racial/ethnic differences develop while they explore the physical world, their own social group, and ego development. Therefore, our goal is not to have the "best" response in moments of racism in the playroom but to be in this process of seeing and accepting the child's experiences through their lens with humility, genuineness, and vulnerability.

Jordan

Jordan, a five-year-old girl, presented for play therapy due to a lack of self-regulation and high anxiety during the COVID pandemic. Imagine the following scenario. Both Jordan and the therapist wore a mask during the session for safety. As she explored the playroom for the first time, she looked at the therapist and said:

JORDAN: "I don't like wearing a mask."
THERAPIST: "You don't like wearing a mask; it makes you uncomfortable."
JORDAN: "Yeah, and now I have to wear a mask everywhere I go."
THERAPIST: "Sounds like you are tired of that."
JORDAN: "Yeah, and the Chinese have the virus. They make people sick."
THERAPIST: "Well, that is not true. It is the virus that makes people sick, not Chinese. And it is hurtful to say things like this, and people's feelings are not for hurting."
JORDAN: "But my mom told me that."

In this example, the therapist responded to the cultural opportunity of racism by correcting Jordan's racist comment and setting a limit with a positive intention. However, this response may not only invalidate the child's experience in the moment but also imply that the child's mother is wrong. In addition, the therapist may be at risk of imposing their own opinion that seems to conflict with the opinion expressed by the mother to the child. Imagine you were the therapist in this situation and consider the following questions:

1   How might your personal and professional experiences and cultural identities affect your reactions and how you would respond?
2   What is your view of Jordan, and how would it affect your acceptance of her and your relationship?
3   What is your view of Jordan's mother, and how would it affect your relationship and working together moving forward?
4   The race/ethnicity of the child is not presented in the example. Would you change your response if the racial/ethnic identity of the child differs (i.e. if the child were Asian or Black, etc.)?

Consider the following alternative responses:

JORDAN: "I don't like wearing a mask."
THERAPIST: "You don't like wearing a mask; it makes you uncomfortable."
JORDAN: "Yeah, and now I have to wear a mask everywhere I go."
THERAPIST: "Sounds like you are frustrated by that."
JORDAN: "Yeah, and the Chinese have the virus. They make people sick."
THERAPIST: "Sounds like you have heard that from somewhere, that the Chinese have the coronavirus and make people sick."
JORDAN: "My mom told me that. People are dying."
THERAPIST: "Oh, so you have heard that from your mom, and that seems very scary for you."
JORDAN: "Um-hum."

The alternative responses from the play therapist are primarily a reflection of feelings and content that center on cultural humility, an openness and desire to strive to understand the child's reality and convey this understanding to the child. Most importantly, the therapist goes beyond the racist comment and recognizes the underlying *why* and *how* of the comment (i.e. the intention behind making the racist comment and the verbal, nonverbal, and other mannerisms exhibited when commenting). In this case example, the *why* would be that Jordan uses the moment in the playroom to share with the therapist how her world has been shaken by the pandemic and how much she believes in her mother's words. The desire to connect with the therapist through sharing is also evident. The *how* would be that Jordan says the racist comments in a matter-of-fact manner based on her interpretation of and feelings regarding the pandemic, that is the "figuring out." Such self-focused expression does not seem rooted in the intention to be hurtful to others in the moment; rather, it seems to be a demonstration of a young child's race/ethnic identity development from which she operates as egocentric in thinking and starts to internalize perspectives from others (Dillman Taylor, 2016). Nevertheless, if the play therapist experiences and conceptualizes that hurting people's feelings is the intention behind the racist comment of the child, it would be therapeutic and important to reflect this meaning.

We would like to take a step further with Jordan's example. Consider the following situation where the therapist is Chinese:

JORDAN: "I don't like wearing a mask."
THERAPIST: "You don't like wearing a mask; it makes you uncomfortable."
JORDAN: "Yeah, and now I have to wear a mask everywhere I go."
THERAPIST: "Sounds like you are frustrated by that."
JORDAN: "Yeah, and my mom told me that Chinese have virus. They make people sick."
THERAPIST: "So you have heard that from your mom and you seem worried about that. [Pause.] I am Chinese."

In this scenario, the therapist uses reflection of content to express understanding of the child's view of the world; furthermore, the therapist discloses her ethnicity. This way of responding may present a risk in the play therapy situation but also has a potential to deepen the relationship by being congruent. It is crucial to note that a therapist would not self-disclose as a teaching moment or to deny the child's experience. Rather, this response is rooted in the therapist's intentionality and expression of being culturally vulnerable and genuine regarding her ethnicity without blame or confrontation, as she experiences a sense of congruence within herself and the relationship with the child in the moment. This response may also present the child with dissonance (i.e. Mom says Chinese make people sick but I really like my Chinese play therapist) that may further facilitate opportunities where both the child's and the therapist's acceptance of self and of each other can be explored and deepened. Obviously, the play therapist would have to be emotionally prepared for the child's unpredictable reaction and remain self-aware in their responses and reactions to the child following the self-disclosure.

Mateo

Mateo and I (DR) walked down the school hallway toward the playroom. We had seen each other in play therapy for approximately 15 sessions and had a close therapeutic relationship. Mateo was Mexican-American and six years old. As we walked side by side, I noticed him looking at my hand by my side. He stopped and extended his arm forward. I instinctively extended my arm to be beside his. Originally, when he extended his arm, his hand was palm-down and mine was the same. He then flipped his palm up and said, "There! Now we're the same color." Mateo was referring to the darker tone of his skin on his upper hand as compared to my much lighter skin tone. When he flipped his hand to show his palm, our skin tones matched almost perfectly. He was super proud when he made his announcement. Without thinking, I immediately responded, "You wanted us to look just alike." I then flipped my hand over and said, "This way we look the same and [flipping again] this way we look different and you're telling me that I'm important to you." I also went further based on our long-term relationship and my own authenticity in the moment and said, "You're important to me too." I considered this a cultural opportunity to respond specifically to how Mateo equated skin color with relationship. Developmentally, it made sense that Mateo concluded that if we looked the same, we were closer in relationship. However, I wanted to reflect that we can be the same and different and the relationship is strong in both cases. I did not want to deny that Mateo felt that it was important to look like me but I also did not want to confirm that looking like me was better. Instead, I chose to reflect on the whole interaction and the meaning behind his observations (i.e. I am important to him).

Throughout the preceding examples, the play therapist is engaged in an ongoing internal dialogue regarding cultural humility and engaging in the opportunity. As mentioned in Aaron's case, the play therapist may be shocked, or possibly hurt, by the child's play or verbalizations. It would only be natural for the play therapist to take a breath or disengage for a second to regulate emotions. The therapist's ability to regulate their own emotions is essential to expression of cultural humility through focusing on the other, the child's world. We also recommend that when play therapists engage in cultural opportunities with children, they benefit from processing the experience with a colleague or supervisor. Play therapists are better able to care for their clients and continue to engage in cultural opportunities when they engage in their own self-care and are provided support for their cultural experiences.

Cultural Opportunities with Families

Cultural opportunities in play therapy begin with a child's caretakers or family members. From the initial interaction with the adult who is referring a child, the play therapist initiates a relationship in which parents or care-takers feel safe to share their cultural identities and trust the play therapist to embrace their child's cultural being. Best practices for intakes include asking parents/caretakers questions regarding the saliency of their cultural identities. Intake questions such as, "Is there anything you would like me to know about your culture?" or "Is there anything you would like to share about your beliefs or values that you feel will be helpful in working with you and your child?" sends the message that the play therapist is open to cultural conversations and values the parent/caretakers' culture while allowing the parent/caretaker the safety to share or not share. The therapist can then follow up in consultations with the parent/caretaker to have conversations about family values and salient identities. Ongoing consultations often present opportunities for the play therapist to continue to deepen their understanding of the parent/caretaker's values regarding culture, as well as the opportunity for the therapist to check in regarding the parent/caretaker's level of safety in working with the play therapist.

A Story of Missed Cultural Opportunities with Families

Whenever I (YO) think about cultural opportunities with families, there is a particular family that I think about, and whenever I think about them, I bite my lip because I missed many cultural opportunities with them.

Maria, an eight-year-old, was referred to play therapy by a school counselor because the mother suddenly returned to her home country permanently without any notice, and Maria was left with her father. I met her father at the intake session for the first time. He was an older gentleman with a cowboy hat and boots. He was very polite and shared that he did not know anything about counseling but he came to seek support for Maria because he was told to do so by Maria's school. Maria's mother was a migrant overseas worker from an Asian country and her father was a farmer. They lived a frugal life. The father was not emotional when sharing the mother's disappearance but he was clearly committed to supporting and taking care of Maria. At the end of the intake session, when we were saying goodbye in the waiting room, the father tried to give me a couple of dollars as a tip. For a second, it took me off guard, and I needed another couple of seconds to figure out what was going on. I just said, "Thank you but we do not accept tips here." He accepted my response without being offended. I remember feeling very confused with what had just happened and with what I had said.

However, I believe the father was confused as much as or more than I was, not knowing what counseling really was. And how about the fact that his wife who just disappeared was an Asian and now he had an Asian female therapist working with her daughter? I was a novice graduate student intern who was too nervous to attend to such a vital fact. If I could go back to the moment, I would have enough cultural comfort to address the elephant in the room (cultural opportunities may often feel like an elephant in the room) and ask the father: "I know your wife who just left you and Maria is an Asian. I am also an Asian and I wonder how you feel about working with me and letting me work with Maria… I would like to be sensitive to any thoughts and reactions you may have toward me." In addition, this was a story from almost 20 years ago. I remember I shared this story in my supervision. My supervisor and my classmates were surprised but we did not discuss the cultural implications of the incident. The importance of attending and addressing cultural issues in play therapy was not emphasized as much as it should have been back then.

Luckily, the father trusted me and I worked with Maria until termination with positive results. However, the unaddressed cultural gap between the father and me remained. I know I could have worked more effectively, particularly with the father, if I did not miss the cultural opportunities. This is why I bite my lip when I think about them.

Bigger Picture of Cultural Opportunities

In the multicultural orientation framework, cultural opportunities are conceptualized as therapeutic encounters between therapist and client. We heartily embrace this conceptualization as a pathway to deepen play therapy relationships. We provided examples of ways in which the play therapist seizes cultural opportunities by reflecting the child's deeper meaning and responding to how culture can be addressed within the relationship. However, seeking cultural opportunities within the therapeutic relationship does not absolve the play therapist's responsibility to take advantage of cultural opportunities on a broader scale. Because play therapists work systemically, accountability extends to providing awareness and education through advocacy in children's systems. In each of the provided examples, children were struggling with confusion regarding racism. From a child-centered play therapy perspective, there is an assumption that children are engaging in these play scenes and verbalizations because they are attempting to figure out what they are being told to believe and how the world works. As children are trying to figure out these complex issues, play therapists can support educational and experiential initiatives in schools and other formal settings that promote empathic understanding and the questioning of systemic traditions of oppression. We would even venture to say that play therapists are accountable for providing support to systems of care for children by facilitating broader advocacy efforts to enhance culturally safe environments for children at home and school.

Cultural Comfort

The likelihood of effectively navigating cultural opportunities is directly mediated by a play therapist's cultural comfort. Cultural comfort, the third pillar of multicultural orientation, is defined as "the feelings that arise before, during, and after culturally relevant conversations in session between the therapist and client. The emotional states of feeling at ease, open, calm, and relaxed are hallmarks of cultural comfort" (Hook et al., 2017, p. 38). Cultural comfort is facilitated by an emotional state marked by the therapist's ability to engage with the clients' various cultural identities in an open, fluid, relaxed, and connected manner (Hook et al., 2017). Furthermore, cultural comfort is seen as a behavioral manifestation of cultural humility, demonstrated through the therapist being less guarded, anxious, or defensive when a client shares a salient part of their cultural identity. In other words, cultural comfort is internally experienced yet externally expressed to clients through a willingness to enter into cultural opportunities. Some studies with racial/ethnic minority clients suggest that they can detect signs of cultural comfort in therapists, and they use these signs to evaluate therapists' attitudes, abilities to address racial/ethnic differences, and whether therapists seem safe and trustworthy (Pérez-Rojas et al., 2019).

Cultural Comfort in Play Therapy

In play therapy, cultural comfort is manifested through the play therapist's awareness of cultural opportunities and the ease with which the therapist engages with these opportunities. Play therapists with high levels of cultural comfort are more likely to allow a child's cultural play and verbalizations into their awareness and respond to this expression directly. Increased cultural comfort also allows the play therapist to see the more subtle forms of cultural expression, such as a child's silence in play therapy when English is their second language but it is the first language of the therapist. A therapist who has high cultural comfort may reflect, "You're not sure if it's okay to talk just like you normally do. In here, you get to decide how you talk." Increasing levels of cultural comfort allow a play therapist to experience and express increased levels of unconditional positive regard for the child. Cultural comfort sends the message that I honor and accept all of you which includes your cultural identities, thus fostering a safe, trusting, and positive therapeutic relationship.

Cultural comfort exists on a continuum for each play therapist and can be at different levels based on the therapeutic relationship or the topic that emerges. It is common for a play therapist to experience some level of anxiety around cultural opportunities in play therapy. A therapist's anxiety might develop due to general discomfort with acknowledging cultural aspects of the client and the therapeutic relationship or may be related to a therapist's sincere desire to handle cultural issues with care. Play therapists often appreciate that a child trusted us enough to share their cultural experiences and we may experience anxiety around how to respond with empathic care. Anxiety may result from self-imposed pressure such as, "I do not want to mess this opportunity up." Wherever on the continuum of cultural comfort, a play therapist benefits from being attuned to feelings of discomfort and making intentional efforts to address such discomfort through consultation or supervision, or possibly personal counseling.

In addition, being comfortable enough to witness or listen to cultural opportunities or cultural themes in play therapy does not necessarily mean that the content shared by a child is comfortable. Past and current situations of child clients are likely to stimulate uncomfortable feelings in therapists. I (YO) have been working with unaccompanied and undocumented children for the last few years. Lucas, an eight-year-old Latinx boy, witnessed his family member being killed by a gang member in his home country, crossed the border with his sister in order to be reunited with an aunt in the United States but was separated from her at a detention center. He was then detained for three months in the center, struggling with intense fear every day. Building relationships with children like Lucas will likely raise some discomfort in a play therapist. This type of discomfort can be a motivating force for advocacy as well as deepen a therapist's empathy toward clients who are the victims of injustice. It is important for counselors to be comfortable with being uncomfortable while listening to clients' stories of their painful experiences of racial violence, injustice, and discrimination (Phillips, 2020). This ability to comfortably sit with discomfort can be also considered an indicator of cultural comfort.

Cultural opportunities that children bring to their play therapy sessions are often unpredictable and/or blunt (verbally or/and symbolically), and they sometimes catch the play therapist off guard. Furthermore, some of the cultural opportunities that children present in play therapy can be emotionally triggering for play therapists based on their own cultural background. Responding to such moments in a therapeutic way while simultaneously being overwhelmed by the discomfort can be a source of incongruence for the therapist. Similar to the concept of congruence, cultural humility, in which cultural comfort is looped in, encompasses the therapist's whole way of being. Hook et al. (2017) report that practicing cultural humility might be described as other-centered self-growth because such commitment facilitates a therapist's professional and personal growth. Developing cultural comfort is not a mere acquisition of knowledge, skills, or techniques, but rather it is dynamic development of a way of being. How we strive to facilitate our cultural comfort as play therapists is individualized due to many factors such as our cultural identity development, our own specific biases, and areas and sources of our cultural discomfort.

Going back to my (YC) experience with Aaron, the seven-year-old boy building a wall in a play session, it was apparent that my cultural comfort level in the moment was low. More specifically, I was upset, confused, and shocked. Therefore, I stayed silent to protect myself. For me, it was uncomfortable because his statement conflicts with my values; it was challenging because I started wondering what he thinks of me, an Asian who has an international cultural background and speaks with an accent. As I was not able to hold a space within myself that would allow further connection and understanding between Aaron and me, I missed the cultural opportunity. If I were able to embrace this discomfort comfortably, I probably would be more able to access to my empathic understanding and acceptance for Aaron and his process of exploring his world by saying, "Sounds like you are worried about Mexicans coming to the U.S."

Ways to Address Personal Level of Cultural Comfort

Because cultural comfort is an attitude from which to engage in cultural opportunities, methods of exploring cultural comfort involve personal and introspective work. We recommend that play therapists engage in a journey toward developing greater levels of cultural comfort. This journey requires that play therapists intentionally explore and seek experiential activities for the purpose of growing their cultural comfort.

Cultural Comfort Scale: Personal Experiences

Hook et al. (2017) adapted the Therapist Comfort Scale (TCS; Slone & Owen, 2015), a tool developed to measure clients' perceived comfort exhibited by their therapists, and proposed to use it as an exercise for therapists to explore their cultural comfort with different cultural identities by watching a series of videos covering cultural topics. They renamed it as the Cultural Comfort Scale (CCS), which asks therapists, "Overall, how comfortable did you feel watching the video?" on ten items using a five-point scale ranging from 1 (strongly disagree) to 5 (strongly agree) (Hook et al., 2017). These ten feeling items include comfortable, awkward, tense, nervous, confident, uneasy, relaxed, calm, edgy, and genuine (Hook et al., 2017; Owen et al., 2016). The video assignment and CCS are useful tools in helping play therapists explore their cultural comfort. We recommend that play therapists select social media clips, videos, or movies that depict children of various identities and then self-rate on how comfortable they felt watching the video. I (DR) recently watched the movie *Cuties*, which brought up quite a bit of cultural discomfort for me regarding the main character's felt pressure to reject her traditional culture to take on the values of the internet culture. Regarding the CCS rating of this experience, I felt tense, nervous, uneasy, and uncomfortable throughout the movie. The experience prompted me to explore the origins of my discomfort and encouraged me to sit with my discomfort without trying to escape from it.

As an additional exercise for self-reflection, we recommend that play therapists use the many play therapy examples presented throughout this book as stimuli for CCS ratings. As chapter authors share stories of cultural encounters and experiences and discuss various ideas and perspectives, we encourage readers to pause, be self-reflective, and use the CCS to rate their level of comfort.

Finally, play therapists can actively seek to structure cultural conversations and experiences within safe relationships as they are building cultural comfort. Hook et al. (2017) adapted Locke and Bailey's (2013) list of questions to explore self-identity as prompts for "practice cultural conversations" with colleagues. We go one step further to suggest that these questions can be used as prompts for expressive arts (e.g. drawings, sandtray, collage, clay) between two play therapist colleagues to practice integration of cultural comfort and play expression. Examples of prompts include create a scene of your cultural heritage, draw a picture of cultural identities that are most salient to you, create a collage of beliefs, values, and attitudes that you hold that are consistent with dominant culture or inconsistent with the dominant culture. As play therapists practice the processing of expressive arts mediums in a cultural context, they are likely to increase their cultural comfort in both conversation and play.

Cultural Comfort Scale: Professional Experiences

In addition to assessing personal reactions and relative comfort levels with news, social media, videos, books, and texts on multicultural, diversity, or social justice issues, we invite play therapists to assess and rate their comfort levels in order to intentionally gain self-awareness and expand cultural comfort based on professional interactions. Following play therapy sessions or parent/teacher consultations, play therapists may use the CCS to explore, "Overall, how comfortable did I feel in this session/moment of the session?" We suggest that play therapists examine the overall comfort level and each specific feeling item, such as uneasy, calm, edgy, genuine, and others (Hook et al., 2017). In particular, play therapists can cultivate their self-awareness of cultural comfort by posing such questions as "What parts about the child's culturally related play expressions (both verbal and nonverbal) exhibited today were more/less comfortable for me to experience and respond to?" "What parts about the parent/caregiver's culturally related sharing were more/less comfortable for me to respond to and have further discussion with?" "What might be the sources of my comfort level?" "How did my comfort level affect my genuine way of being and access to convey empathic understanding and unconditional positive regard for the client?" "How did my comfort level affect my ability to respond to the moment therapeutically?" "What does my comfort level tell me about my strengths and areas for growth while continuing working with this client?" "In addition to the ten feeling items listed in the CCS, what other salient feelings or thoughts was I experiencing?" For play therapists who are able to video-record their sessions, observations of body posture, facial expressions, and voice tone can be especially helpful in exploring levels of cultural comfort.

We also encourage play therapists to share this processing with a supervisor or colleague to further explore the interpersonal and intrapersonal dynamics embedded in these cultural experiences and discuss ways to maintain being therapeutic while being comfortable in moments of discomfort.

Increasing Cultural Comfort through Professional Interactions

The Association for Play Therapy (APT) as well as other mental health professional organizations are rising up to use this moment to not only address structural racism in the United States but also attend to the disparities in the mental health field. It is inspiring that many experienced fellow play therapists initiated more workshops on cultural issues in play therapy as a response to the recent and cruel emergence of structural injustice. A crucial part of nurturing our cultural comfort as play therapists is to expand our own bubble by welcoming opportunities which bring disconfirming information to our existing perspectives, values, beliefs, and convictions. It was more than 60 years ago when Gordon Allport (1954) proposed the contact hypothesis in his book *Nature of Prejudice*. We seek inspiration from this hypothesis to create an environment where play therapists can increase their cultural comfort and develop cultural humility. Allport postulated that positive effects of intergroup contact occur in an environment characterized by four essential conditions: equal status, inter-group cooperation, common goals, and support by social and institutional authorities. Play therapy organizations, approved play therapy training providers, university professors, and individual play therapists can recruit fellow play therapists with various cultural backgrounds to form groups under Allport's guidelines: equal status of play therapists; intergroup cooperation of sharing and learning; the common goal of creating cultural opportunities among play therapists to develop and nurture our cultural comfort and cultural humility; and accomplishing these guidelines through the support of APT. Such groups may provide us with invaluable opportunities to learn and deepen relationships surrounding our cultural identities which will enhance our cultural comfort and cultural humility.

Conclusion

In this chapter, we introduced two other important pillars of the multi-cultural orientation (MCO) framework, cultural opportunities and cultural comfort, and how they can be applied to play therapy practice. The three ingredients of MCO – cultural humility, opportunities, and comfort – work in tandem. Cultural humility is comprised of attitudes, beliefs, and motivations, while cultural opportunities are comprised of observations and actions (seizing and engaging in opportunities), whereas cultural comfort is personal reaction. All three pillars form an imperative for play therapists in order to facilitate children's organic way of addressing their lived cultural experiences and deepening authentic relationships with children in play therapy. We hope that readers use this practical framework to enact the principles of the MCO and feel motivated to engage in work preparing for future cultural opportunities that children bring to us.

References

Allport, G. W. (1954). *The nature of prejudice*. Addison-Wesley.

Danso, R. (2018). Cultural competence and cultural humility: A critical reflection on key cultural diversity concepts. *Journal of Social Work*, 18, 410–430. doi:10.1177/1468017316654341.

Dillman Taylor, D. L. (2016). The extraordinary 5-year-old. In D. C. Ray (Ed.), *A therapist's guide to child development: The extraordinarily normal years* (pp. 71–82). Routledge.

Hook, J. N., Davis, D. E., Owen, J., & DeBlaere, C. (2017). *Cultural humility: Engaging diverse identities in therapy*. American Psychological Association.

Locke, D., & Bailey, D. (2013). *Increasing multicultural understanding* (3rd ed.). Sage.

Owen, J. (2013). Early career perspectives on psychotherapy research and practice: Psychotherapist effects, multicultural orientation, and couple interventions. *Psychotherapy*, 50, 496–502. doi:10.1037/a0034617.

Owen, J., Drinane, J. M., Davis, D. E., Tao, K. W., Hook, J., & Kune, N. F. (2016). Client perceptions of therapists' multicultural orientation: Cultural (missed) opportunities and cultural humility. *Professional Psychology: Research and Practice*, 47, 30–37. doi:10.1037/pro0000046.

Pérez-Rojas, A. E., Lockard, A., Bartholomew, T. T., & Gonzalez, J. M. (2019). Development and initial validation of the therapists cultural comfort scale. *Journal of Counseling Psychology*, 66(5), 534–549.

Phillips, L. (2020, July 27). *Black mental health matters*. https://ct.counseling.org/2020/07/black-mental-health-matters.

Quintana, S. M. (1998). Children's developmental understanding of ethnicity and race. *Applied and Preventive Psychology*, 7, 27–45. doi:10.1016/S0962-1849(98) 80020-80026.

Quintana, S. M., & McKown, C. (2008). Introduction: Race, racism, and the developing child. In S. Quintana & C. McKown (Eds.), *Handbook of race, racism, and the developing child* (pp. 1–15). John Wiley & Son.

Ray, D. (2011). *Advanced play therapy: Essential conditions, knowledge and skills for child practice*. Routledge.

Rogers, L. O., Moffitt, U., & Foo, C. (2021). "Martin Luther King fixed it": Children making sense of racial identity in a colorblind society. *Child Development*, 1–19. doi:10.1111/cdev.13628.

Ross, L. (2010). Notes from the field: Learning cultural humility through critical incidents and central challenges in community-based participatory research. *Journal of Community Practice*, 18(2–3),315–335. doi:10.1080/10705422.2010.490161.

Slone, N. C., & Owen, J. (2015). Therapist alliance activity, therapist comfort, and systemic alliance on individual psychotherapy outcome. *Journal of Psychotherapy Integration*, 25(4), 275–288. doi:10.1037/a0039562.

Spencer, M. B. (2008). Lessons learned and opportunities ignored since Brown v. Board of Education: Youth development and the myth of a color-blind society. *Educational Researcher*, 37, 253–266. doi:10.3102/0013189X08322767.

3 Integrating Advocacy in Play Therapy

Peggy L. Ceballos and Tamara Iliff

As societies continue to experience the process of globalization, mental health professionals are called to respond to the needs of culturally diverse clients (Ceballos et al., 2021). This call includes an ethical responsibility to advocate for removal of oppressive factors as well as address in therapy the negative effect these factors have on clients' socioemotional wellbeing (Ratts et al., 2016). Attending to social justice issues and integrating advocacy in the work play therapists do is important given recent statistics that show 50% of children in the United States are identified as racially or ethnically minoritized (Forum on Child and Family Statistics, 2020) and approximately 11 million children live in poverty, with children of color experiencing more poverty than their White counterparts (Haider, 2021).

In the field of play therapy, attention has been given to providing culturally responsive services (e.g. Davis & Pereira, 2014; Gil & Drewes, 2005; Post & Tillman, 2015) and increasing knowledge about specific cultural groups (Agarwal & Meany-Walen, 2019; Killian et al., 2017; Post et al., 2019). However, less emphasis has been given to the applications of social justice advocacy in the work play therapists do (e.g. Ceballos et al., 2012). This is alarming given the bearing of oppressive factors on the socioemotional well-being and physical development of children (Berry et al., 2021). In response, it is pivotal for play therapists to gain a deeper understanding of the effects of oppression on children and their caregivers, the meaning of social justice, and the application of advocacy into the therapeutic process.

Oppression

In order to understand the detrimental effects of oppression on the development of children, we must first understand the meaning of oppression and ways in which it manifests in the everyday lives of children and their caregivers. According to David & Derthick (2014),

> Oppression occurs when one group has more access to power and privilege than another group, and when that power and privilege is

DOI: 10.4324/9781003190073-5

used to maintain the status quo (i.e., domination of one group over another). Thus, oppression is both a state and a process, with the state of oppression being an unequal group access to power and privilege, and the process of oppression being the ways in which inequality between groups is maintained.

(p. 3)

The process of oppression can occur through imposition or deprivation (Hanna, et al., 2000). Imposition occurs as privileged groups, or those in power, impose conditions on oppressed groups. An example of how imposition works for minoritized children is the constant exposure to stereotypes and discriminatory messages that confirm they are less than their White counterparts. This imposition process is seen in the daily micro-aggressions that children are exposed to such as "you throw like a girl" as a negative description of someone's physical strength (indicating males' superiority over females), "that is so gay" as a derogatory term to refer to someone's mannerism (indicating heterosexism as the norm), or "illegal aliens" to refer to immigrants who do not have documentation (implying they are criminals). Deprivation occurs when the system robs oppressed groups of equal access to living conditions such as shelter, high-quality education, or social support, among others (Hanna et al., 2000). Two examples of social deprivation for children include lack of access to high-quality educational opportunities and lack of access to healthcare. As these examples show, oppression is reinforced at the individual level through discrimination and stereotypes and at the institutional level through policies, customs, laws, and practices. Scholars in the field have identified three specific types of oppression that were previously defined as types of racism: interpersonal, institutional, and internalized (Jones, 2000).

David and Derthick (2014) define interpersonal oppression as "driven by and expressed as stereotypes (biased thoughts or Cognitions), prejudices (biased attitudes or Affect), and discrimination (biased actions or Behaviors)" (p. 77). Interpersonal oppression is reinforced everyday through "isms" (e.g. racism, sexism, ableism). Institutional oppression is defined as oppressive policies, laws, and customs used to privilege one group over others (David & Derthick, 2014). For example, the cycle known as school-to-prison pipeline that disproportionately affects minoritized children is driven by inadequate resources for schools in low-income areas and harsh disciplinary policies (Barnes & Motz, 2018). The final type of oppression is internalized oppression, defined as the process that occurs when oppressive messages from the environment are internalized by oppressed individuals, thus affecting one's self-concept (David & Derthick, 2014).

Paulo Freire (2017) explained the process of internalized oppression in his landmark work, *Pedagogy of the Oppressed*. The author contended that due to the lack of opportunities for oppressed groups to critically examine their position in society, they become unknowingly complicit with dominant group dogmas and practices, resulting in adopting these dogmas into their self-concepts. For example, a child who grows up in a bilingual home and experiences negative reactions from people when speaking Spanish in public unwillingly internalizes that speaking Spanish is a negative trait. As a result, the child stops using the second language, sometimes at the expense of losing the ability to be fully bilingual as well as the consequences of losing part of one's heritage and identity.

A key concept to understanding the effects of oppression on clients' socioemotional well-being is the concept of intersectionality of identities. Crenshaw (1991) first introduced the concept of intersectionality to refer to the way in which social identities (e.g. gender, race, age, social class, sexuality) can be understood in terms of power and privilege. Crenshaw argued that these identities are inseparable and non-hierarchical. Thus, in order to understand the effects of oppression on children, play therapists first have to understand how the child's intersectionality of identities exposes the child to various oppressive and privileged experiences. For example, a Black child with a visible disability who lives in an upper middle-class home is exposed to ableism and racism while social class gives him access to certain privileges that children in poverty do not have. In this way, the more oppressed identities one has, the greater the exposure to oppressive deprivation and imposition.

Effects of Oppression on Children and Caregivers

Berry et al. (2021) conducted a review of studies published over the last five years that looked at the effects of oppressive factors on early childhood mental health. The authors found that structural and personally mediated racism (Jones, 2000) known also as interpersonal and institutionalized types of oppression had the most detrimental effects on young children's development. Barry et al. noted that children's primary exposure to these types of oppressions was through witnessing and suffering the effects of their caregiver's direct exposure to it. Given the importance of the caregiver-child relationship, the authors concluded that caregivers' exposure to racism and lack of access to important resources had a direct effect on children's development. This conclusion is supported by numerous longitudinal and cross-sectional studies done to examine the effects of racism on children's well-being.

Rosenthal et al. (2018) explored intergenerational effects of socioeconomically disadvantaged Black and Latinx women's experiences of discrimination during pregnancy on their infants' socioemotional development in the first year of life. Results indicated that incidents of discrimination related to the mothers' intersectionality of marginalized identities reported during pregnancy were positively correlated to greater separation problems and greater negative emotions among infants at six months and one year of age, even after controlling for some medical and sociodemographic factors.

Similarly, studies done in the United States and other countries have found that caregivers' exposure to discrimination were associated with a range of detrimental physical and mental health outcomes in children 5–11 years old (Bécares et al., 2015; Cave et al., 2019; Shepherd et al., 2017). These detrimental effects included greater adolescent disruptive behavior (Savell et al, 2019), negative impact on mental health, sleep difficulties, and obesity (Shepherd et al., 2017), and higher risk for trying cigarettes (Cave et al., 2019). While these studies focused on the effects of primarily institutionalized and personally mediated oppression, other scholars have examined the process of internalized oppression.

Research shows that the process of internalized oppression starts at an early age. The famous doll experiment by psychologists Kenneth and Mamie Clark showed that as early as five years old, children were already unconsciously internalizing negative views about their race (Legal Defense and Educational Fund, 2021). A growing body of research continues to support the theory that members of oppressed groups involuntarily learn to link negative traits with their oppressed identities (e.g. Chae et al., 2014; David, 2010; David & Okazaki, 2010; Hatzenbuehler, 2009). For children and adolescents, internalized oppression occurs through daily exposure to discriminatory messages and interactions, especially in schools (Monzó, 2016; Muller & Boutte, 2019).

Schools play a pivotal part in children's racial/ethnic identity development and as such become a primary institution that form part of the oppressive cycle. Several authors have identified different factors that contribute to schools being part of the oppressive system; these include: (1) schools' emphasis on testing and on English-only training at the expense of developing critical thinking (Gutiérrez et al., 2009); (2) instruction based on an Eurocentric curriculum that reinforces the lack of representation from people of color making them invisible to children (González et al., 2005); (3) the numerous policies and practices within the educational system that contribute to the criminalization and subsequent incarceration for minoritized youth (McGrew, 2016); and (4) school practices that contribute to the internalization of oppression such as the way in which minoritized parents are viewed and treated from a "deficit framing" (Monzó, 2016, p. 156).

Due to the effects of these oppressive factors on children's physical and socioemotional well-being (Saleem et al., 2020), it is imperative for play therapists to work from a social justice and advocacy framework. In fact, continuing to work as if the problems exhibited by children are happening in a vacuum with no influence from these outside stressors can be detrimental, especially for children of color. Working without awareness of the impact of oppression on our clients can lead to inadvertently using play therapy as a way to deepen internalized oppression on our clients by helping them to adjust to the oppressive factors. In response, we must change our framework when working with children to ensure we are attending to the role that oppression has played in their lives. This new framework requires us to understand our role in seeking social justice as well as our role as advocates through the work we do.

Social Justice

Social justice is used as an "umbrella term" (Furman, 2012, p. 193) involving a range of concepts related to the meaning of justice within society (Capeheart & Milovanovic, 2020). Social justice involves a consideration of what is just for society overall (Capeheart & Milovanovic, 2020). Gewirtz and Cribb (2002) suggested that social justice is multidimensional as it involves concepts related to distributive, cultural, and associational justice. Distributive justice refers to equitable access to resources within society (Furman, 2012; Capeheart & Milovanovic, 2020; Chung & Bemak, 2011; Gewirtz & Cribb, 2002; Ibrahim & Heuer, 2016). Cultural justice refers to ensuring no cultural groups oppress other groups, and that all cultural groups are visible, acknowledged, and respected (Gewirtz & Cribb, 2002). Associational justice refers to all members of a society being able to fully engage in societal decision-making processes and having power to make choices over their lives (Gewirtz & Cribb, 2002).

The history of social justice within mental health fields in the United States can be traced back to Frank Parson's work during the vocational guidance movement of the early 1900s (Ratts & Pedersen, 2014). Around the same time, Clifford Beers published his memoir, *A Mind That Found Itself: An Autobiography*, which documented the abuses he experienced from the mental health profession as a psychiatric patient (Kiselica & Robinson, 2001). This early work was followed by social unrest during the 1960s which underscored the need for increased attention to multicultural issues within the mental health profession (Ratts & Pedersen, 2014). Emphasis on the importance of multiculturalism within mental health professions brought increased attention to research and conceptualization from a multicultural lens, prompting what has been labeled the "fourth force" in counseling (Pedersen, 1991).

With increased attention to multicultural competence came increased awareness of the role of oppression and privilege in the lives of clients (Ratts & Pedersen, 2014). Consequently, counselors became aware of the need to become actively engaged in confronting oppressive factors at the root of client problems (Ratts & Pedersen, 2014). Recognition of the need to consider the impact of societal oppression and discrimination on the psychological well-being of clients prompted a shift towards a focus on social justice within the mental health professions, which has been identified as the fifth force in counseling (Ratts, 2009).

The fifth force in counseling calls for mental health professionals to understand how issues of power, privilege, and oppression interact to impact clients' mental health and development (Chang et al., 2010; Odegard & Vereen, 2010). To this end, social justice involves mental health professionals working to ensure equitable distribution of opportunities and resources for clients, as well as engagement in social action to change unjust systems and policies that impact clients' well-being and socioemotional development (Fouad et al., 2006).

Social Justice and Play Therapy

In its "Play Therapy Best Practices" document (APT, 2020), the Association for Play Therapy emphasizes the importance of multicultural competence and providing culturally responsive services in play therapy practice. Play therapists are encouraged to engage in self-examination and reflection related to their own identities and biases, and to engage in ongoing education related to the roles of culture and bias in the lives of clients (APT, 2020). While cultural competence is certainly essential for play therapy practice, cultural competence without attention to issues of social justice is insufficient to meet the needs of marginalized clients (Ceballos et al., 2012).

Practicing from a social justice framework requires play therapists to consider how the intersections of their own identities impact the therapeutic relationship as well as a commitment to ongoing self-reflection regarding their own values, beliefs, and biases (Post & Tillman, 2015). Additionally, social justice work in play therapy practice requires play therapists to consider negative impacts of oppression and inequality on children's socio-emotional well-being and development (Ceballos et al., 2012). This requires an understanding of how institutions, policies, and global issues privilege certain communities while marginalizing others (Furman, 2012; Ratts et al., 2016). By considering the role of oppression in the lives of marginalized children and families, play therapists can cultivate greater empathy and understanding for their clients through conceptualizing their clients from a systemic perspective (Ceballos et al., 2012).

Additionally, practicing from a social justice paradigm requires that play therapists move beyond awareness of issues of power and oppression, and take action to confront systemic barriers and oppressive social and political forces that negatively impact their clients' well-being (Ceballos et al., 2012; Ceballos et al., 2021). Conceptualization from a social justice perspective can assist in identifying needed advocacy interventions to remove oppressive environmental factors in the lives of clients.

Advocacy

Inherent in practicing from a social justice framework is the understanding that mental health services must be accompanied by advocacy in order to fully address the roots of clients' problems (Ratts et al., 2016; Ratts et al., 2010). Chang et al. (2010) define social justice advocacy as "the act of arguing on behalf of an individual, group, idea, or issue to achieve social justice" (p. 84). Advocacy within the mental health professions involves taking action with and/or on behalf of clients to promote equitable access to power and resources (Chang et al., 2010). From this perspective, play therapists operating from a social justice perspective advocate both with and for clients at the individual, community, and systemic levels in order to effect change and confront oppressive social and environmental factors that impact their clients' psychological health and socioemotional development.

Marshall-Lee and colleagues (2020) suggested a three-tiered model of advocacy based on interventions at the micro, meso, and macro levels. The micro level, or individual level, consists of a client, as well as the client's, family, friends, and immediate community (Marshall-Lee et al., 2020). In the American Counseling Association Advocacy Competencies, Toporek and Daniels (2018) suggest that advocacy at this level may involve a focus on client empowerment through helping clients identify oppressive factors in their lives, gaining skills to confront oppression and systemic barriers, and evaluating and processing their experiences in advocating for themselves. Additionally, advocacy at the individual level may also at times require taking action on behalf of clients in situations in which the therapist has the power to navigate systems and services which are inaccessible to the client, or when client is unable to advocate due to potential personal risks or other reasons (Toporek & Daniels, 2018).

The meso level, or community level, consists of systems and organizations within a client's community, such as educational and healthcare systems (Marshall-Lee et al., 2020). Advocacy at this level involves working with groups within the community to alleviate systemic oppression (Toporek & Daniels, 2018). Rather than entering into a community as an expert, therapists serve alongside organizations and marginalized communities and offer their skills and expertise as a supportive ally (Marshall-Lee et al., 2020; Toporek & Daniels, 2018). Additionally, advocacy at the community level may involve advocating on behalf of groups within a community to address systemic concerns that are negatively impacting clients. Therapists may engage in advocacy on behalf of client groups at the systems level by using their power to advocate for change within systems in their community, such as within schools or organizations (Toporek & Daniels, 2018). Therapists may also choose to advocate on behalf of client groups at the community level when they have access to organizations and systems that are inaccessible to client and community groups (Toporek & Daniels, 2018).

The final level is the macro or public level. The macro level consists of economic, social, cultural, and political systems that impact clients' day to day lives (Marshall-Lee et al., 2020). Advocacy at the public level involves partnership with advocacy groups to confront broader systemic barriers and oppressive factors in society (Toporek & Daniels, 2018). Therapists at this level engage in collective action by offering their expertise and abilities to advocacy efforts such as public education campaigns and calling for legislative change (Toporek & Daniels, 2018). Additionally, advocacy at the macro level may involve advocating for clients by engaging in social and political action to address systemic issues, such as by testifying at legislative hearings and utilizing media to spread awareness of systemic issues impacting clients (Toporek & Daniels, 2018). Through using a socioecological framework, play therapists can work with clients to identify areas of needed advocacy interventions at various levels within the systems in which clients live (Ratts et al., 2016).

Applications for Play Therapists

Decisions regarding how to incorporate social justice advocacy into practice begins with clients (Ratts et al., 2016). By considering the role of the client's culture, intersectionality of identities, and oppressive environmental factors on their client's presenting problems, play therapists can gain a deeper understanding of their clients' needs (Ceballos et al., 2021). Furthermore, through conceptualizing clients through a social justice framework, play therapists can identify areas in need of advocacy interventions at the individual, community, and public levels (Ceballos et al., 2021). In order to illustrate social justice advocacy within play therapy practice at various systemic levels, we offer the following case study example.

Case Example

In order to protect clients' confidentiality, the following case study is a fictional compilation of several clients that the authors have worked with from a social justice framework. Maria is a seven-year-old Latinx bilingual student who came to counseling presenting with anxiety. The school referred Maria to play therapy because she was having extreme anxiety when it was time to stay at school and at times had panic attacks during the school day. These behaviors had resulted in Maria being exposed to some bullying from classmates who made fun of her behaviors. The intake revealed that both parents immigrated with Maria and currently they did not have the required documents to be in the United States. The father had been suffering from an illness for the last couple of months and due to not having access to health care, he was unable to get the surgery he needed. As a result, for the past few months, there had been several trips to the hospital that resulted in quick short-term fixes to the underlying medical problem. Maria's mother had picked up several extra jobs to make up for the lack of income that the father's illness had caused.

The play therapist used the following questions (Ceballos et al., 2021) to complement her conceptualization of the case:

- *How do clients' cultural identities contribute to their experience of privileges versus oppressive factors?*

In the case of Maria, there are several identities that need to be explored for her and for her parents:

1   Identifying ethnically as Latinx brings exposure to stereotypes and micro-aggressions that reinforce negative perceptions about one's ethnic identity. For example, through her play, Maria expressed having confusing feelings about speaking in Spanish. One time she sang Spanish songs as she played and it appeared to be soothing, while in a different session, she played a puppet show where she told some puppets they were not allowed to speak in Spanish.

2   Not having documentation and lack of financial resources. When examined as an identity, not having documentation to be "legal" in the United States prevented Maria and her family from accessing basic resources such as health care insurance. This was further complicated by their lack of financial resources. One of the ways in which this was playing a factor in Maria's case can be seen in how the father was unable to afford the surgery he needed to solve the underlying medical condition. Instead, because it was not a life-or-death situation, the only medical care he was able to get was a non-permanent fix that resulted in him having multiple trips to the hospital in a short period of time. This identity also prevented Maria's parents from finding better paying jobs, even though both of them had previous work experience as administrators and both had undergraduate degrees.

3   Both parents identified as Christians which is considered a privileged identity in the United States. As a result, they did not have to hide their religious affiliations or be exposed to microaggressions related to this identity. Also, their link to their local church allowed them to have access to some resources other families do not have.

4   Maria's racial identity was Black, the same as her father's identity. Their race exposed them both to more microaggressions in society. For example, exposure to jokes that reinforce Whites are superior to Blacks. Because Maria's mother had White skin, Maria was also exposed in her daily interactions to witnessing how people treated her mother differently than her father or her.

- *Have clients been exposed to discriminatory messages? Have they internalized these messages?*

In the case of Maria, it was observed through therapy that she was trying to make sense of her identity as a Black Latinx female. In the playroom she expressed ambivalence around speaking Spanish, being Black (e.g. sometimes she said she wanted to be like her mom while playing with the White doll). She had also internalized the undocumented status as a negative identity and one that she needed to hide from others to protect her family. For example, her play had a theme of mistrust toward strangers. On one occasion, she said to the play therapist she had to protect her family from the police that came to send them back to their countries.

- *How are oppressive factors challenging children's abilities to fully engage in the self-actualization process?*

Being an immigrant without documents prevented Maria and her family from accessing basic needs such as medical care. Similarly, due to the challenges of finding better paying jobs, the family was not economically stable, which caused lack of access to other resources. This primary lack of security made it hard for Maria to be able to realize her full potential. Similarly, exposure to bullying related to her racial and ethnic identity and bilingualism caused an internal struggle for Maria that prevented her from fully accepting herself. Similarly, as a seven-year-old, Maria is forming her own identity by becoming significantly more aware of individual differences and by comparing herself to others (Stulmaker, 2016). Developmentally, she is also more likely to process her experiences internally (Stulmaker, 2016), which can make it hard for her to externalize these oppressive experiences.

- *Who has the power to remove or mitigate the effects of the identified oppressive factors?*

The power to remove these barriers can be found at different levels. At the macro level, sociopolitical change that calls for immigration integration instead of criminalizing immigrants is needed to eradicate some of these oppressive factors. Similarly, continuing to advocate for institutional policies and customs that end racism and White supremacy are needed to make long-lasting change. At the micro level, advocating for changes in Maria's school, seeking resources to help the family find the medical care they needed, and addressing Maria's racial identity development to prevent the continued internalization of oppressive factors are some of the actions that reside within the play therapist. Some of these actions could also be done in collaboration with Maria and her parents as a way to empower them.

- *What advocacy actions does the play therapist need to take outside of the work done in the playroom?*

Through attending to the previous questions in conceptualizing Maria, the play therapist was able to identify areas of needed advocacy interventions at the micro, meso, and macro levels and develop a treatment plan that addressed Maria's presenting concerns from a systemic perspective. In the following section, we outline the advocacy steps the play therapist took to work toward alleviating systemic barriers that were negatively impacting Maria and her family.

Micro Level

Advocacy at the micro level involved the play therapist taking direct action to advocate for Maria, as well as supporting and empowering Maria and her parents in advocating for themselves. The following advocacy interventions were developed in collaboration with Maria and her parents and were incorporated into Maria's treatment plan.

1   The play therapist reached out to the school counselor to develop a better action plan for when Maria experienced panic attacks. This new plan included training the teacher on how to recognize signs and immediate actions she could take to de-escalate the situation. Maria and her parents were also part of creating this plan. Maria's parents were present during the meeting that took place between the play therapist and the school counselor and they were able to express their opinions as well as offering ideas on how to help Maria; this was empowering for them. It is important to mention that prior to this school meeting, the play therapist had an opportunity to let Maria's parents know about their rights within the school system (e.g. asking for a 504 if needed, requesting an explanation on how the situation was currently being handled, soliciting an interpreter if needed) and process how they wanted to handle the meeting.
2   The play therapist found several resources in the community that could easily be accessed by immigrants who do not have documentation. Among the resources was a referral to a community clinic that worked specifically with immigrant families and who had the resources to help Maria's father get the medical attention he needed.
3   The play therapist talked to Maria's parents about Maria's racial/ethnic identity development and provided free resources and activities the parents could do to start countering internalized oppression. These included reading children's books that highlighted the Latinx culture as well as important Latinx role-models. Similar resources were given to address Maria's racial identity.

Meso Level

Advocacy at the meso, or community, level involved the play therapist collaborating with groups within the community to address systemic factors that negatively impact Maria and her family, as well as other clients like Maria. Additionally, advocacy at the meso level involved taking action to advocate on behalf of children like Maria within organizations in the community. The play therapist continued to engage in her own reflection regarding her role as an activist outside of the playroom. To this end, she engaged in the following advocacy interventions within her own community:

1   The play therapist continued to volunteer for organizations in the local community that help immigrants.
2   The play therapist provided pro-bono multicultural trainings for teachers regarding immigrant families as well as interventions such as Child-Parent Relationship Therapy (Landreth & Bratton, 2020).

Macro Level

Advocacy at the macro, or sociopolitical, level involved the play therapist engaging in political action to address systemic oppression and barriers that negatively impact children's well-being and self-actualization abilities.

1   The play therapist remained active in supporting policies and laws that helped dismantle racism and anti-immigrant views.
2   The play therapist partnered with an advocacy organization to advocate for immigrant rights to state legislators.
3   The play therapist offered free educational workshops through various institutions in the area (e.g. churches, nonprofit pro-immigrant organizations) to educate the public on immigration, especially the challenges that immigrant families face.

For the purpose of this chapter, we focused on the social justice framework and the advocacy plan. As can be seen, these principles and the addition of these questions to a case conceptualization and treatment plan can be implemented regardless of the theoretical approach of the play therapist. In this case, both authors practice from a child-centered approach, thus, in the playroom, the work with Maria focused on providing her with a relationship characterized by the core conditions (Rogers, 1961). We truly believe that allowing Maria to feel completely accepted without any conditions was the therapeutic factor that eventually allowed her to learn to accept herself and to reject internalized oppressive messages. Similarly, in providing this therapeutic environment, Maria was empowered to find her own ways to deal with the anxiety she was feeling. This empowerment piece was essential not to become another oppressive force that imposed values on her. Because Maria had no power over many of the experiences she was living, giving her control during the play sessions was important to release her potential for growth and self-actualization. For play therapists who practice from other theoretical orientations, it is important to conceptualize what other theoretically sounded techniques or interventions can be used inside the playroom and in parent consultations to counter the effects of the oppressive factors on the clients as well as to empower clients who are already disenfranchised.

Importance of Ongoing Self-Awareness

Working from a social justice framework requires play therapists' commitment to an ongoing self-awareness process regarding one's intersectionality of identities as well as awareness of clients' intersectionality of identities. This type of ongoing self-reflective process is captured in the meaning of cultural humility. Tervalon and Murray-García (1998) pioneered the work on cultural humility within the medical field and defined it as "a lifelong commitment to self-evaluation and critique, to redressing the power imbalances in the physician patient dynamic, and to developing mutually beneficial and non-paternalistic partnerships with communities on behalf of individuals and defined populations" (p. 123). Foronda et al. (2016) conducted a concept analysis of the term cultural humility and found the following attributes: (1) openness to exploring new ideas and concepts; (2) self-awareness regarding one's "strengths, limitations, values, beliefs, behavior, and appearance to others" (p. 211); (3) egoless, defined as one's ability to be humble and to view others as equal; (4) engagement in supportive interactions or meaningful and positive human interchanges; (5) willingness to engage in critically assessing one's attitudes, actions, and feelings; (6) awareness of cultural diversity and power differentiations; and (7) the achievement of mutual empowerment through engaging in cultural humility. We consider these attributes to be the base for play therapists who want to work from a social justice framework and engage in advocacy work. While these attributes are necessary, they do not automatically guarantee one's ability to become a social advocate.

Kiselica and Robinson (2001) outlined skills necessary for developing one's advocacy identity: (1) an emotional appreciation for clients' suffering; (2) commitment to ending such suffering; and (3) the ability to intervene at the organizational, group, and individual level. In order to gain an emotional appreciation for clients' sufferings, it is not enough to understand oppression at an intellectual level, we must be willing to empathize and offer unconditional acceptance for clients' worldview and suffering. This type of empathy can be developed through interacting with the communities we work with in a way that allows us to engage in meaningful experiences, discussions, and relationships with individuals from these communities. Such a level of engagement with clients' current exposure to oppression has to be turned into commitment to end oppression. As play therapists, we must engage in a process of examining our own level of commitment to social justice and equality and we must work tirelessly to increase the level of commitment. Once we have this commitment, we need to ask ourselves what actions we will take to become advocates in the work we do as play therapists. The goal is to come up with specific actions that allow us to evolve from being culturally responsive to integrating understanding of oppression on case conceptualizations to becoming activists who seek to end inequality and oppression.

For both of us, our commitment to social justice work as play therapists started as part of our personal experiences. We both have had many experiences working with minoritized clients; based on our own experiences of oppression and discrimination in our personal lives and on the experiences that our clients explore in counseling, we strengthen our emotional understanding of the challenges minoritized clients face in the United States. For example, as the first author, I am a bilingual Latinx immigrant, which has exposed me to many discriminatory experiences while also affording me the wonderful opportunity to work primarily with Spanish-speaking immigrant families. Although constantly living and hearing these experiences can be very painful for us, it is a reminder of the work that needs to be done. We both seek to advance our work by engaging in a constant self-discovery journey to understanding in more depth our identities and how their intersectionality affords us many privileges as well as oppressive experiences. We believe that working towards social justice is a never-ending process and although it can be challenging at times, the impact that it has on the children we see and their families is important and very significant.

Conclusion

The negative effects of oppressive factors on the socioemotional well-being and physical development of children (Berry et al., 2021) makes it pivotal to deliver play therapy services within a social justice framework that leads to the integration of advocacy in treatment plans. In fact, not doing it can inadvertently turn the therapeutic process into helping clients adjust to the oppressive factors rather than empowering them to fight them. To change the working framework, play therapists must commit to a self-reflection process regarding their own values, beliefs, and biases (Post & Tillman, 2015). In addition, play therapists need to commit to developing one's advocacy identity though acquiring a deep understanding and emotional appreciation for clients' oppressive experiences, committing to end oppression and developing the ability to take action (Kiselica & Robinson, 2001). By practicing from a social justice framework, play therapists are intentional in considering the role of the client's culture, intersectionality of identities, and oppressive environmental factors on the presenting problem and can identify areas in need of advocacy interventions at the individual, community, and sociopolitical levels (Ceballos et al., 2021).

Positionality Statements

Peggy

I identify as a cisgender, heterosexual, middle-class, Latinx first-generation immigrant from Venezuela. The intersectionality of my identities affords me many privileges as well as oppressive experiences in my daily life. My desire to engage in advocacy and to seek social justice comes from these personal experiences and from my hope to leave a better society for all children, including my two beautiful daughters. As a Latinx immigrant, I suffer first-hand the pain caused by discrimination and prejudice, yet I am aware that my privileged identities allow me to mitigate the impact of these experiences on my well-being. Thus, I remain committed to continuously engaging in a self-awareness journey. I believe engagement in self-reflection is essential if I want to open myself to understanding others' experiences and to feel the pain caused by social injustices and historical trauma in so many minoritized communities all around the world. In response, I have remained committed to using my privileged identities to be a voice for change. I plan to continue to use my voice as a counselor educator and the work I do in schools with children and parents as means to enact change. It is my belief that if each of us do our part, the combined efforts can have a significant impact on the lives of children worldwide.

Tamara

As a White, middle-class, first-generation college graduate and able-bodied person, I recognize the privilege I hold in the various intersections of my identities. I am also keenly aware that my White and privileged identities have impacted my worldview and continue to shape my experiences in the world. I am incredibly thankful for access to education, mentorship, and community that have both challenged and affirmed me in my own multicultural awareness and cultural identity development. While I recognize that examining and unlearning my own unconscious biases will be a life-long, intentional, and at times uncomfortable process, the kindness and grace I have received from my mentors serve as my motivation to continue to commit myself to engaging in cultural humility and advocacy within and outside of my play therapy practice. It is my hope that this chapter will support and inspire play therapists in their growth as social justice advocates, so that together we may work toward building a more just, affirming, and compassionate world for children.

References

Agarwal, S. M., & Meany-Walen, K. (2019). Application of Adlerian play therapy with multiracial children. *International Journal of Play Therapy*, 28(4), 207–217.

Association for Play Therapy (2019). *Play therapy best practices: Clinical, professional, and ethical issues.* https://cdn.ymaws.com/www.a4pt.org/resource/resmgr/publica tions/best_practices_-_sept_2019.pdf.

Barnes, J.C., & Motz, R. T. (2018). Reducing racial inequalities in adulthood arrest by reducing inequalities in school discipline: Evidence from the school-to-prison pipeline. *Developmental Psychology*, 54(12), 2328–2340. doi:10.1037/dev0000.

Bécares, L., Nazroo, J., & Kelly, Y. (2015). A longitudinal examination of maternal, family, and area-level experiences of racism on children's socioemotional development: Patterns and possible explanations. *Social Science & Medicine*, 142, 128–135. doi:10.1016/j.socscimed.2015.08.025.

Berry, O. O., Tobón, A. L., & Njoroge, W. F. (2021). Social determinants of health: The impact of racism on early childhood mental health. *Current Psychiatry Reports*, 23(5), 1–10. doi:10.1007/s11920-021-01240-0.

Capeheart, L., & Milovanovic, D. (2020). *Social justice: Theories, issues, and movements* (Revised and expanded edition). Rutgers University Press.

Cave, L., Cooper, M. N., Zubrick, S. R., & Shepherd, C. C. (2019). Caregiver-perceived racial discrimination is associated with diverse mental health outcomes in Aboriginal and Torres Strait Islander children aged 7–12 years. *International Journal for Equity in Health*, 18(142), 1–10. doi:10.1186/s12939-019-1045-8.

Ceballos, P. L., Parikh, S., & Post, P. B. (2012). Examining social justice attitudes among play therapists: Implications for multicultural supervision and training. *International Journal of Play Therapy*, 21(4), 232. doi:10.1037/a0028540.

Ceballos, C. L., Post, P., & Rodríguez, M. (2021). Practicing child-centered play therapy from a multicultural and social justice framework. In E. Gil & A. A. Drewes (Eds.), *Cultural issues in play therapy* (pp. 13–31). Guilford Press.

Chae, D. H., Nuru-Jeter, A. M., Adler, N. E., Brody, G. H., Lin, J., Blackburn, E. H., & Epel, E. S. (2014). Discrimination, racial bias, and telomere length in African-American men. *American Journal of Preventive Medicine*, 46(2), 103–111. doi:10.1016/j.amepre.2013.10.020.

Chang, C. Y., Crethar, H. C., & Ratts, M. J. (2010). Social justice: A national imperative for counselor education and supervision. *Counselor Education and Supervision*, 50(2), 82–87. doi:10.1002/j.1556-6978.2010.tb00110.x.

Chung, R. C. Y., & Bemak, F. P. (2011). *Social justice counseling: The next steps beyond multiculturalism*. Sage Publications.

Crenshaw, K. (1991). Mapping the margins: Intersectionality, identity politics, and violence against women of color. *Stanford Law Review*, 43(6), 1241–1299. www.jstor.org/stable/1229039.

David, E. J. R. (2010). Testing the validity of the Colonial Mentality Implicit Association Test and the interactive effects of covert and overt colonial mentality on Filipino American mental health. *Asian American Journal of Psychology*, 1(1), 31–45. doi:10.1037/a0018820.

David, E. J. R., & Derthick, A. O. (2014). What is internalized oppression, and so what? In E. J. R. David (Ed.), *Internalized oppression: The psychology of marginalized groups* (p. 1–30). Springer Publishing Company.

David, E. J. R., & Okazaki, S. (2010). Activation and automaticity of colonial mentality. *Journal of Applied Social Psychology*, 40(4), 850–887. doi:10.1111/j.1559-1816.2010.00601.x.

Davis, E. S., & Pereira, J. K. (2014). Child-centered play therapy: A creative approach to culturally competent counseling. *Journal of Creativity in Mental Health*, 9(2), 262–274. doi:10.1080/15401383.2014.892863.

Foronda, C., Baptiste, D. L., Reinholdt, M. M., & Ousman, K. (2016). Cultural humility: A concept analysis. *Journal of Transcultural Nursing*, 27(3), 210–217. doi:10.1177/1043659615592677.

Forum on Child and Family Statistics (2020). *America's children in brief: Key national indicators or well-being*.

Fouad, N. A., Gerstein, L. H., & Toporek, R., L. (2006). Social justice and counseling psychology in context. In R. L. Toporek, L. H. Gerstien, N. A. Fouad, G. Roysicar, & T. Israel (Eds.), *Handbook for social justice in counseling psychology: Leadership, vision, and action* (pp. 1–16). Sage.

Freire, P. (2017/1970). *Pedagogy of the Oppressed*. Bloomsbury Academic.

Furman, G. (2012). Social justice leadership as praxis: Developing capacities through preparation programs. *Educational Administration Quarterly*, 48(2), 191–229. doi:10.1177/0013161X11427394.

Gewirtz, S., & Cribb, A. (2002). Plural conceptions of social justice: Implications for policy sociology. *Journal of Education Policy*, 17(5), 499–509. doi:10.1080/02680930210158285.

Gil, E., & Drewes, A. A. (Eds.). (2005). *Cultural issues in play therapy*. Guilford Press.

Gil, E., & Pfeifer, L. (2016). Issues of culture and diversity in play therapy. In K. J. O'Connor, C. E. Schaefer, & L. D. Braverman (Eds.), *Handbook of Play Therapy*. Wiley.

González, N., Moll, L. C., & Amanti, C. (Eds.). (2005). *Funds of knowledge: Theorizing practices in households, communities, and classrooms*. Routledge.

Gutiérrez, K. P., Zitlali, M., & Martinez, C. (2009) Re-mediating literacy: Culture, difference, and learning for students from non-dominant communities. *Review of Research in Education* 33, 212–245.

Haider, A. (2021, January 12). *The basic facts about children in poverty*. Center for American Progress. www.americanprogress.org/issues/poverty/reports/2021/01/12/494506/basic-facts-children-poverty.

Hanna, F. J., Talley, W. B., & Guindon, M. H. (2000). The power of perception: Toward a model of cultural oppression and liberation. *Journal of Counseling & Development*, 78(4), 430–441. doi:10.1002/j.1556-6676.2000.tb01926.x.

Hatzenbuehler, M. L. (2009). How does sexual minority stigma "get under the skin"? A psychological mediation framework. *Psychological Bulletin*, 135(5), 707–730. doi:10.1037/a0016441.

Ibrahim, F. A., & Heuer, J. R., (2016). *Cultural and social justice counseling: Client-specific interventions*. Springer.

Jones, C. P. (2000). Levels of racism: A theoretic framework and a gardener's tale. *American Journal of Public Health*, 90(8), 1212–1215. doi:10.2105/ajph.90.8.1212.

Killian, T., Cardona, B., & Hudspeth, E. F. (2017). Culturally responsive play therapy with Somali refugees. *International Journal of Play Therapy*, 26(1), 23. doi:10.1037/pla0000040.

Kiselica, M. S., & Robinson, M. (2001). Bringing advocacy counseling to life: The history, issues, and human dramas of social justice work in counseling. *Journal of Counseling & Development*, 79(4), 387–397. doi:10.1002/j.1556-6676.2001.tb01985.x.

Kiselica, M. S. (2004). When duty calls: The implications of social justice work for policy, education, and practice in the mental health professions. *The Counseling Psychologist*, 32(6), 838–854. doi:10.1177/0011000004269272.

Kranz, P. L., Ramirez, S. Z., Flores-Torres, L., Steele, R., & Lund, N. L. (2005). Physical settings, materials, and related Spanish terminology recommended for play therapy with first-generation Mexican-American children. *Education*, 126(1), 93–100.

Landreth, G., & Bratton, S. (2020). *Child parent relationship therapy (CPRT): An evidence-based 10-session filial therapy model*. Routledge.

Lee, R. M., & Darnell, A. J. (2002) Theory and method of multicultural counseling competency assessment. In K. S. Kurasaki, S. Okazaki, and S. Sue (Eds.), *Asian American Mental Health*. International and Cultural Psychology Series. Springer. doi:10.1007/978-1-4615-0735-2_19.

Legal Defense and Educational Fund (2021). A revealing experiment: Brown v. board and "the doll test". Retrieved from: www.naacpldf.org/ldf-celebrates-60th-anniversary-brown-v-board-education/significance-doll-test.

Marshall-Lee, E. D., Hinger, C., Popovic, R., Miller Roberts, T. C., & Prempeh, L. (2020). Social justice advocacy in mental health services: Consumer, community, training, and policy perspectives. *Psychological Services*, 17(1), p. 12–21. doi:10.1037/ser0000349.

McGrew, K. (2016). The dangers of pipeline thinking: How the school-to-prison pipeline metaphor squeezes out complexity. *Educational Theory*, 66(3), 341–367.

Monzó, L. D. (2016). "They don't know anything!": Latinx immigrant students appropriating the oppressor's voice. *Anthropology & Education Quarterly*, 47(2), 148–166. doi:10.1111/aeq.12146.

Muller, M., & Boutte, G. S. (2019). A framework for helping teachers interrupt oppression in their classrooms. *Journal for Multicultural Education*, 13(1), 94–105. doi:10.1108/JME-09-2017-0052.

National Association of Social Workers (2017). *Code of ethics of the National Association of Social Workers*. www.socialworkers.org/About/Ethics/Code-of-Ethics/Code-of-Ethics-English.

Odegard, M. A., & Vereen, L. G. (2010). A grounded theory of counselor educators integrating social justice into their pedagogy. *Counselor Education and Supervision*, 50(2), 130–149. doi:10.1002/j.1556-6978.2010.tb00114.x.

Pedersen, P. B. (1991). Multiculturalism as a generic approach to counseling. *Journal of Counseling & Development*, 70(1), 6–12. doi:10.1002/j.1556-6676.1991.tb01555.x.

Post, P., Phipps, C. B., Cam, A. C, & Grybush, A. L (2019). Effectiveness of child-centered play therapy among marginalized children. *International Journal of Play Therapy*, 28(2), doi:88-97. http://dx.doi.org/10.1037/pla0000096.

Post, P. & Tillman, K. S. (2015). Cultural issues in play therapy. In D. Crenshaw & A. L. Stewart (Eds), *Play therapy: A comprehensive guide to theory and practice*. Guilford Press.

Ramirez, S. Z., Flores-Torres, L. L., Kranz, P. L, & Lund, N. L. (2005). Using Axline's eight principles of play therapy with Mexican-American children. *Journal of Instructional Psychology*, 32(4), 329–337.

Ratts, M. J. (2009). Social justice counseling: Toward the development of a fifth force among counseling paradigms. *The Journal of Humanistic Counseling, Education and Development*, 48(2), 160–172. doi:10.1002/j.2161-1939.2009.tb00076.x.

Ratts, M. J, Lewis, J. A., & Toporek, R. L., (2010). Advocacy and social justice: A helping paradigm for the 21st century. In M. L. Ratts, R. L. Toporek, & J. A. Lewis (Eds.), *ACA advocacy competencies: A social justice framework for counselors*. American Counseling Association.

Ratts, M. J., & Pedersen, P. B. (2014). *Counseling for multiculturalism and social justice: Integration, theory, and application*. John Wiley & Sons.

Ratts, M. J., Singh, A. A., Nassar-McMillan, S., Butler, S. K., McCullough, J. R., & Hipolito-Delgado, C. (2015). *Multicultural and social justice counseling competencies*. American Counseling Association. www.counseling.org/docs/default-source/competencies/multicultural-and-social-justice-counseling-competencies.pdf?sfvrsn=8573422c_22.

Ratts, M. J., Singh, A. A., Nassar-McMillan, S., Butler, S. K., & McCullough, J. R. (2016). Multicultural and social justice counseling competencies: Guidelines for the counseling profession. *Journal of Multicultural Counseling and Development*, 44(1), 28–48. doi:10.1002/jmcd.12035.

Rogers, C. R. (1961). *On becoming a person: A therapist's view of psychotherapy*. Houghton Mifflin Company.

Rosenthal, L., Earnshaw, V. A., Moore, J. M., Ferguson, D. N., Lewis, T. T., Reid, A. E., Lewis, J. B., Stasko, E. C., Tobin, J. N., & Ickovics, J. R. (2018). Intergenerational consequences: Women's experiences of discrimination in pregnancy predict infant social-emotional development at 6 months and 1 year.

62   *Peggy L. Ceballos and Tamara Iliff*

Journal of Developmental and Behavioral Pediatrics, 39(3), 228–237. doi:10.1097/DBP.0000000000000529.

Saleem, F. T., Anderson, R. E. & Williams, M. (2020). Addressing the "myth" of racial trauma: Developmental and ecological considerations for youth of color. *Clinical Child and Family Psychology Review*, 23, 1–14. doi:10.1007/s10567-019-00304-1.

Savell, S. M., Womack, S. R., Wilson, M. N., Shaw, D. S., & Dishion, T. J. (2019). Considering the role of early discrimination experiences and the parent–child relationship in the development of disruptive behaviors in adolescence. *Infant Mental Health Journal*, 40(1), 98–112. doi:10.1002/imhj.21752.

Shepherd, C. C., Li, J., Cooper, M. N., Hopkins, K. D., & Farrant, B. M. (2017). The impact of racial discrimination on the health of Australian Indigenous children aged 5–10 years: Analysis of national longitudinal data. *International Journal for Equity in Health*, 16(116). doi:10.1186/s12939-017-0612-0.

Stulmaker, H. L. (2016). The extraordinary 7-year-old. In D. Ray (Ed), *A therapist's guide to child development: The extraordinarily normal years* (pp. 95–108). Routledge.

Tervalon, M., & Murray-García, J. (1998). Cultural humility versus cultural competence: A critical distinction in defining physician training outcomes in multicultural education. *Journal of Health Care for the Poor and Underserved*, 9(2), 117–125. doi:0.1353/hpu.2010.0233.

Toporek, R. (2006). *Handbook for social justice in counseling psychology: Leadership, vision, and action.* Sage.

Toporek, R., & Daniels, J. (2018). *American Counseling Association advocacy competencies.* ACA. www.counseling.org/docs/default-source/competencies/aca-advocacy-competencies-may-2020.pdf?sfvrsn=85b242c_6.

Part 2

Cultural Opportunities in Play Therapy Across Populations

4 Cultural Opportunities with LGBTQIA Populations

Kimberly M. Jayne and Cody T. L. Wehmeier

COLE (CHILD): "You sound weird."
CODY (THERAPIST): "You noticed something about how I talk seems different."
COLE: "Yeah – why do you talk like a girl?"
CODY: "Hmmm, my voice sounds a bit more like a girl's than a boy's to you."
COLE: "Mhm."
CODY: "Well, this is just the way my voice sounds."
COLE: "Oh, okay."

Following this early interaction in our play therapy relationship, Cole accepted my answer with ease before seemingly forgetting his question and returning his focus to the sand box. Several sessions later, Cole moved from his typical play in the sand to exploring the dress-up corner for the first time. He laughed as he picked up and discarded several clothing items before finally placing the pink boa on himself. Cole paused, made an expression of uncertainty, and quickly turned to me.

COLE: "It's okay if I wear this one, right?"
CODY: "Correct – in here, you get to decide if you want to wear that one."
COLE: "Yeah, in here you and I can say and wear what we want!"

Cultural Considerations for LGBTQIA Children and Their Families

LGBTQIAP2S+ is an acronym that describes children and the adults in their lives who identify as Lesbian, Gay, Bisexual, Transgender, Queer, Questioning, Intersex, Asexual, Pansexual, and Two-Spirit with the plus denoting the multitudes of identities and experiences of individuals across gender and sexuality. Across this dynamic web of sexual and gender diversity, individuals and community members use and reclaim language to more fully and authentically reflect their experiences and identities. Terms and

DOI: 10.4324/9781003190073-7

their meanings shift within the LGBTQIA community over time and are used uniquely and expansively by individuals within the LGBTQIA community. Additionally, children and individuals may not find themselves represented within current or popular categories and terms used to reflect sexual and gender diversity. Gender-expansive, -creative, and non-binary (gender identity does not correspond with sex assigned at birth and does not identify as male or female) children may use a variety of ways to describe themselves. As terms are used differently and shift over time, we will use the specific acronyms the cited authors, researchers, and organizations have used to identify people within the LGBTQIA community.

There are approximately 11.3 million LGBTQ adults in the U.S. (Conron & Goldberg, 2020). Between 2 and 3.7 million children under age 18 in the U.S. have an LGBTQ parent and 29% of LGBTQ people are raising children. It is estimated that there are 1,994,000 LGBT youth ages 13–17 in the United States (Conron, 2020). Accurate data for LGBTQIA children ages 3–12 are harder to know based on limitations of self-report surveys with children those ages and the dynamic developmental processes of gender and sexual identity development from preschool to early adolescence. Gender identity development and development of one's sexual orientation are independent and interacting developmental processes. Children are typically able to identify and articulate their gender identity as early as three years of age (Rafferty, 2018). While children ages nine and ten often experience and develop awareness of their romantic and sexual attraction across sexual orientations, LGBQ youth typically self-identify or disclose their sexual orientation between ages 16 and 17 (Boxer et al., 1993). Before disclosure of sexual identity, many LGBQ individuals report knowing their sexual orientation as early as seven or eight years of age. Over the past 25 years, the average age of "coming out" or disclosure of sexual orientation has increasingly become earlier as children and youth have experienced more supportive social environments and representation of LGBTQ individuals and families in society. However, the pervasive social and legal context of discrimination, homophobia, and transphobia in the United States presents profound barriers, increased vulnerability, and risk for LGBTQIA children and families to openly disclose their sexual and gender identities (Family Equality Council, 2020). There are currently no comprehensive federal nondiscrimination laws, or parenting, foster, and adoption laws in the United States for LGBTQ individuals or families, with legal rights and protections for LGBTQ youth and families varying widely from state to state. Additionally, hate crimes against LGBTQ people (US Department of Justice, 2019) and anti-LGBTQ legislation are increasing nationwide (Ronan, 2021).

Because of the discrimination, stress, inadequate support and resources, and risks to their psychological and physical safety from living and developing in environments that are oppressive based on their gender and sexual identities, LGBTQ youth are at greater risk for suicidal ideation and suicide attempts, non-suicidal self-injury, substance abuse, depression, anxiety, houselessness, family rejection, involvement with child welfare, incarceration, harassment and bullying, trauma, and physical violence (GLSEN, 2019; The Trevor Project, 2021a). LGBTQ youth also report higher rates of discrimination and lack of safety in schools. In a national survey of over 40,000 LGBTQ youth, nearly half of respondents reported that they did not receive wanted mental health care due to concerns related to parental permission and financial barriers and nearly half of transgender (gender identity does not correspond to sex assigned at birth) youth did not receive wanted mental health care due to concerns related to the LGBTQ competence of providers (The Trevor Project, 2021a). While research with younger gender-diverse and transgender children is more limited, researchers working with preschool transgender children and their siblings have found that socially transitioned young transgender children were just as likely as gender-typical children to (a) show preferences for peers, toys, and clothing culturally associated with their expressed gender, (b) dress in a stereotypically gendered outfit, (c) endorse flexibility in gender stereotypes, and (d) say they are more similar to children of their gender than to children of different genders (Fast & Olson, 2018) which indicates that trans children who are supported in expressing their gender identity follow similar gender identity development patterns as their gender-typical or cisgender (gender identity corresponds with sex assigned at birth) peers. Socially transitioned transgender children also showed the same rates of depression and anxiety as gender-typical children (Olson, 2016) and LGBTQ youth who are supported in their identities and social environments show similar rates of anxiety, depression, and suicidal ideation and attempts as their gender-typical and heterosexual peers (The Trevor Project, 2021a) pointing to the reality that impairment and pathology are not inherent to gender or sexual diversity but rather a reflection of cultural and social environments that do not support LGBTQIA children. Additionally, transgender and gender nonconforming children and their siblings show more flexibility in thinking about gender, hold fewer gender stereotypes, and demonstrate greater tolerance of gender nonconformity than gender-typical children (Olson & Gülgöz, 2018).

Play Therapy Considerations for LGBTQIA Children and Families

Although no child truly emerges from early life without having encountered some degree of perceived rejection or judgment, the cultural context in which children's early experiences are embedded can, and often do, have a profound impact on their development. In general, people who possess marginalized identities face increased rejection and harm from others, often at the hands of those from a contrasting privileged group. These messages are often echoed and/or influenced by layers of negative systemic and cultural biases, and can be seen in stereotypical, harmful views depicted in media or in institutional structures, such as rigid, binary-based student dress codes. For most gender-expansive or -creative children, growing up in a hetero- and cis-normative culture involves frequent reminders of the ways in which others deem their natural experience and personhood as incorrect, bad, or threatening. Many gender-creative children may likely endure direct efforts from caregivers to change or modify behaviors. For a young child, such critical messages would understandably serve to undermine their organismic valuing process, especially when such harmful societal messages are not being countered with ones of radical affirmation and active protective intervention in critical relationships.

From an early age, I (Cody) was often described as a very effeminate boy, and it terrified my parents. I was not turning out to be what a young boy was *supposed* to be. Many, if not most, of my behaviors were coded as girly, feminine, or gay by others. These characteristics always felt natural and powerful to me. They were deemed deviant, inappropriate, and even dangerous to others. My mother and I encountered much conflict as she worked harder and harder to redirect or extinguish my various feminine mannerisms, particularly as I started kindergarten and bullying increased in likelihood. And indeed, I remember that the last embers of my internal sense of defiance against this onslaught to my personhood seemed to finally burn out around second grade, the time I was first called a particular three-lettered slur by a classmate. At that point, I had already encountered endless messages insisting my experiences which felt natural and enhancing to me were in actuality wrong, distorted, and greatly risking my chance at acceptance. By fifth grade I had begun to keep a journal whereby I tracked notes analyzing my behavior. I looked for what would give the gay away, and then aggressively sought to extinguish it like a cancer. I now understand I was directly at war with my own organismic valuing (Rogers, 1951), and the resulting incongruence extended into a turbulent depression- and anxiety-laden adolescence. In reflecting back, I understand my mother was gripped with fear over the bullying she anticipated I would face starting grade school (and her predictions did not turn out wrong). She loved me very much. However, even with loving intention, fear-based approaches from my caregivers which aimed at changing me, rather than the things or people hurting me, simply added to my struggles with incongruence and self-loathing.

The Gender Affirmative Model and Humanistic Play Therapy

Given the growing onslaught of social stressors LGBTQIA children and families face, there is an ever-increasing demand for accessible and affirming therapeutic services to support this population's unique needs. However, the prevailing methods through which gender-expansive children have received clinical support have evolved throughout the last decade as collective understanding of gender health has expanded (Ehrensaft, 2016; Hidalgo et al., 2013). Outdated clinical approaches to addressing gender diversity in children typically focused on shaping the behaviors of gender-creative children to reflect their sex assigned at birth in hopes of ultimately fostering self-acceptance. Such methods disregard gender-expansive children's self-understanding by erroneously pathologizing gender variations, and as illustrated above, likely cause harm even when fueled by caring intentions. In fact, approaches aimed at altering gender expression and behaviors are classified as conversion or reparative therapies, and have widely been condemned for being ineffective, harmful, and unethical (Chang et al., 2018; SAMHSA, 2015).

Conversely, the gender affirmative model, a transtheoretical clinical guide developed through direct clinical practice, represents much of the positive growth within helping professions in regard to collective understanding of gender identity and gender health in children. The core principles of the gender affirmative model include:

a   Gender variations are not disorders; they are not pathological
b   Gender variations are healthy expressions of infinite possibilities of human gender
c   Gender presentations are diverse and varied across cultures, therefore requiring cultural sensitivity
d   Gender involves an interweaving of biology, development and socialization, and culture and context, with all three bearing on any individual's gender self
e   Gender may be fluid, and is not binary, both at a particular time and if and when it changes within an individual across time
f   If people suffer from any kind of emotional or psychiatric problem connected to their gender, this is most likely because of negative reactions to them from the outside world
g   If there is pathology, we will find it *not* in the child but in the culture (e.g. transphobia, homophobia, sexism)

(Ehrensaft, 2016, p. 15; Hildago et al., 2013, p. 285)

Within this model, gender health is defined as the opportunity for children to live in the gender that feels most real and/or comfortable to them; and for children to be able to express gender without experiencing restriction, criticism, or ostracism (Hidalgo et al., 2013). The model serves to recontextualize the disaffirming environment as the "problem," and never the gender-creative child.

Upon review of the gender affirmative model, clinicians may likely note an internal sense of familiarity, as many of the tenets of the model parallel humanistic sentiments. Indeed, Carl Rogers (1951, 1959), often considered the father of the humanistic approach to therapy, gave extensive emphasis towards radically respecting clients as the experts within the therapeutic process and empathically relating to the entirety of clients' fluctuating experiences. By extension, child-centered play therapy (CCPT), based on Rogers' person-centered approach, represents one path for affirmingly working with gender-creative children given its child-led nature and emphasis on facilitating children's innate ability to move towards self-understanding and self-enhancement.

Cultural Opportunities in the Play Therapy Environment

Children and families experience a play therapist's affirming practice before they enter the playroom. Play therapists provide safety and build trust by considering how their marketing materials and their office or clinical environment provide a sense of welcoming and safety to LGBTQIA children and families. Play therapists may foster an affirming environment by examining what gender identities, sexual orientations, and family compositions are represented through artwork, literature, media, and signs in spaces including waiting rooms, lobbies, hallways, bathrooms, counseling offices, and playrooms. Additionally, they may consider how gender stereotypes and/or heteronormative assumptions reinforced or conveyed in these entry and community spaces. For gender-diverse children and families, having access to an all-gender or family bathroom reduces additional stress and provides psychological and physical safety for the child around one of their basic needs and primary developmental processes. One of the many ways that a play therapist can convey acceptance and broach gender identity in play therapy is by sharing their pronouns with clients through their marketing and educational resources and when they introduce themselves to the child and their family. Additionally, sharing their training and experience working with LGBTQIA children and families with parents and caregivers at the beginning of the play therapy relationship can provide a context for families to feel safe and understood and further demonstrate the play therapist's commitment to competent practice.

Toys and Materials

In the playroom, play therapists can be intentional about including toys that represent the experiences of LGBTQIA children and their families and support the exploration and expression of their gender identity and sexual identity. For example, including doll families and animal families that allow for children to represent and explore their family composition in their play, such as two moms or two dads, provides a foundation for children to perceive empathy and acceptance from the play therapist. Play therapists can support children in their gender and sexual identity development by providing dress-up clothes that allow for a wide range of gender expression (feminine, masculine, neutral, androgynous, and beyond) and being intentional about the colors and branding of toys that are typically associated with gender stereotypes or roles. Having a play kitchen in natural tones or colors rather than one that is bright pink or including play cars and vehicles in a variety of colors may allow children to explore play that is not traditionally associated with their assigned sex or perceived gender more freely and authentically. While it is common for children to explore play and demonstrate play behaviors that reflect their gender socialization and gender stereotypes or roles (Stutey et al., 2020), it is helpful to consider how the playroom environment inhibits or frees children of all genders in expressing themselves. Children need toys and materials that are traditionally feminine, traditionally masculine, and that transcend the gender binary to allow for exploration, creativity, and full expression of their experiences and perceptions of gender.

Play Therapist Knowledge and Attitudes

Understanding research and developmental knowledge specific to the experiences of LGBTQIA children and families is also critical for providing competent and empathic care to play therapy clients and students. Knowledge of gender identity development (Bockting & Coleman, 2007; Fast & Olson, 2018; Gülgöz et al., 2019; Levitt & Ippolito, 2014; Martin & Ruble, 2010) and sexual identity development models (Cass, 1979; D'Augelli & Patterson, 1995, 1994; Jamil et al., 2009; Troiden, 1988; Rosario et al., 2006) is critical for more fully understanding and empathizing with the experiences of gender and sexually diverse children and their families. Beyond professional knowledge for working with LGBTQIA children, it is essential that play therapists explore their own gender and sexual identity, socialization, and biases while developing routines and structures in their practice and professional communities that support ongoing growth, critical reflection, and actions towards becoming more affirming of children's diverse gender and sexual identities.

Language

A critical aspect of affirming play therapy practice is the language a play therapist uses in their communication with a child. Pursuing education and experience with accurate terminology used within the LGBTQIA community is important for being responsive to the child and families' experiences in and out of the playroom. Several authors and organizations provide updated glossaries and infographics with definitions for sex, gender, gender expression, sexual orientation, and other essential terms for play therapists to build comfortability and competency when working with LGBTQIA children and their families (Angello & Bowman, 2016; Ehrensaft, 2016; GLSEN, 2021; Trans Student Educational Resources, 2021). Additionally, many resources exist for providing developmentally responsive definitions and terms for gender diversity for children (Chinn-Raicht, 2021; Parr,

2021; Pessin-Whedbee, 2017; Storck, 2018; Thorn, 2019). Using a child's pronouns, and not gendering or using gender labels for toys until the child does are some of the ways that a play therapist may use language to facilitate the child's authentic and whole expression of themselves. Following the child's lead for how they express their gender and use language to describe their gender identity and sexual orientation while also demonstrating openness and ease with broaching gender and sexuality in the play therapy relationship provide the child with the freedom and context to explore, question, express, and disclose their authentic self. For languages where feminine and masculine cases are used for nouns, pronouns, verbs, and/or adjectives, play therapists can employ gender-neutral endings and gender-neutral alternatives that are developing as advocates and linguists work to create more inclusive and representative ways of representing gender and sexual diversity (Berger, 2019).

Nonverbal and Verbal Skills

Play therapists' use of nonverbal and verbal communication in the play therapy relationship with LGBTQIA children provides the opportunity to convey empathy, acceptance, and facilitate the child's exploration and expression of their experiences and identities. While many of the nonverbal and verbal skills a play therapist uses may be consistent across therapeutic relationships, it is important for play therapists to consider and examine how their own beliefs, values, and biases may impact their nonverbal and verbal communication and how to be more intentional in their use of skills with gender and sexually diverse children. Play therapists may reflect on sessions, video record sessions, or seek supervisory feedback to explore patterns in how they relate to children of different genders and sexual orientations. For example, is a play therapist more or less likely to lean towards, make eye contact, receive physical contact or play from the child, join in the child's play, or be comfortable with a child playing or being in close physical proximity based on their own and/or the child's gender and sexual identity? Is the play therapist more comfortable with play behaviors that match gender norms or stereotypes? Are they more willing to join in or respond to gender-typical or gender-diverse play activities or role-play with the child?

The play therapist's values, beliefs, attitudes, and biases similarly extend to their use of verbal skills in the play therapy relationship with LGBTQIA children. Play therapists work to reflect the child's whole experience and honor the child's self-awareness of their gender and sexual identities. Play therapists demonstrate empathy and acceptance by responding to the full range of the child's experiences, expression, play behaviors, and themes within the play therapy relationship. By working not to privilege or respond primarily to gender and sexual stereotypes and roles, or rather cis- or heteronormative expectations, the play therapist attends to and accepts experiences of the LGBTQIA child that are expansive and reflect their whole, genuine self. For example, if a child assigned female at birth (AFAB) engages in more physical or aggressive play like punching the bop bag, throwing toys, or hitting the play therapist with a sword, or a child assigned male at birth (AMAB) engages in more nurturing play such as rocking and feeding the baby doll or brushing and styling the play therapist's hair, the play therapist seeks to respond to the child actively, openly, and with acceptance. If a play therapist seems more withdrawn, less responsive, or becomes silent to specific play behaviors, they may communicate conditional regard to the child. Affirming play therapists are also intentional in not setting limits on children's play based on gender expectations or stereotypes or their exploration of sexual orientation and to use tracking, reflections of content, feeling, and meaning across gender and sexual identities. For example, being mindful about any tendencies to reflect more feelings or setting limits on risk-taking to female-appearing or AFAB children. With critical reflection, observation, and consultation, play therapists may explore how their values, beliefs, experiences, and biases may impact their nonverbal and verbal responses to children based on gender, gender expression, and sexual orientation.

Cultural Opportunities in the Therapeutic Relationship

Through the therapeutic relationship, cultural opportunities arise as LGBTQIA children and play therapists interact from their own cultural experiences and identities, and as the play therapist actively seeks to create an environment where the child may experience and express their full selves. These opportunities are numerous, dynamic, and often mutually transforming, for in the play therapist's endeavors to remain truly open to the moment-to-moment becoming of the child, they are also open to their own growth and becoming in the play therapy relationship. As Ehrensaft (2016, p. 25) describes, "The job of the adults is to allow a wide berth for this spinning and weaving, mirroring the children's artistic creations – their gender self – back to them, rather than controlling the motion of the threads and imposing their own gender images on the child."

Exploration of Gender Socialization

Children often explore gender and sexual stereotypes and their own gender and sexual socialization through the play therapy process. Children are socialized by how significant others behave and relate to them, the models of gender and sexuality they are exposed to through childhood, and through their social and cultural environments (Ehrensaft, 2016; Derman-Sparks et al., 2020; Martin & Ruble, 2004). Children internalize these norms, roles, and stereotypes and apply them to themselves and others with periods of more rigidity and flexibility throughout development. A child may study the crayons in the playroom, pick one up and then set it back down suddenly while emphatically declaring, "Pink is a girl's color!" The play therapist may provide acceptance of the child's experience while also recognizing the child's development, socialization, and individual context by responding, "You think pink is a girl's color, and you want to use it even though you are a boy." A child with gay parents may repeatedly arrange dolls in the sand and put family units together with a male parent and a female parent that do not reflect their family structure. The play therapist may respond, leaning towards the child, "Mmm. You're putting the families together like that." The child continues setting up hetero-normative family units. "Your family has a papa and a daddy, and you're thinking a lot about different kinds of families right now." The play thera-pist seeks to acknowledge the child's direct experiences and their potential struggles with heteronormative expectations for families.

Exploration of Family Structure and Dynamics

Children additionally explore their family relationships, structure, and dynamics in the play therapy process. It is essential for LGBTQIA children to experience acceptance and understanding as they express their own feel-ings and experiences related to their families. LGBTQIA children may play out experiences of rejection, isolation, or punishment in their families rela-ted to their gender or sexual identity. They may also explore their family structure in comparison to other families. Following the child's lead, the play therapist has the opportunity to respond and facilitate the child's play by honoring the child's experiences related to the identities they hold and the identities of their family members and their family structure. For example, a child whose family is struggling to accept and support their transgender or gender-expansive identity may choose giraffes to represent their parents and siblings, and then choose a whale for themselves. The child creates a home environment for the animals to live, and lays all the giraffes down in the sand, but narrates that the whale does not fit. The play therapist may respond, "That one feels different. Like they don't belong with the others," reflecting on the whale's experience of being othered and feelings of rejection.

Exploration of Gender and Gender Identity

Children of all gender identities may explore their gender identity in their play behavior, trying out and exploring different gender roles and norms, and expressing their gender in new ways. Many children may feel inhibited in their play early in the play therapy relationship, hesitant to choose or use toys and materials that are typically associated with a gender identity differ-ent from their own or their assigned sex at birth. Play therapists' empathy and acceptance for this struggle and for the child's desire and need to play outside of gender norms and express their gender more expansively and holistically becomes a context for freedom. For gender-expansive and transgender children, being able to express their true gender authentically and dynamically in an accepting and affirming play therapy relationship is liberating and allows for deeper integration of their true experience of their gender. The play therapy environment and materials, and the play therapist's attitudes and responses to the child as discussed previously, both facilitate children's exploration and expression of their gender and their experiences related to gender socialization. For example, a child who was assigned male at birth, puts on a sparkly tutu and tiara, looks in the mirror and states with excitement and pleasure, "I'm a beautiful mommy." Rather than paraphrasing what the child says, such as, "You feel really beautiful," or "You think you look like a mommy," it may be more empathic and impactful to reflect back, matching the child's tone and affect, "You're a beautiful mommy!" Using the child's exact words in this instance conveys trust in their self-experience and resists qualifying their experience of their gender or gender expression. Beyond reflecting the child's gender expression and identity, the play therapist also has the opportunity to express their gender holistically and congruently in the play therapy relationship. A female play therapist may dress in a typically masculine way or be more athletic than a child may expect. The play therapist's own acceptance of their identities allows them to be more fully present and responsive to the child's experiences and identities, and allows the child to experience adults with different or similar gender identities and sexual orientations as authentic and integrated in the relationship.

Play therapists may also choose to self-identify or disclose their own identities as part of their introduction to children and families or throughout the therapeutic process. As with all self-disclosure, the play therapist considers the therapeutic benefit and risks of sharing personal information, and how self-disclosure promotes or inhibits the attitudinal conditions (i.e. genuineness, unconditional positive regard, and empathic understanding). For play therapists who are LGBTQIA, self-disclosure also involves consideration of the play therapist's own sense of vulnerability and safety and the visibility of their identities based on their gender expression, community involvement and relationships, and/or work setting. The play therapist's self-disclosure is similarly impacted by the conditions in their environments and the degree to which they experience true empathy and acceptance personally and professionally. For example, as children explore their own identities and experiences in the world and seek to connect with their play therapist, they often ask about the therapist's identities, families, and experiences.

A child may ask a play therapist, "Are you a boy or a girl?" A non-binary play therapist may respond, "You're wondering what gender I am."

CHILD: I'm a girl.
THERAPIST: You're a girl. And you're wondering about me, if I'm the same or different than you.

CHILD: Are you a girl?

THERAPIST: You think I may be a girl like you. I'm neither a boy or a girl. I'm non-binary.

Exploration of Romantic Relationships

Children in play therapy often explore their understanding of romantic and sexual relationships related to their own development and their identities. In early childhood, children will explore the more physical or modeled aspects of gender and sexuality and romantic relationships (Derman-Sparks et al., 2020; Martin & Ruble, 2004; Rafferty, 2018). A child may talk about or act out how they see people kissing on the mouth or ask if they can marry a parent or teacher. They are also focused on the physical aspects of their bodies that are often associated with gender and sexuality. As children move into middle childhood and early adolescence, they more frequently explore what they know and understand about sexual and romantic relationships in their peer relationships. A younger child may declare in play therapy, "When you're a grown up, you get married and have babies," reflecting their socialization related to the structure and purpose of romantic/sexual relationships. Pre-adolescents may share more about their feelings and interactions with peers related to their own awareness of developing more romantic and sexual attractions. A pre-adolescent may ask the play therapist, "Do you think it's okay if girls date girls?" The play therapist has the opportunity to reflect the child's questioning and with some experience with the child over time and knowledge of their context, to respond in a manner that supports the child in their own self-understanding and self-acceptance. The play therapist may respond, "Hmm. You're thinking about dating relationships, and it seems like you've noticed that some people think it's okay and some people think it's not okay. I wonder how you feel about girls dating girls."

Responding to Trans/Homophobia in the Playroom

As children express their gender and sexual socialization, and their own gender identity and orientation in play therapy, they may use language or express ideas that are sexist, homophobic, and/or transphobic in the play-room. Children may also misgender or make assumptions about the play therapist's sexual orientation or family composition, and project gender stereotypes/roles onto the play therapist. The play therapist has the oppor-tunity to respond to the child based on their understanding of the child's socialization experiences and worldview. How the play therapist responds may be connected to the context in which they are practicing such as a school environment or a clinical environment or in individual or group play therapy; if the child is directing the language or idea towards the play therapist directly; the child's identities; the play therapist's identities; and the play therapist's theoretical orientation and philosophy related to limit-setting. Children need to be able to express aspects of their experience and self-understanding that may be harder for the play therapist to accept, and for LGBTQIA children it is essential that they can explore their own internalized sexism/homophobia/transphobia as well as ways they have experienced bias and discrimination from others. Children in play therapy often repeat what they have heard or experienced in their social environments, and it may be helpful to reflect their socialization in these instances, "That's something you've seen on television before," or "It seems like you've heard other people saying those things about gay people before." Understanding the child's need or motivation for expressing sexist, homophobic, and/or transphobic language or ideas provides the play therapist the opportunity to personalize their response to the child and their therapeutic process. Meeting all of these opportunities and many others allows the play therapist to be fully present to the child's experience of themselves through their development and socialization.

Working with Families

The family environment is critical to LGBTQIA children's health and development, and play therapists are positioned to play a central role in supporting LGBTQIA children and families. LGBTQ youth who experience greater parental acceptance and support have less suicidal ideation and attempts, decreased depression, lower levels of psychological distress and post-traumatic stress disorder, higher self-esteem, higher life satisfaction, and better overall mental health (Travers et al., 2012; Wilson et al., 2016). Familial support has been shown to have the strongest association with fewer symptoms of depression and anxiety and greater resilience for trans youth than other types of social and community support and protective factors (Puckett et al., 2019).

Beginning the Play Therapy Process with Families

When play therapists begin their relationship with families of LGBTQIA children, it is important that they include exploration and discussion of the child's gender and sexual development as part of their developmental interview or intake process. Understanding the child's developmental experiences related to gender identity, sexual development, and sexual orientation allows the play therapist to more fully understand the context of the child and to begin to assess the family's values, beliefs, attitudes, and perceptions related to their child's gender and sexuality. Including opportunities for parents/caregivers to disclose their own and the child's pronouns and chosen name(s) and asking questions that explore the child's history related to how they have articulated and expressed their gender and sexuality is important for providing an affirming environment, and also being able to understand these central aspects of a child's development and social experience.

Parent/Caregiver Consultation and Family Therapy

Beyond intentional intake procedures, consistent family and parent/caregiver consultation provide the opportunity for play therapists to understand how family members are experiencing the child's gender and sexual development and to provide systemic support and resources. While the experiences of families of LGBTQIA families are unique and varied based on family members' own histories and experiences related to gender and sexuality, their identities and cultural experiences, and their social contexts, it is common for family members (especially gender-typical or heterosexual parents/caregivers) to encounter feelings of uncertainty, ambiguity, loss, and grief when a child articulates, discloses, or expresses their gender or sexual diversity (Ehrensaft, 2016). Many parents/caregivers may experience fears related to their child experiencing discrimination or challenges in life and concerns related to how their extended families, social, educational, and/or religious communities may respond to the child or the family because of the child's gender identity and/or sexual orientation. Parents and caregivers may question if they did something wrong or have feelings of guilt of self-blame. Play therapists strive to convey understanding and empathizing with the parents/caregivers' experiences and provide unconditional positive regard for parents/caregivers' experiences, perspectives, and own developmental process related to their child's gender identity and/or sexual orientation. Only after parents/caregivers experience the acceptance and empathy of the play therapist are they ready for the play therapist to provide education and resources related to gender identity and sexual development, supporting and affirming their child in their identities. Connecting with other parents and families of LGBTQIA children and the broader LGTBQIA community can help families experience greater social support and provide opportunities for connection, mentorship, and advocacy.

Through parent/caregiver consultation and family therapy, play therapists work within the family system to promote an accepting and supportive home and family environment. Coolhart (2018) provides a helpful model for supporting parents/caregivers in moving from initial distress towards acceptance of their child's gender that has applications for children across gender identities and sexual orientations. In the beginning of therapy, Coolhart recommends starting with separate sessions for caregivers/parents to buffer the child from parents' intense emotions, views, thoughts, and feelings that may be harmful to the child while also allowing the parent to freely express and explore their own experiences, values, and beliefs related to their child's gender and/or sexual identity in an accepting environment. Separate child sessions also allow the play therapist to provide an environment where the child may express and explore their true self and experience empathy, acceptance, and support directly from the therapist. Throughout this process the therapist is transparent with parents/caregivers about their gender-affirming approach while also striving to meet family members where they are at and avoid alienating them from the therapeutic process.

As play therapists continue to work with parents/caregivers, they provide accurate education on children's gender identity and sexual development, gender and sexual diversity, and address questions and concerns that parents/caregivers may have related to their child's gender and/or sexual identity (Coolhart, 2018). This often includes normalizing gender and sexual diversity and helping parents/caregivers develop familiarity and comfortability with key terminology related to gender and sexuality. In addition to providing direct support to parents/caregivers, the play therapist supports the parent in listening, empathizing, and more fully understanding their child's experience. This often includes teaching parents/caregivers specific attitudes and skills that are consistent with play therapy, filial, and child-parent relationship therapy (CPRT; Landreth & Bratton, 2020; e.g. following the child's lead, reflections of content, reflections of feeling, etc.), sharing observations from play therapy sessions with the parent that expand their understanding of the child, and listening attentively to how the parent describes the child that allows the therapist to amplify and illuminate the parent's perspective and understanding of the child and the child's world. Helping parents/caregivers understand that the child's identity is not a "problem to be fixed," illuminating the child's pain, distress, and the risks to the child in not being able to live into their true self, and in parallel, identifying the child's happiness and progress when they are able to express their gender and/or sexuality congruently and authentically all promote parents' attunement and movement towards greater acceptance of the child. This may also include helping the parent/caregiver reflect on and identify threads of the child's gender or sexual diversity throughout their development and helping them explore the protective and risk factors related to the parents' behaviors towards the child. The Family Acceptance Project (2020) provides comprehensive resources on parental/familial behaviors that increase LGBTQ children's health and wellbeing and behaviors that increase LGBTQ children's risk for serious physical and mental health problems (https://familyproject.sfsu.edu).

Play therapists consider the impact of and on the LGBTQIA child's siblings, close family members, and extended family and/or friends and help parents/caregivers navigate communication and relationship dynamics with other family members. Co-parents may also need support as they often have different values, beliefs, and experiences related to their child's gender and sexual identity; move towards acceptance in different ways or on different timelines; and also may need support navigating conflicts and stress related to different parenting approaches for their LGBTQIA child.

When working with LGBTQIA children and families of color, play therapists strive to honor all aspects of their identities, acknowledge the multiple sources of oppression and discrimination that they may experience, and avoid focusing on the child's gender or sexual identity to the exclusion of their racial or ethnic identity. Play therapists understand that sexuality and gender are experienced and understood uniquely across cultures. Many children and families of color may find that mainstream LGBTQ communities and representation socially and in the media are predominantly White (Brown & Mar, 2018). For LGBTQIA children of color, they may feel pressure to choose between identifying with their racial/ethnic group or with the predominantly White LGBTQIA community resulting in a type of cultural splitting that diminishes the experience and person of the child. As the play therapist works with children and families of color, they prioritize cultural representation in and out of the playroom, language accessibility, mentorship and peer relationships with other LGBTQ people of color, and community support and resources that are culturally specific (Brown & Mar, 2018). LGBTQIA children with disabilities, who are undocumented, Black, Indigenous, Latinx, of color, immigrants, and/or economically under-resourced experience more discrimination and systemic oppression. Play therapists must consider how to promote a truly psychologically and physically safe environment that honors the full humanity, intersectional identities, and cultural selves of LGBTQIA children of color.

As parents/caregivers become more attuned to their LGBTQIA child's experiences, they often move towards advocacy for their child. Play therapists support parents in this process by helping them understand their rights and explore options to improve their child's support in specific environments and systems. For gender-expansive and trans children specifically, this primarily includes helping parents as they support their children in social, medical, and legal transitions, and for sexually diverse children this often includes supporting children in when/if, who to, and how they disclose their sexual orientation and how they navigate romantic and sexual relationships. Familial advocacy also includes protecting the child from discrimination and harassment and working to create environments and relationships that are safe and supportive for the child. Advocacy may also extend to the community, local, state, and national level, as parents seek structural and systemic changes that protect and support their child in their identities.

For gender-expansive, non-binary, and transgender children, social transition provides them the opportunity to let others know their true gender identity and for them to live in their gender authentically. Social transition is often a critical and first intervention for young transgender children in and out of the playroom and may include changing one's pronouns and/or name; changing one's appearance and dress to reflect one's gender identity (including binding, tucking, padding, etc.); expressing new behaviors, engaging in new activities, and using facilities that correspond to one's gender rather than one's sex assigned at birth. Before puberty, social transition is the most accessible option for trans children to live in their true gender. Play therapists can help parents/caregivers and children explore the ways in which they may want to socially transition and the risks and benefits of social transition within specific environments. Play therapists also support parents/caregivers in understanding and navigating their child's dynamic, fluid, and developmental exploration of gender as a child's decision to socially transition or express their gender in a specific way may change or remain stable over time.

Key factors to consider when identifying when social transition best serves the child include: (a) gender identity is not a symptom of some other underlying problem (e.g. trauma, cultural advantage, resolves a different challenge); (b) the central issue is gender identity not gender expression; (c) the child expresses the need and desire to socially transition to another gender; and (d) caregivers/parents can offer positive support for their child transitioning (Ehrensaft, 2018). Families and children may choose for the child to transition in some social environments and not others. Children may also choose to express their gender differently in different environments or at different times. For prepubertal children who "insistently, persistently, and consistently" articulate their gender as different than their sex assigned at birth (e.g. "I *am* a _____ boy/girl/other)," social transition reduces their risk for negative mental health outcomes and often resolves gender distress and dysphoria (Ehrensaft, 2016). If parents/caregivers are unable to support a child's social transition, the play therapist would work to increase the parents/caregivers' acceptance of the child and understand the impact of not socially transitioning on the child, and support the child in navigating their experiences of not being supported in transitioning socially.

Medical treatments that affirm a child's true gender including puberty and hormone blockers are available for children at the onset of puberty. Puberty blockers delay the development of secondary sex characteristics in children and reduce potentially increasing gender dysphoria. Other medical treatments including hormone therapy and gender confirmation surgeries are not typically available until youth are well beyond the age most children would be engaged in play therapy. Play therapists may support parents/caregivers in navigating decisions about medical treatment by allowing them to process their feelings and concerns, providing referrals to trans-competent health and medical professionals, and supporting parents in their advocacy efforts for their child to receive affirming healthcare.

Working with Systems

Schools and Educational Settings

Educational settings are often a primary social environment for children ages 3–12 and play a significant role in socialization and in physical and mental health outcomes for LGTBQIA children. LGBTQ students report school absences due to feeling unsafe and uncomfortable at school; avoiding gender-segregated spaces in schools such as bathrooms and locker rooms; experiencing verbal and physical harassment based on their gender identity and/or sexual orientation; and being prevented from using bathrooms, locker rooms, names, pronouns, and dressing in ways that align with their gender identity (GLSEN, 2019). LGBTQ students in affirming school environments (e.g. gender-affirming policies allowing students to engage in the school environment in their true gender, Gender and Sexuality Alliances, a comprehensive anti-harassment and bullying curriculum, students having access to 11 or more supportive adults, etc.) are less likely to experience discrimination and to miss school, are more likely to pursue post-secondary education, have higher GPAs, and feel a greater sense of safety and belonging to their school community (GLSEN, 2019).

Play therapists need to understand the impact of the child's school or educational environment on the child specifically, while also learning specific school, district, and state policies and legislation impacting LGBTQIA children and families where they practice. Play therapists have the opportunity to help parents/caregivers advocate for their child in the educational environment and support their decisions about how to navigate transitions and discrimination or harassment in the school setting. Consultation with a child's teachers, school counselor, school social worker, and/or other school staff allows the play therapist to work systemically to better understand the child's experience and impact change in their social environments. Play therapists can provide professional development and work with teachers and staff to overcome barriers to the child's acceptance and success in the school environment. Play therapists can also advocate for clients through participation in meetings related to an LGBTQIA client's Individual Education Plan or 504 meeting and planning. In the playroom, the child's social experiences in school, like home and family, will often be part of their play and therapeutic process. The play therapist can respond to the child's experiences while working with the family and school system to improve the individual and systemic supports and resources available to the child.

Child Welfare Systems

LGBTQ youth are more likely to be involved in the foster care system, with transgender and LGBTQ youth of color even more likely than cisgender or White LGBQ youth (The Trevor Project, 2021b) to be in foster care. LGBTQ youth in foster care are at higher risk for attempting suicide and experiencing victimization and abandonment/rejection than LGBTQ youth who are not in foster care. Play therapists working with children who are involved with child welfare systems and foster care often engage across multiple complex systems that impact the child's development and well-being, serving as a bridge between caregivers, case and social workers, guardian ad litems and court-appointed special advocates, educational and healthcare systems, and as an advocate with the child in all of these systems.

Because children who are involved with child welfare have typically experienced maltreatment or potentially traumatic events, the play therapist works directly with the child to actively support the child in their integration and healing of any trauma, working to support them in their gender and sexual identity development while also working systemically to strengthen and reduce barriers to affirming relationships and environments with which the child engages.

Conclusion

Play therapists can play a critical role in supporting and facilitating children's exploration and development of their gender identity and sexual orientation in play therapy and through their work with family, educational, and other core systems in the child's life as they foster affirming relationships and environments that support the child beyond the play therapy relationship. The work of meeting the cultural opportunities and responsibilities of play therapy with LGBTQIA children and their adults begins with the person of the play therapist, exploring their own identities, socialization, and biases; being open to learning and pursuing education on the experiences of LGBTQIA children; and committing to action in how they create environments and develop relationships that honor the full humanity and experience of the LGBTQIA child. This work is best supported and sustained in community and in relationship with others who are committed and actively pursuing a play therapy practice that affirms children's gender and sexual diversity.

Positionality Statements

Kimberly

I (Kimberly, she/her/hers or they/them/theirs) am a White, cisgender, non-disabled woman in a long-term monogamous relationship with a man. I hold privilege based on my economic status, education, and U.S. citizenship. I understand my own and other's gender identity and sexuality as dynamic, fluid, and lifelong developmental processes. I feel incongruent identifying myself in a single category of gender or sexual orientation beyond questioning, exploring, growing, and a process of becoming. I have had the great privilege of working and growing with many LGBTQIAP children and their adults, clients, and students. Through those opportunities as a play therapist and counselor educator, and through my own therapeutic process and development, I have experienced greater freedom and healing in my own experience and understanding of my gender and sexual development and identities. As a parent to young children, I have also had the amazing gift and responsibility of supporting them in being and expressing their true selves, as I strive to support their exploration and creative weaving of their gender identities and sexual orientations with openness, attunement, empathic understanding, and unconditional positive regard. They teach me and help me become more me every day.

Cody

I (Cody, he/him/his) am a gay, White, cisgender, non-disabled man in a long-term monogamous marriage with another man. I, too, hold privilege based on my economic status, education, and U.S. citizenship. My sexual orientation and gender expression have always been my greatest sources of strife or oppression, with most of the additional facets of my identity holding privilege. Although I have always identified as cisgender, many of my mannerisms and ways of being are typically coded as feminine. As such, I have walked through life often being presented with the notion that I am not what a man should be, and at times I have put much effort into altering myself to present more masculine. My process of becoming a play therapist has been complicated. As I have moved towards increased personal congruence and integration, I have sought to reclaim the pieces of me that feel natural and self-enhancing, including my femininity. At times, this presents a challenge, particularly when working in Texas. However, my own experience of working to heal and embrace my whole self has only served to enhance my desire to support children in their own processes of becoming.

References

Angello, M., & Bowman, A. (2016). *Raising the transgender child: A complete guide for parents, families, and caregivers.* Seal Press.

Berger, M. (2019, December 15). A guide to how gender-neutral language is developing around the world. *The Washington Post.* www.washingtonpost.com/world/2019/12/15/guide-how-gender-neutral-language-is-developing-around-world.

Bockting, W. O. & E. Coleman (2007). Developmental stages of the transgender coming-out process: Toward an integrated identity. In R. Ettner, E. Coleman, & S. Monstrey (Eds.), *Principles of transgender medicine and surgery* (pp. 209–232). Routledge.

Boxer, A. M., Cohler, B. J., Herdt, G., & Irvin, F. (1993). Gay and lesbian youth. In P. H. Tolan & B. J. Cohler (Eds.), *Handbook of clinical research and practice with adolescents* (pp. 249–280). John Wiley & Sons.

Brown, E. & Mar, K. (2018). Culturally responsive practice with children of color. In C. Keo-Meier & D. Ehrensaft (Eds.), *The gender affirmative model: An interdisciplinary approach to supporting transgender and gender expansive children* (pp. 55 70). American Psychological Association.

Cass, V. C. (1979). Homosexual identity formation. *Journal of Homosexuality,* 4(3), 219–235. doi:10.1300/J082v04n03_01.

Chang, S. C., Singh, A. A., & Dickey, L. M. (2018). *A clinician's guide to gender-affirming care: Working with transgender and gender nonconforming clients.* Context Press.

Chinn-Raicht, H. (2021). *A kids book about being non-binary.* A Kids Book About, Inc.

Coolhart, D. (2018). Helping families move from distress to attunement. In C. Keo-Meier & D. Ehrensaft (Eds.), *The gender affirmative model: An interdisciplinary approach to supporting transgender and gender expansive children* (pp. 125–140). American Psychological Association.

Conron, K. J., & Goldberg, S. K. (2020). Adult LGBT population in the United States. The Williams Institute, UCLA. https://williamsinstitute.law.ucla.edu/p ublications/adult-lgbt-pop-us.

Conron, K. J. (2020). LGBT youth population in the United States. The Williams Institute, UCLA. https://williamsinstitute.law.ucla.edu/publications/lgbt-youth-pop-us.

D'Augelli, A. R., & Patterson, C. J. (1995). *Lesbian, gay, and bisexual identities over the lifespan.* Oxford University Press.

Derman-Sparks, L., Edwards, J. O., & Goins, C. M. (2020). *Anti-bias education for young children and ourselves* (2nd ed.). National Association for the Education of Young Children.

Ehrensaft, D. (2016). *The gender creative child: Pathways for nurturing and supporting children who live outside gender boxes.* The Experiment.

Ehrensaft, D. (2018). Exploring gender expansive expressions versus asserting gender identity. In C. Keo-Meier & D. Ehrensaft (Eds.), *The gender affirmative model: An interdisciplinary approach to supporting transgender and gender expansive children* (pp. 37–54). American Psychological Association.

Family Equality Council (2020). LGBTQ family fact sheet. www.familyequality.org/wp-content/uploads/2021/01/LGBTQ-Families-2020-Sheet-Final-clean-version.pdf.

Fast, A. A., & Olson, K. R. (2018). Gender development in transgender preschool children. *Child Development*, 89(2), 620–637. doi:10.1111/cdev.12758.

GLSEN (2019). The 2019 national school climate survey: The experiences of lesbian, gay, bisexual, transgender, and queer youth in our nation's schools. www.glsen.org/research/2019-national-school-climate-survey.

GLSEN (2021, June 29). Gender terminology. Retrieved from: www.glsen.org/activity/gender-terminology.

Gülgöz, S., Glazier, J. J., Enright, E. A., Alonso, D. J., Durwood, L. J., Fast, A. A., Lowe, R., Ji, C., Heer, J., Martin, C. L., & Olson, K. R. (2019). Similarity in transgender and cisgender children's gender development. *Proceedings of the National Academy of Sciences – PNAS*, 116(49), 24480–24485. doi:10.1073/pnas.1909367116.

Hidalgo, M. A., Ehrensaft, D., Tishelman, A. C., Clark, L. F., Garofalo, R., Rosenthal, S. M., Spack, N. P., & Olson, J. (2013). The gender affirmative model: What we know and what we aim to learn. *Human Development*, 56(5), 285–290. doi:10.1159/000355235.

Jamil, O. B., Harper, G. W., & Fernandez, M. I. (2009). Sexual and ethnic identity development among Gay-Bisexual-Questioning (GBQ) male ethnic minority adolescents. *Cultural Diversity & Ethnic Minority Psychology*, 15(3), 203–214. doi:10.1037/a0014795.

Landreth, G., & Bratton, S. (2020). *Child-parent relationship therapy: An evidence-based 10 session filial therapy model.* Routledge.

Levitt, H. M., & Ippolito, M. R. (2014). Being transgender: The experience of transgender identity development. *Journal of Homosexuality*, 61(12), 1727–1758.

Martin, C. L., & Ruble, D. (2004). Children's search for gender cues: Cognitive perspectives on gender development. *Current Directions in Psychological Science: A Journal of the American Psychological Society*, 13(2), 67–70. doi:10.1111/j.0963-7214.2004.00276.x.

Martin, C. L., & Ruble, D. N. (2010). Patterns of gender development. *Annual Review of Psychology*, 61, 353–381. doi:10.1146/annurev.psych.093008.100511.

Olson, K. R. (2016). Prepubescent transgender children: What we do and do not know. *Journal of the American Academy of Child and Adolescent Psychiatry*, 55(3), 155–156. doi:10.1016/j.jaac.2015.11.015.

Olson, K. R., & Gülgöz, S. (2018). Early findings from the TransYouth project: Gender development in transgender children. *Child Development Perspectives*, 12(2), 93–97. doi:10.1111/cdep.12268.

Parr, G. (2021). *A kids book about being transgender*. A Kids Book About, Inc.

Pessin-Whedbee, B. (2017). *Who are you? The kid's guide to gender identity*. Jessica Kingsley.

Puckett, J. A., Matsuno, E., Dyar, C., Mustanski, B., & Newcomb, M. E. (2019). Mental health and resilience in transgender individuals: What type of support makes a difference? *Journal of Family Psychology*, 33(8), 954–964. doi:10.1037/fam0000561.

Rafferty, J. (2018, September 18). Gender identity development in children. Retrieved from: www.healthychildren.org/English/ages-stages/gradeschool/Pages/Gender-Identity-and-Gender-Confusion-In-Children.aspx.

Rogers, C. R. (1951). *Client-centered therapy*. Houghton Mifflin.

Rogers, C. R. (1957). The necessary and sufficient conditions of therapeutic personality change. *Journal of Consulting Psychology*, 21(2), 95.

Rogers, C. R. (1959). *A theory of therapy, personality, and interpersonal relationships: As developed in the client-centered framework* (Vol. 3, pp. 184–256). McGraw-Hill.

Ronan, W. (2021, April 22). 2021 slated to become worst year for LGBTQ state legislative attacks. Human Rights Campaign. www.hrc.org/press-releases/2021-slated-to-become-worst-year-for-lgbtq-state-legislative-attacks.

Rosario, M., Schrimshaw, E. W., Hunter, J., & Braun, L. (2006). Sexual identity development among lesbian, gay, and bisexual youths: Consistency and change over time. *The Journal of Sex Research*, 43(1), 46–58. doi:10.1080/00224490609552298.

Storck, K. (2018). *The gender identity workbook for kids: A guide for exploring who you are*. Instant Help Books.

Stutey, D. M., Klein, D. E., Henninger, J., Crethar, H. C., & Hammer, T. R. (2020). Examining gender in play therapy. *International Journal of Play Therapy*, 29(1), 20–32. doi:10.1037/pla0000108.

Substance Abuse and Mental Health Services Administration (2015). *Ending conversion therapy: Supporting and affirming LGBTQ youth*. HHS Publication No. (SMA) 15-4928. Rockville, MD: Substance Abuse and Mental Health Services Administration.

Thorn, T. (2019). *It feels good to be yourself: A book about gender identity*. Henry Holt and Company.

Trans Student Educational Resources (2021, June 29). The gender unicorn. Retrieved from: https://transstudent.org/gender/tr.

Travers, R., Bauer, G., Pyne, J., Bradley, K., Gale, L., & Papadimitriou, M. (2012). *Impacts of strong parental support for trans youth*. Trans Pulse Project, 1–5.

The Trevor Project (2021a). National survey on LGBTQ youth mental health 2021. www.thetrevorproject.org/survey-2021.

The Trevor Project (2021b, May 12). Research brief: LGBTQ youth with a history of foster care. www.thetrevorproject.org/2021/05/12/research-brief-lgbtq-youth-with-a-history-of-foster-care.

Troiden, R. R. (1988). *Gay and lesbian identity: a sociological analysis*. General Hall.

US Department of Justice (2019). FY 2019 Hate crimes statistics report. www.jus
tice.gov/crs/highlights/FY-2019-Hate-Crimes.

Wilson, E. C., Chen, Y. H., Arayasirikul, S., Raymond, H. F., & McFarland, W.
(2016). The impact of discrimination on the mental health of trans*female youth
and the protective effect of parental support. *AIDS and Behavior*, 20(10), 2203–
2211. doi:10.1007/s10461-016-1409-7.

5 Cultural Opportunities with Religious Populations

Hayley L. Stulmaker and Katherine E. Purswell

Olivia, a play therapist, met with a parent of an eight-year-old for the first time because of the parent's concern about specific gendered behaviors. Olivia made an assumption that the parent wanted to help support their child in their gender identity, and they were looking forward to this opportunity. Olivia greeted the parent and went through standard intake procedures, reviewing informed consent, gathering typical background information, etc. Olivia perceived the intake as going smoothly until she learned that the parent held fundamentalist religious beliefs that differed strongly from her own. When Olivia asked about the client's pronouns, the parent espoused their negative views on same-sex relationships and gender identity development, attributing their views to their religion and citing scripture. Immediately, Olivia felt a wave of judgment towards the parent crash over her. Olivia worried about her ability to help the child when the parent held such strong beliefs that were very deeply intertwined with their identity and directly against the beliefs of Olivia. In that moment, Olivia had to take a deep breath and find a way to recalibrate to be empathic and accepting of the parent where they were, including their religious beliefs. Olivia quickly assessed for any shift in dynamics between herself and the parent and then moved forward as usual in the intake, taking into account the parent's religious background as part of the context of the child to best support them in their journey.

Despite recent declines in the number of adults who identify as religious (Pew Research Center, 2015), religion is an important component of identity for many families play therapists serve. In fact, 77% of adults in the United States said that religion was very important or somewhat important to them and 36% noted they attended religious services at least once per week (Pew Research Center, 2015). The same survey cited that the importance of religion increased for Black (91%) and Latino (84%) adults. Yet, literature on sensitivity to religious issues in play therapy is limited. In this chapter we will discuss how clients' and parents' communication around religion can provide humanistic play therapists opportunities to respond warmly and empathically to deepen their work with clients.

Religion refers to an "organized set of beliefs and values shared by a group of people related to sacred things, such as a higher power" while

DOI: 10.4324/9781003190073-8

spirituality is a more intrapersonal process connected to ideas of values, meaning, and purpose (Gladding & Crockett, 2019, p. 153). We think that most humanistic play therapists feel comfortable facilitating an intrapersonal process of clarifying values and meaning, while understanding and responding to issues around religion may be further outside some people's comfort zones. In addition, the organized nature of religion creates systems that impact children in ways that are beyond children's control, thus requiring the play therapist to have skill in working with systemic constructs outside the playroom and to develop accepting and empathic attitudes toward those with varied religious beliefs. For these reasons, we will focus on the topic of religion and religious diversity.

The role of religion can vary substantially from one family to another, and we think it is helpful to think of religious activity on a continuum from people who engage in religious practices primarily as a cultural expression to people with fundamentalist beliefs about their religion. Examples from the cultural side of the continuum could be a person of Mexican heritage who celebrates *Día de los Muertos* even though they do not believe in the spirit world or a Jewish person who celebrates Passover with their family, but otherwise does not have a strong connection to the faith. On the fundamentalist side of the continuum are those who hold their beliefs to be infallible methods for obtaining salvation, enlightenment, or right living and see themselves as separate, righteous, and chosen (Kossowska et al., 2018). A child in a fundamentalist setting may believe they should avoid playing with others outside their group so that they are not negatively influenced or may fear divine retribution for small misdemeanors. Fundamentalist settings tend to exhibit higher levels of control over group members, and in extreme cases may demonstrate characteristics of a cult. Of course, there are many families who fall somewhere between a cultural understanding of religion and fundamentalism.

Research on the impact of religion in children's lives is limited, but existing studies indicate parent religiousness tends to be associated with more positive parenting and child outcomes except when the child and parent disagree (Howell Kelley et al., 2020). From a developmental perspective, parental religiousness may have a more protective effect on younger children who are more likely to identify with their parents' views and a more divisive effect on older children and adolescents who may be more attuned to peer and social values that conflict with their family's religious beliefs and practices (Bornstein et al., 2017). These findings fit with previous research suggesting that parental religiousness can result in more effective parenting and can also have a maladaptive impact in some situations. For example, religious parents may have more access to community support (Bornstein et al., 2017) and may be more likely to believe that the parent-child relationship is a sacred responsibility while they may also have higher expectations for behavioral control and conformity (Mahoney et al., 2013).

Systems

Bronfenbrenner's ecological systems model (Berk, 2018) can be helpful for understanding how religion may impact the lives of play therapy clients regardless of their religious affiliation. The microsystem involves the contexts in which the child is directly involved on a regular basis. For example, family, school, daycare, and place of worship could all be part of a child's microsystem. The microsystem would have the most influence on a child's specific religious beliefs and practices. The mesosystem, or interactions between aspects of the microsystem could substantially impact how a child views their religion in context. For example, a child whose caregivers and school personnel have alignment about how religion should be addressed and expressed at school will likely have a very different experience than a child in the opposite situation. For many children with minoritized identities the religious community may provide a safe space when other microsystems may not feel safe.

The exosystem (Berk, 2018) includes laws, which impact children's expression and experience of religion, and broader religious systems. As of 2014, about 65% of adults in the United States categorized themselves as a category of Christian (including Catholic). About 22% of adults reported they were unaffiliated with a religious belief system, and the remaining identified with other religions. These data demonstrate the United States continues to be overwhelmingly religious and Christian, suggesting that most children probably experience the influence of Christian holidays and theology as part of their exosystem, whether they know it or not.

Bronfenbrenner's macrosystem (Berk, 2018) includes broader cultural values and norms in the society in which the child lives. In the United States, a country founded on Judeo-Christian values, children whose family religion aligns with those values are more likely to feel their religious values are accepted than a child whose religion is less similar (i.e. Hinduism and its deities; indigenous polytheistic beliefs). Bronfenbrenner's final system, the chronosystem, can be defined as historical influences that may impact a child, even if the child has no knowledge of them. Some of these influences may be the use of Christianity to colonize indigenous peoples, the use of Christianity to justify slavery, the Holocaust, and the impact of the terrorist attack of 9/11 in the U.S. on the perception of Islam.

Common Religious Groups in the U.S.

Protestant Christians make up the largest religious group in the U.S. with about 46% of adults belonging to one of the many Protestant Christian denominations (Pew Research Center, 2015). Broadly speaking, Protestant Christians hold the Holy Bible to be scripture, believe in one triune God made up of God the Father, God the Son (Jesus), and God the Holy Spirit. Their religion centers on the divine birth, death, and resurrection of Jesus

Christ as well as the belief that salvation comes through faith in Jesus, not by good deeds. Protestants from different denominations differ in their literal interpretations of these faith tenets (Worthington et al., 2014). Mainline Protestant Christians (18% of U.S. adults) are more likely to emphasize advocacy related to social issues, de-emphasize literal interpretations of the Bible, and be more open to scientific advances and understandings of the world (Worthington et al., 2014). Evangelical Christians (26% of U.S. adults) can range from moderate to fundamental (Stiehler Thurston & Seegobin, 2014), and as their name suggests, they place a stronger emphasis on salvation through faith and on evangelizing the world. They follow a more literal understanding of the Bible and are likely to believe hell is a physical place. Fundamentalist Evangelicals may see themselves as separate and doubt that other types of Christians are truly saved. Historically Black churches (7% of U.S. adults) may be mainline, evangelical, or other, and throughout American history they have served a key role in the African American/ Black community by promoting a healthy conception of self, a sense of community, and emphasizing the existence of spiritual powers that can provide protection and direction in one's life (Cook & Wiley, 2014).

Children who are raised in Protestant Christian circles may experience religious education through private Christian schools, Sunday School (short classes that usually occur before church services), or Vacation Bible School (often a week-long morning or evening summer program). In some Protestant denominations, children may be baptized as babies and in others, they may choose to be baptized as a declaration of their belief in Jesus.

Catholics make up about 20% of the adult population in the U.S. (Pew Research Center, 2015) and represent a diverse set of beliefs, but generally experience a shared identity of being Catholic in addition to identifying as Christian (Shafranske, 2014). Catholics hold similar beliefs about Jesus and the virgin birth as Protestants, and also emphasize prayer and the Eucharist, or Holy Communion, which is traditionally believed to be the body and blood of Christ transformed into bread and wine that is ingested as an act of remembrance of Christ's sacrifice. The Virgin Mary is also a more central figure for Catholics than for Protestants, particularly for immigrants from Latin America. For many Latinx immigrants who practiced Catholicism in their home countries, the Catholic church can serve a protective function in a society that may not welcome them (Shafranske, 2014). There, they may find a sense of belonging, continuity, and social network of other immigrants as well as shared language or values. Children being raised in the Catholic church will most likely experience infant baptism, and First Holy Communion when they first participate in the Eucharist around age seven. Some older children may prepare for and participate in confirmation, a sacrament that indicates the young person is now old enough to take responsibility for their own faith (BBC, 2021).

Many people who identify as Jewish tend to do so culturally rather than religiously, making it difficult to determine a true estimate of the Jewish population. Religiously identifying Jews comprise 1.9% of the United States population (Pew Research Center, 2015). Basic tenets of Judaism come from the Ten Commandments, listed in the Torah, which are believed to have been given to Moses from G-d (Jews do not write or even say the name fully without intent to worship). The first three commandments are concerned with there being only one G-d and worshipping and respecting G-d appropriately and solely. The fourth commandment is to keep the Sabbath, a day of rest and reflection. The remainder of the commandments are related to codes of conduct; honor your parents and do not commit murder, adultery, stealing, lying, or jealousy. Jews are expected to follow these covenants and use them as a guide for praying and living. Jews can be described as on a spectrum, ranging from culturally identifying Jews to ultra-Orthodox Jews. Ultra-Orthodox Jews adhere strictly to Jewish law, keeping strict dietary restrictions (Kosher), and immersing themselves in studying holy texts and learning from rabbis, religious leaders. Ultra-Orthodox Jews tend to value family, have many children, and live in insular communities (Serfaty et al., 2020). When Jewish children are born, they have a baby naming (female) or a bris (ceremony that involves a circumcision, male) when they are given their Hebrew name. Jewish children typically participate in Sunday school for religious education and oftentimes Hebrew school during the week. At age 12 (female)/13 (male) Jewish children take on the responsibility of leading a service at their synagogue and become a bar(male)/bat(female) mitzvah, officially becoming an adult in the Jewish religion. This is typically accompanied by a community service project (mitzvah project) and a large party.

Approximately 1.5% of adults in the U.S. identify as Mormon or the Church of Jesus Christ of Latter-Day Saints (LDS; Pew Research Center, 2015). LDS members consider themselves Christians and hold many of the beliefs of mainstream Protestants but also consider the Book of Mormon to be scripture, along with the Holy Bible (Ulrich et al., 2014). Latter-Day Saints believe the Book of Mormon was revealed to John Smith in upstate New York in 1820 and consists of the writings of early Christians who traveled from Jerusalem to America in search of a new promised land, making Mormonism a distinctly American religion in origin. Even so, the early Latter-Day Saints faced severe persecution that drove them west, a fact that is helpful in understanding their status as a minority religion in the U.S. today and tendency to value self-reliance and personal agency. Religious leaders are a key part of the LDS community and lay leaders play a critical role in spiritual guidance. Children raised in the LDS community may participate in Primary, a spiritual education program that takes place while parents are in weekly worship meetings (LDS, 2021). In the LDS church, children are not able to be baptized until they reach the age of accountability (eight years old), and are usually baptized shortly thereafter. Baptism is followed by a confirmation ceremony in which the child is conferred the Holy Spirit (Ulrich et al., 2014).

Muslims represent 0.9% of the United States; however, this religious group is projected to continue increasing in its presence (Pew Research Center, 2015). There are five basic pillars of Islam (1) Iman: the belief in one God and his final prophet Muhammed, (2) Salat: prayer occurring five times daily, (3) Zakat: donating money, around 2.5% of yearly income to relieve social inequities, (4) Sawm: fasting during Ramadan, and (5) Hajj: pilgrimage to Mecca (Ali et al., 2004). These pillars are the foundation of the beliefs of Muslims, specifically the first pillar, and some of the actions taken to fulfill these beliefs. Muslims follow the Qu'ran as a guide in prayer and ways to enact the religion. One custom is not consuming pork and alcohol. Men and women are expected to dress modestly, and in some sectors women are expected to wear a Hijab, a head covering. Men tend to be more dominant. With regards to marriage, there is an expectation to marry within the faith, heterosexual marriage only, and divorce is discouraged. Muslim communities are collectivist in nature, resulting in children (even adult children) deferring to parents and considering the larger Muslim community in decision-making. People who are Muslim also tend to keep concerns within the family (Ali et al., 2004). Muslim children do not have an official coming of age ceremony; however, they are expected to follow religious practices and customs at the age of puberty.

Play Therapy Considerations for Religious Populations

The four religions that we are highlighting in this chapter all have similar tenets at their core that can relate to play therapy principles. While these populations might be less likely to engage in therapeutic services, play therapists can work with clients in a way that supports rather than driving them away from their beliefs. Play therapists can emphasize these connections in creating buy-in for parents and provide more attuned care for the families.

When working with religious populations, play therapists need to be aware of potential scheduling concerns. Christians tend to have their holy day of the week on Sundays, while Jews have their Sabbath on Friday night through Saturday night. Furthermore, scheduling sessions without awareness of religious holidays can be seen as insensitive. As Christians are the dominant religious group in the United States, most play therapists will be aware of Christmas and Easter and schedule around them. When working with Muslim clients, a play therapist might want to be sensitive to a client's exhaustion during Ramadan as they might be staying up late to celebrate. Jews celebrate many holidays throughout the year in which they do not engage in anything considered work and might need to be flexible in scheduling during these holidays.

Physical appearance, including attire, and instances of touch might influence the therapeutic experience. Most fundamentalist religions encourage modesty of some sort, specifically of women. I (Hayley) wore a sleeveless maxi dress as it was extremely hot that day for a parent consultation with a fundamentalist client. I realized I forgot my sweater, and although the dress was not revealing in a way that most would consider provocative, I was aware of my client, who glanced at my uncovered arms in this setting, and thought she might be offended. I apologized for forgetting my sweater and she was comfortable; however, if it had been her husband, it could have had much more of a negative impact therapeutically. Play therapists who express themselves outside of the traditional professional attire for their assumed sex also might inadvertently be disrupting fundamentalist clients' level of comfort. This can be addressed directly by the play therapist with the client (i.e. "I know I sometimes dress differently than what many might expect. How might that impact our work together?") as a point of processing so that a play therapist can still be who they are while also being sensitive to concerns parents might have. Furthermore, many fundamentalist religions also have guidelines around touch, specifically with people of another sex. For example, Ultra-Orthodox Jewish men are not supposed to have any physical contact with adult females, including handshakes, hugs, etc. Play therapists can defer to the client in instances regarding touch, allowing them to initiate, or ask directly prior to engaging in one of these forms of contact.

Protestants, Catholics, and Jews all espouse God's unconditional love for people, and this belief can help a humanistic play therapist explain the role of unconditional positive regard in play therapy. Further, instilling values of responsibility and hard work are important for many Jewish, Muslim, and Protestant and Catholic caregivers, and play therapists can explain how humanistic play therapy can help children develop these characteristics. The belief in the divine worth of human beings which is present in LDS, Islam, and Judaism, and the emphasis on personal agency and personal development (Ulrich et al., 2014) fit well with a philosophy of play therapy that allows children space to make their own decisions and take responsibility for their own behavior and growth. Further, family is a very important structure in fundamentalist religions (Casey et al, 2020; Serfaty et al., 2020) and children are highly valued (Ulrich et al., 2014), increasing the chances that a caregiver who brings their child to play therapy will be highly invested and engaged in the process. For Muslim children, there is a large emphasis placed on play until around age seven when the focus shifts towards education (Casey et al., 2020), aligning well with young children participating in play as a therapeutic modality.

However, fundamentalists may tend to be more resistant to therapy, and instead, seek out support through their institution of worship. When venturing out to see mental health professionals, fundamentalists will be more likely to seek out therapists who match their religious beliefs (Casey et al., 2020; Stiehler Thurston & Seegobin, 2014; Ulrich et al., 2014) and might be more suspicious of mental health professionals due to the concern that they may be misdirected with secular ideas. Additionally, fundamentalists tend to have more rigidity in their thinking, creating an "us versus them" dynamic that can be disruptive to the therapeutic relationship (Serfaty et al., 2020; Stiehler Thurston & Seegobin, 2014).

Many fundamentalists see value in authority, which can work to play therapists' advantage as the authority figure for the change process. Muslims identify tending to mental health as aligning with their religious principles of tending to overall health which can help combat the stigma of receiving mental health services (Casey et al., 2020). These connections philosophically may help with other fundamentalist groups as well.

Therapist and Client Match

When the play therapist and client match in their religion and degree to which they believe and practice, this creates a seemingly easier therapeutic experience. The play therapist might be able to pick up on nuances or terminology more easily that apply to the shared religion, increasing their accurate empathic expression towards the client. Additionally, the child and/or family's knowledge of the play therapist's similar belief system may inherently create more trust within the therapeutic relationship. This can help the therapeutic process progress more quickly as there is already an unspoken understanding that they are connected.

While a fundamentalist client-therapist match can be therapeutically beneficial, there is also the opportunity for a therapist to assume similarities that do not exist, and the play therapist needs a high level of self-awareness. The play therapist's religious experience may be different from that of the client. They need to be monitoring their own reactions to the client so as to not project their beliefs or experiences onto the client, or to have the focus be religiously driven if that is not what the child is bringing to the therapeutic process.

Therapist and Client Do Not Match

The play therapist and client may not match, either in their religious affiliation or their level of practicing. Some very religious clients may seek out "secular" counselors because they feel ashamed to admit their problems within their religious community. Play therapists are likely to be more effective if they know how to work with families who hold vastly different religious beliefs and values. Furthermore, understanding personal biases developed about certain religions and common assumptions that might be made about fundamentalist groups is central to the therapeutic work. Play therapists might hinder the therapeutic process through their own biases and assumptions, discounting a therapeutically valuable goal in lieu of respecting a stereotype about a certain religion (i.e. female deference to males, and not helping them assert themselves in certain situations; Casey et al., 2021). Furthermore, play therapists can fall into the trap of not fully understanding children's motivation, thoughts, feelings, and behaviors from being clouded by their own understandings of the religion, and may misdiagnose or incorrectly conceptualize and treatment plan for children. In rare cases, the play therapist may not be able to work with a family for ethical reasons (e.g. the family insists that the play therapist help ensure a child is not gay), but we believe that the majority of the time we can continue to work with and express empathy and care for clients whose religious beliefs are very different from ours.

Tension sometimes exists between fundamentalist groups which can inhibit the therapeutic relationship from both sides. When growing up in a fundamentalist religion, many children receive negative messages about other religions and people who practice them. Play therapists need to be aware of their biases that they have been told growing up so as to not impede the therapeutic relationship and potentially pass judgment onto the client. Furthermore, if a client becomes aware of the play therapist's differing beliefs, this might also negatively impact the therapeutic relationship.

Cultural Opportunities

The more religious a family is, the more religion will likely come up in play therapy as it is something that is vital to who children are and their lived experiences. These instances can present unique opportunities to help them continue to develop their identity, integrating their religious beliefs in a way that feels congruent with their self-structure.

Fundamentalist Client Concerns

Children within fundamentalist religions may present with similar concerns within the therapeutic relationship, across religions. As these issues arise, they are wonderful opportunities to help clients process and integrate their self-structure further.

Juggling Multiple Identities

Religion is only one piece of children's identity, and it is often something that you cannot identify solely by looking at them. Yet, for fundamentalists, religion is hugely central to their sense of identity. Children may have more pressures to identify with their sex, race, or ethnicity, and may be treated differently based on those categories as a more central identifying cultural component. When outside of the religious group, this identity may be overlooked at times as it is not something that others may be aware of. These messages can be confusing for children in fundamentalist families, causing stress within their sense of who they are at their core. Play therapists can respond with empathy regarding the identity confusion.

Anxiety/Fear

Highly religious children in counseling may express fear or anxiety within their counseling sessions. These children may experience Islamophobia, anti-Semitism, and other negative judgments on a consistent basis. This may lead children to feeling fearful for their physical safety, while also internalizing messages of anxiety about their worth as people. As children communicate this anxiety in play therapy, the play therapist can respond with empathy (i.e. "You're worried something might happen to you or your family," "You don't think you are as good as Christian kids") to help them feel less isolated and accepted as they are. Unconditional positive regard for children expressing these feelings can be immensely healing, especially from a play therapist with unknown religious beliefs. It is easy to want to rush in quickly and negate children's experience when they are in pain; however, being accepting of this pain is how children can express it and process through what these experiences mean for them as people.

Another fear that may be expressed by fundamentalist children is a fear of being judged or rejected by the play therapist, especially when the child knows the play therapist has a different set or level of beliefs. When this comes up in session, it can be addressed directly, using congruence and unconditional positive regard. For example, if a child says, "No one likes Muslims, everyone thinks they are trying to kill everyone, even you do," the play therapist can respond in a few different ways: "You feel like no one likes you," "You're confused by what you've heard about your religion," or "You're worried I don't like you or I'm scared of you." The last one can be followed by "I'm not scared of you, and I do like you," as long as that is a sincere feeling from the play therapist and it seems to be facilitative for the child within the therapeutic relationship, not just a statement to help make the play therapist feel better.

Locus of Control

Sometimes children may express beliefs that contradict those of the play therapist, and in these situations, it can be helpful to think about facilitating an internal versus external locus of control as illustrated in the following example. Mia, a five-year-old and a member of a religious Christian family, is drawing a picture of a cross and states that people who don't accept Jesus into their hearts are going to hell. The play therapist, who also identifies as Christian, does not believe in a literal hell and personally thinks the idea of hell is harmful.

In this example, the play therapist will be best served by first acknowledging their own belief and/or bias. Then, the therapist can assess what the child is trying to communicate through this statement. If Mia seems confused or saddened, then the play therapist could reflect that feeling and continue to process through whatever else comes up for the client. If Mia does not seem upset and is just sharing a part of her life, then the play therapist could emphasize Mia's internal locus of control by saying, "You believe that people will go to hell if they don't accept Jesus." The use of "you believe" can emphasize the child's internal locus of control and help the client center the statement as a belief, not a fact. Over time, these statements that emphasize an internal locus of control help emphasize that a variety of beliefs exist and that the individual is free to choose their own beliefs. In many religious families, the child will likely continue to choose the beliefs by which they are surrounded, but, with a stronger internal locus of control, their adherence to those beliefs will be less likely to be tied to their self-worth and they will have the tools to question those beliefs if the beliefs are no longer serving them in the future.

Other Considerations to Maximize These Opportunities

Play therapists will be able to work most effectively with fundamentalist religious populations with the above-mentioned areas of focus and knowledge. Additionally, it is helpful to understand what the experience is of their respective communities and the potential hardships they face and unique aspects of their religions. Play therapists can become familiar with various religious texts, especially those geared towards children (i.e. a children's Bible). In some cases, it might be appropriate for the play therapist to attend religious services, separately from the client, and observe the culture within the institution specifically towards children. Play therapists should adopt a curious stance when it comes to clients' religions, not making assumptions about how they believe religion impacts the client or not asking questions for fear of being judged for not understanding. For example, when a parent begins discussing the client's First Holy Communion, the play therapist should not already assume the significance this has for this specific client. Instead, the play therapist can ask how the parent is feeling about this event approaching? How does the child seem to be responding to the upcoming communion? Furthermore, if the play therapist is not exactly sure what communion means, they should not shy away from asking.

Working With Caregivers and Families

Talking with caregivers and families about religion is useful because religion may be a key meaning-making system in the family's life (Hathaway, 2013). Parents and caregivers pass down the teachings from their clergy to their children in a more consistent and daily manner. This is where children learn the day-to-day practices of the religion and the values that are upheld within their families. Further, religion may be both part of the problem and part of the solution (Mahoney et al., 2013). Fundamentalist families may promote positive values for children's mental health and wellbeing such as family, love, comfort in a higher power, etc. These are excellent joining-in points for play therapists to continue to connect with religion and promote emotionally healthy messages. However, the family system may have a negative influence on some children's emotional states with issues of female oppression, control of sexuality, homophobia, etc. Therefore, understanding the role of religion in a family's life will help the play therapist be more empathic and accepting.

Parent/Caregiver Consultations

Many parents/caregivers (P/C) may believe religion and spirituality are things they should keep private and are not relevant to play therapy, so asking explicitly about religion in the initial parent consultation can yield valuable information about the family system. However, for many religious families, their goals for play therapy and parenting strategies may be impacted by their religion (Mahoney et al., 2013). Further, understanding the role of religion in a family's life can help the play therapist develop a stronger understanding of the child's context and thus potentially deepen empathy. The following questions are adapted from Hodge (2013, p. 70) and may be useful for an initial parent consultation:

1   I am wondering how important spirituality or religion is to you and your family.
2   Do you and your family happen to attend religious services in a church or some other type of religious or spiritual community?
3   Are there certain spiritual or religious beliefs and practices that you and your family find particularly helpful in dealing with difficulties?
4   I am wondering whether [presenting problem] has affected your family spiritually or religiously.

The latter questions would be modified depending on how the P/C answered the first question. Understanding the answers to these questions can help the play therapist better understand the context for certain parenting practices and the P/C's understanding of the presenting problem.

The following dialogue illustrates the benefit of addressing religion from a stronger relationship and working alliance with the P/C. In this example, the client has been having behavioral difficulties at school and will be receiving school-based services. The child was referred to play therapy by the school counselor as a requirement for his continued attendance at the school. We were intentionally vague in the terms we used so that this dialogue could be relevant to P/Cs from multiple religions, but of course in real life the play therapist would use the terms the P/C used to describe their religion and spirituality.

PLAY THERAPIST (PT): I am wondering about the importance of religion/ spirituality for your family.
CAREGIVER (C): Well, it's very important. It's not just religion to us, but something we try to live every day. We go to religious services once or twice a week, but we also try to do stuff at home with the kids to help them see that it's not just about going to a place.

PT: It's important to you to instill those values in your kids

C: Yeah, I think it's good for them to have the community and develop the self-discipline.

PT: You want it to be more than just a set of beliefs for them. Are there certain practices your family finds especially helpful in dealing with challenges like the one your child is experiencing?

C: I guess prayer is a big one for us. I know everyone may not agree, but I think that prayer changes things. I've been encouraging my child to pray about his behavior, and I think it's helping some, but he's not very consistent with it, and sometimes he doesn't want to admit what he's done is wrong, even in prayer.

PT: Prayer is generally helpful for you, and you're frustrated with your child's lack of prayer. I'm wondering how else your child's difficulties have impacted your family spiritually.

C: For us, getting along in the family is really important, and my child's behavior has been causing stress between my husband and I, and it's not good for the kids to see that. But it's not causing us to doubt our faith or anything! I know we'll get through this. We've started talking to a religious leader, and I think that's going to help my child's behavior.

PT: It sounds like you might be worried that I'm calling into question your spiritual beliefs and that seeking help through your religious institution is helpful for you. I'm wondering what it's like to have to come and seek play therapy in this non-religious space.

C: To be honest, I'm a little nervous. It's really important to us that our kids rely on our higher power, not on people to learn how to solve their problems. I mean, you seem really nice, and I know you're a professional, so I'm sure everything will be fine.

PT: Yeah, but there are still some concerns there that what I'm doing with your child in play therapy might not be a good fit with how your family does things.

C: I guess so.

PT: I can hear how important those things are to you and also how important your faith is to you. It's also important to me that I understand your family values and your concerns. I can explain a little more about play therapy so you can have some more information about what it actually is, and then we can discuss any remaining concerns you have.

[Therapist goes into an explanation of play therapy that emphasizes the child-directed nature of the play within certain limits, that the therapist will not directly teach coping strategies but will facilitate the child developing ones that work for the child within their cultural and religious context, that the child is free to express their religion in play, that the play therapist will not try to get the child to change their thinking, and that goals of play therapy are more self-control, self-esteem, and more empathy for others, goals that will probably fit with some of the caregiver's values.]

Religious beliefs can impact parenting practice in both positive and negative ways. Often when people think of religious parents the phrase "Spare the rod, spoil the child" associated with Proverbs 13:24 in the Bible comes to mind. However, research suggests that, for many parents, religious beliefs about their responsibility to raise healthy children who will contribute to the community encourage the development of warm parent-child relationships, and they may receive support from their faith community that supports this goal (Mahoney et al., 2013). Yet, religious individuals and communities certainly exist where control is much more highly emphasized than warmth, resulting in negative effects on children. Understanding the role of religion in a family's life can help a play therapist begin to assess the extent to which the P/C's parenting strategies are influenced by religious beliefs and where they fall on the warmth and control continua.

Understanding the role of religion and spirituality in the presenting problem can also be helpful. For example, for a family heavily involved in a faith community with strong beliefs that the parent's role is to teach the child how to behave in the community, a presenting problem of externalizing behavior may have both practical and spiritual significance to the family, potentially increasing the P/C's attempts to exercise control over the child, likely resulting in the child increasing acting out behaviors. When a P/C feels the play therapist truly understands them, they will probably be more likely to consider exploring the possibility that their religious community's expectations may be too strong or that different parenting behaviors might be more effective (Mahoney et al., 2013). When assessing the role of religion in the presenting problem, play therapists need to be aware of their own beliefs and biases so that they do not err in assuming religion is not relevant or that religion is the primary problem (Hathaway, 2013). For example, an eight-year-old who has started refusing to attend a place of worship with the family may be doing so as a way to assert power, may not feel emotionally or physically safe in those spaces (e.g. in a homophobic environment), or may not want to be a part of that religion anymore.

Once the play therapist has a workable understanding of the parenting practices and the role of religion in the presenting problems of religious clients, the play therapist may need to use education about development as well as a thorough explanation of humanistic play therapy to help the P/C revise some of the goals. For example, if a goal is that a seven-year-old will stop lying because lying is a sin that impacts the client's relationship with the parent and with God, then a play therapist might work to help the parent understand the cognitive development of seven-year-olds and why lying at this age is rarely accompanied by the same intent as lying at age 15, for example. Then, in subsequent parent-consultations, the play therapist could work with the P/C to find developmentally appropriate ways to address the child's lying. However, if the play therapist does not understand and acknowledge the severity of the P/C's concern (i.e. that lying is a sin), the parent may not be as willing to consider alternate ways of viewing and addressing the problem (Mahoney et al., 2013).

In our experience, children from fundamentalist families do not seem to struggle as much with social issues when they are children as they have been steeped in these beliefs and do not know that there are other ways to view these issues. However, once they are adults they are able to understand how these belief systems contribute to their struggles in adulthood around sex and sexuality, marriage, and religion. It might be appropriate for play therapists to teach caregivers more about specific taboo topics and find ways for this information to fit in to their religion. For example, a play therapist could teach a caregiver about sexual development and gender identity development when they are concerned about their six-year-old engaging in masturbation. Caregivers might be more open when they understand that masturbation for a young child is self-soothing and not sexual in nature. However, a follow-up might need to happen to explain that masturbation is a normal part of sexual health and wellness and will likely be encountered as the child hits puberty and adolescence. Planting those seeds now can pave the way for children to develop more in line with what research shows is healthy sexual development instead of developing shame and guilt around sex. These types of ideologies can be noticed by play therapists and inter- cepted as they are being introduced to young children, hopefully stopping the cycle of promoting potentially problematic beliefs that may impact them well into adulthood.

Often, working with these clients means finding the pieces of the P/C's beliefs that play therapists can support and emphasizing those. For example, letting a P/C know the play therapist sees how hard they are working to make sure their child grows up into a caring, contributing member of society, and then offering some professional ideas to help the child get there. Oftentimes, demonstrating empathy for P/Cs involves looking past the play therapist's own pre-conceived notions about religion or religious dogmatism to see the fear or pain the P/C is experiencing when their child engages in the problematic behavior for which they are seeking play therapy. Sometimes, work with P/Cs, especially those with belief sys- tems that seemingly contradict the values of play therapy, can be slow, but empathy goes a long way in moving the process forward. One key consideration in working toward empathy for very religious parents is understanding the perceived consequences if they fail in their role as parents. For many P/Cs, the eternal state of their child's soul is depen- dent on their ability to teach the child right living, and P/C rigidity and authoritarianism can be empathically reframed as an expression of the caregiver's love for their child. Once the play therapist has that per- spective, they can work with the P/C to gently confront parenting practices and beliefs that may be harming the child. If the play therapist does not understand the stakes, they may be viewed as pushy or a threat to the child's eternal wellbeing.

Working with Systems

Fundamentalists inherently have their religious institution as a prominent system in their lives, which can be a huge opportunity for play therapists to enact change. Additionally, fundamentalists may encounter issues systemically within their schools and communities at large.

Religious Institutions

Fundamentalists will most likely identify their primary system as being their specific religious institution. Many will turn to their religious institution for counsel instead of mental health professionals. This creates a unique opportunity for play therapists to make connections with leaders within the institution to influence change. Play therapists can meet with priests, rabbis, bishops, or imams to help explain what play therapy is and how it is useful. When play therapists have knowledge of the religion, they can tie in foundations of the religion to the underlying tenets of play therapy to demonstrate alignment and create more buy-in from the institution. The goal of building these relationships would be to channel referrals and reduce stigmas associated with seeking mental health services outside of the institution. Hopefully, with clergy support, members within these communities will be more likely to seek out further help.

Part of the previous suggestion seems idealistic rather than realistic, leading us to our next goal of building relationships with members of the clergy. Play therapists can hold trainings for clergy on ways to respond more therapeutically to members who are having mental health struggles. In some institutions, specifically if the play therapist has a similar religious background, there might be some room to partner and have the play therapist provide services on site. This may reduce some of the barriers to accessing services and increase the effectiveness as it is encouraged by the institution.

Unfortunately, in various fundamentalist institutions there are instances of problematic actions or ideology for mental health such as sexual abuse, female oppression, homophobia, and control of sexuality. Play therapists are in a unique position to be able to conduct trainings with clergy or members of the institution to help educate the population on the impact of some of these struggles, as long as it is handled carefully with an understanding of their beliefs. We believe that a play therapist can begin to create awareness about the LGBTQ+ community with knowledge around demographic statistics and their mental health struggles and how to approach people who are in this community with compassion while maintaining their beliefs. Subtle introductions to these concepts might help fundamentalists begin to open their views in a way that is potentially less emotionally harmful around these types of social issues.

Schools and Communities

The first step in advocating within schools and communities is to truly understand what the schools and communities are like for fundamentalists. In schools and communities where they are the dominant culture, there are probably not many struggles for these children as far as being different from the norm. However, when they are in the religious minority, more mental health issues may arise.

Islamophobia hugely increased after the 9/11 attacks, and still remains prevalent today. Muslim children may experience this Islamophobia in their school through teasing by other children, prejudices from their teachers, and other explicit and implicit ways. They may hear slurs as they play sports or may get avoided in the cafeteria. While these examples are concerning Muslim children, all fundamentalist children may experience similar ridicule, isolation, and contempt from both adults and children within these systems based on their beliefs or the ones they have been exposed to. Play therapists can serve as advocates within these systems by understanding the children's experiences, understanding how and why others have these hateful ideas, helping others understand these children's experiences, and trying to promote more accepting attitudes based on factual information about these groups.

Concluding Thoughts

Play therapists are uniquely primed to work with children in religious populations as many of the underlying philosophies of play therapy align with religious tenets. Play therapists need to know how to work with these populations as religion can be hugely foundational to children and their families, directly impacting the work with those children. Furthermore, without direct questioning about religion, play therapists can miss crucial information about the child's context that can inform both their conceptualization of the child/family and the most appropriate ways to intervene. Even worse, play therapists can sometimes make incorrect assumptions about clients' religion and not pursue behaviors or dynamics that are problematic. By being knowledgeable and willing to take a curious stance with clients' religions, play therapists can continue to build stronger relationships with both the children and families that they are working with.

Positionality Statements

Hayley

I am Jewish, although more culturally at this point in my life. Growing up, my family belonged to synagogues of varying degrees of religiosity (from orthodox to conservative), and I attended Sunday School and Hebrew School throughout my childhood. I became a Bat Mitzvah, and we always went to services for the High Holidays and other occasional Shabbats. We celebrated Shabbat every Friday night with my extended family and gathered with them and family friends as well for all major holidays. I went to camps and preschool at the Jewish Community Center in early childhood and went on to Jewish sleepaway camps until High School. I participated in BBYO (Jewish youth group) and joined a Jewish Sorority in college. I consider myself a lucky Jew as I have grown up within a Jewish community.

However, being Jewish also has an ostracizing component to it. I had to miss out on "Fair day," when schools would give each student a free ticket to the State Fair for one day and schools would close down to attend, as they would always schedule it on Yom Kippur. I would be penalized in school for missing for Rosh Hashana with extra make up work, especially if I was gone for two days instead of one (which is customary for observance of that holiday, but something only more religious Jews partake in). I had many of my Christian friends try to bring me to church and try to convert me before the rapture came for me. Growing up and continuing to live in the "Bible Belt" has definitely impacted the culture surrounding me.

I watched our local Jewish Community Center increase security multiple times, as anti-Semitists vandalized the building with swastikas too frequently. I hear slurs constantly being spouted off demeaning Jewish people and had to listen to many Holocaust deniers. Even during the attacks on the Capital on January 6, 2021, people were wearing shirts with slogans saying "Six Million Wasn't Enough." Anti-Semitism always feels present in my life, causing further worry for me with our children who attend a Jewish preschool. A large part of orientation for their school each year is on how they are handling issues of security due to anti-Semitism so our children can be safe as they socialize and build the foundations for their education experiences.

In addition to being Jewish, I am also a White, able-bodied, cisgender, heterosexual woman, brought up in an upper middle-class family, meaning I can and do hide this diverse part of my identity and others never actually know what my religious beliefs are unless they are disclosed. I'm fortunate on some level for this, specifically as a play therapist, as most clients assume I have the same religious beliefs as they do. I typically allow this incorrect assumption to carry on as it does not seem therapeutically beneficial to correct them. I am careful not to purposely misrepresent myself while also not needing to divulge my own beliefs.

I struggle with a few issues surrounding fundamentalist religious clients. The first issue is around clients seeking out support from religious institutions rather than mental health professionals. Not only have I had a negative personal experience from this, but I have also heard about other instances of similar outcomes from clients who have gone this route. I also have biases against clients who tend to be very religious due to a personal conflict in values that tend to be held with more fundamentalist religious groups. I see how these values have afflicted people close to me and my clients, making it hard for me to be accepting when parents want children to take in these types of values (strong gendered roles, homophobia, etc.). I work hard to try to be empathic to the parents' adherence to these beliefs as they clearly serve an important purpose in their lives. I also try to see if there is a way to help broaden their perspective if it is seemingly causing problems for their child. Another perspective that I know I have to actively work to hold is that these beliefs can also possibly be helpful for the child. Even though I do not identify as being a fundamentalist within my religion, I can very much relate to the prejudice against these groups, inherently building empathy for their experience.

Katie

I grew up as part of the Christian religious majority in the U.S. I could assume that my religious holidays would be acknowledged by others and that I would have time off school or work to celebrate. At the same time, for much of my adolescence I was involved in a youth program with strong fundamentalist leanings, which left me feeling different from my peers outside that small set of people. In this group, behavior, sexuality, dress, gender roles, and beliefs were controlled by strict explicit and implicit norms, and we saw ourselves as set apart and closer to God than most other Christians. Even though it has been almost two decades since I left that group and began to examine and revise my religious belief system, I still find myself discovering ways in which my religious privilege and my time in fundamentalism continue to impact my thinking and my relationships. It has been particularly difficult for me to learn to trust myself and my experience over what others think I should be or do. One protective factor for me was that my parents modeled a healthy questioning of what I was taught that eventually allowed me to develop a stronger sense of self and more of an internal locus of evaluation. As I work with children in more fundamentalist families, I strive to be that person who provides the empathy and unconditional positive regard that facilitates them becoming more attuned to their own experiencing. Despite negative repercussions of some of my early religious experiences, I am also aware of the ways in which these experiences instilled in me the desire to serve those in need, to seek out real community, and to work toward unconditional love for myself and others.

As a play therapist, I find my biggest biases are around families who hold beliefs reminiscent of those that were most harmful to me. I have to be careful not to assume I know their belief system and especially not to assume their beliefs about issues of sexuality and gender. I have to remind myself there are many kinds of Christians and churches, including those that are social justice oriented and affirming of various sexual and gender identities, and I have to regularly combat the fear that Christians are judging me. Although I continue to have to be aware of implicit and explicit biases toward those of other religions, I find it is often easier for me to approach those relationships with an attitude of openness and curiosity. I also think that my own religious development has provided me with a deeper understanding of the way religion can impact a person both positively and negatively, and as a play therapist, I can work to emphasize those positive impacts in the lives of my clients.

References

Ali, S. R., Liu, W. M., & Humedian, M. (2004). Islam 101: Understanding the religion and therapy implications. *Professional Psychology: Research and Practice*, 35 (6), 635–642. doi:10.1037/0735-7028.35.6.635.

BBC (2021, June 23). Seven sacraments of the Catholic church. *BBC*. www.bbc.co.uk/bitesize/guides/zh4f3k7/revision/1.

Berk, L. (2018). *Exploring lifespan development* (4th ed). Pearson.

Bornstein, M. H., Putnick, D. L., Lansford, J. E., Al-Hassan, S. M., Bacchini, D., Silvia Bombi, A., Chang, L., Deater-Deckard, K., Di Giunta, L., Dodge, K. A., Malone, P. S., Oburu, P., Pastorelli, C., Skinner, A. T., Sorbring, E., Steinberg, L., Tapanya, S., Uribe Tirado, L. M., Zelli, A., & Peña Alampay, L. (2017). "Mixed blessings": Parental religiousness, parenting, and child adjustment in global perspective. *Journal of Child Psychology & Psychiatry*, 58(8), 880–892. doi:10.1111/jcpp.12705.

Casey, S., Moss, S. A., & Wicks, J. (2020). Exploring the accessibility of child-centered play therapy for Australian Muslim children. *Journal of Cross-Cultural Psychology*, 51(3–4), 241–259. doi:10.1177/0022022120913117.

Casey, S., Moss, S., & Wicks, J. (2021). Therapists' experiences of play therapy with Muslim families in Western countries: The importance of cultural respect. *International Journal of Play Therapy*. Advance online publication. doi:10.1037/pla0000142.

Cook, D. A., & Wiley, C. (2014). Psychotherapy with members of African American churches and spiritual traditions. In P. S. Richards & A. E. Bergin (Eds.), *Handbook of psychotherapy and religious diversity* (2nd ed, pp. 373–397). American Psychological Association.

Gladding, S. & Crockett, J. (2019). Religious and spiritual issues in counseling and therapy: Overcoming clinical barriers. *Journal of Spirituality in Mental Health*, 21(2), 152–161. doi:10.1080/19349637.2018.1476947.

Hathaway, W. (2013). Ethics, religious issues, and clinical child psychology (pp. 17–39). In D. F. Walker & W. L. Hathaway, *Spiritual interventions for child and adolescent psychotherapy*. American Psychological Association.

Hodge, D. R. (2013). Assessing spirituality and religion in the context of counseling and psychotherapy. In K. Pargament, A. Mahoney, & E. P. Shafranske (Eds.), *APA handbook of psychology, religion, and spirituality (Vol 2): An applied psychology of religion and spirituality* (pp. 93–123). American Psychological Association. doi:10.1037/14046-005.

Howell Kelley, H., Marks, L. D., & Dollahite, D. C. (2020). Uniting and dividing influences of religion on parent-child relationships in highly religious families. *Psychology of Religion and Spirituality*, 61(4), 689–706. doi:10.1037/rel0000321.

Kossowska, M., Szwed, P., Wyczesany, M., Czarnek, G., & Wronka, E. (2018). Religious fundamentalism modulates neural responses to error-related words: The role of motivation toward closure. *Frontiers in Psychology*, 9, 1–9. doi:10.3389/fpsyg.2018.00285.

LDS (2021, 23 June). Children in the church. The Church of Jesus Christ of Latter-Day Saints. https://newsroom.churchofjesuschrist.org/article/children-in-the-church.

Mahoney, A., Leroy, M., Kusner, K., Padgett, E., & Grimes, L. (2013). Addressing parental spirituality as part of the problem and solution in family psychotherapy (pp. 65–88). In D. F. Walker & W. L. Hathaway (Eds.), *Spiritual interventions in child and adolescent psychotherapy*. American Psychological Association. doi:10.1037/13947-004.

Pew Research Center (2015). *America's changing landscape*. www.pewforum.org/2015/05/12/americas-changing-religious-landscape.

Serfaty, D. R., Cherniak, A. D., & Strous, R. D. (2020). How are psychotic symptoms and treatment factors affected by religion? A cross-sectional study about religious coping among ultra-Orthodox Jews. *Psychiatry Research*, 293. doi:10/1016/j/psychres.2020.113349.

Shafranske, E. P. (2014). Psychotherapy with Roman Catholics. In P. S. Richards & A. E. Bergin (Eds.), *Handbook of psychotherapy and religious diversity* (2nd ed, pp. 53–76). American Psychological Association.

Stiehler Thurston, N., & Seegobin, W. (2014). Psychotherapy for evangelical and fundamentalist protestants (pp. 129–153). In P. S. Richards & A. E. Bergin (Eds.), *Handbook of psychotherapy and religious diversity* (2nd ed). American Psychological Association. doi:10.1037/14371-006.

Ulrich, W., Scott Richards, P., Hansen, K. L., & Bergin, A. E. (2014). Psychotherapy with Latter-Day Saints. In P. S. Richards & A. E. Bergin (Eds.), *Handbook of psychotherapy and religious diversity* (2nd ed, pp. 179–205). American Psychological Association.

Worthington, E. L., Berry, J. T. D., Hook, J. N., Davis, D. E., Ripley, J. S., & Greer, C. L. (2014). Psychotherapy with mainline protestants: Lutheran, Presbyterian, Episcopal/Anglican, and Methodist (pp. 103–128). In P. S. Richards & A. E. Bergin (Eds.), *Handbook of psychotherapy and religious diversity* (2nd ed). American Psychological Association. doi:10.1037/14371-005.

6 Cultural Opportunities with Children with Disabilities

Karrie L. Swan and April A. Schottelkorb

Over the past several years, I (KLS) have had the opportunity to serve as a child therapist in a preschool located on an Indian reservation in the Pacific Northwest. One day, I entered the "Buffalo" classroom wherein I was greeted by "Jake," a four-year-old autistic boy who communicated through unconventional modalities. Upon entering the classroom, Jake grabbed my hand and began jumping up and down, showing me that he was excited to go with me to the playroom. I greeted Jake, smiling and engaging with him by stating: "You are happy to see me and have our special playtime today." Following this, we walked to the playroom holding hands. Upon entering the playroom, Jake gleefully and quickly walked towards the mirror and began to look at himself in the mirror. Jake smiled and began to hum. Then, Jake looked at his reflection in the mirror and began to spit on the ground. Jake began to move his body vertically, moving back and forth. In a rhythmic fashion, Jake swayed back and forth, spitting on the ground, carefully watching his reflection in the mirror. In these moments with Jake, I honored Jake's need for sameness and did not attempt to change his behaviors to fit neurotypical expectations. I also provided acceptance of Jake's sensorimotor and proprioceptive needs and attuned to his momentary shifts in affect, intention, and behavior by altering my engagement responses for facilitating safety and coregulation (Porges, 2011). Our hope in providing this therapeutic vignette is to incite reflectivity in how we as therapists competently and sensitively support children with disabilities through the process of play therapy.

Cultural Considerations

Children with disabilities have been noted as the largest and fastest growing minority population in the world (World Health Organization, 2011). The construct of disability includes physical, mental, cognitive, and emotional variations that pose obstacles; thus, childhood disabilities may encompass an array of biopsychosocial uniquenesses such as: Attention Deficit Hyperactivity Disorder (ADHD), Anxiety, Deafness, Blindness, and Autosomal Trisomy. According to the WHO (2011), childhood disability is an

DOI: 10.4324/9781003190073-9

umbrella term that refers to a nuanced relationship between impairment, activity limitation, and participation restriction. Specifically, the WHO (2011) defines an impairment as a characteristic that impacts one's biopsychological functioning; an activity limitation exists when one experiences challenges participating in a task; while participation restriction is an obstacle encountered while engaging in systems. Thus, the WHO acknowledges that childhood disability is a complex interaction between an individual's variabilities and societal responses. Of importance, the disability population is the only marginalized group that one can join at birth, become aware of in childhood or adulthood, or acquire due to life circumstances (i.e. Traumatic Brain Injury), thus disability intersects with all social identities.

Kraus et al. (2018) reported that over 6% of children in the United States had a disability. Over the last decade, prevalence for common childhood disabilities including Attention-Deficit Hyperactivity Disorder (ADHD), learning disability, other developmental delay and autism spectrum disorder (ASD) rose by four percentage points, with one in six children diagnosed with a disability in the United States (US Census Bureau, 2019). Although childhood disability occurs across all cultural groups, research indicates American Indian and Alaska Native (AIAN) children have the highest disability rates of any ethnic group in the U.S. (5.9%), followed by biracial children (5.2%), and Black children (5.1%). There is also evidence that children living in poverty are more likely to have a disability as compared to children living in advantageous environments (US Census Bureau, 2019). Importantly, poverty is a primary influencing factor regarding prevalence rates amongst children. According to the Department of International Development (2000), "poverty is both a cause and consequence of disability. Poverty and disability reinforce each other, contributing to increased vulnerability and exclusion" (p. 2). Many variables influence the relationship between poverty and disability including nutritional deficiencies, limited access to health care, and poor environmental conditions (DIP, 2000).

The consensus is that children with disabilities experience the most inequities of any marginalized population in the world (WHO, 2011). A considerable body of research indicates that children with disabilities are likely to experience abuse (Nettelbeck & Wilson, 2002), sexual exploitation (Byrne, 2018), neglect (Matthias & Benjamin, 2003), segregation, and discrimination (WHO, 2011). In addition, because disability can intersect with any and all social identities, children with disabilities may experience multiple forms of discrimination. Unfavorable societal attitudes towards individuals with disabilities tends to lead to increased social exclusion and isolation, with children with disabilities experiencing high incidence of bullying and having scarcely any peer relationships (Griffin et al., 2019; Rose et al., 2011). Because implicit societal attitudes and beliefs impact children with disabilities and contribute to the perpetuation of stereotypes, bias, rejection, and discrimination, it is important for play therapists to understand models of disability.

Models of Disability

Disability models detail both micro-level and macro-level tenets of understanding disability. Throughout history, models of disability have emerged and disappeared through societal advances and activism. Because models of disability play an important role in how childhood disability is conceptualized, it is important for play therapists to be aware of how models influence their own worldview and their perception of children with disabilities (Brittain, 2004).

Medical Model

The medical model of disability is most prevalent in Western culture. In the medical model, disability is defined as a medical phenomenon that limits functioning and is therefore in need of correcting (Rees, 2017). As articulated by Armstrong (2010), "there is a tendency among us human beings to take people with diagnostic labels and put them as far away from ourselves as possible." (p. 12). Through this lens, impairment and disability are intermixed with illness and in "being sick", therefore it is assumed that children with disabilities are in need of help, remedy, rehabilitation, and intervention (Bingham et al., 2013; Blustein, 2012; Roush & Sharby, 2011). As a result, the medical model view of disability tends to perpetuate inequities, stigma, and ableism.

Ableism

Childhood disability can intersect with any and all social identities, thus children with disabilities may experience multiple forms of discrimination and ableism. Ableism refers to macro-level oppression, prejudice, and discrimination towards individuals with disabilities (Bogart & Dunn, 2019). According to Fiona Kumari Campbell (2001),

> ableism refers to a network of beliefs, processes and practices that produces a particular kind of self and body (the corporeal standard) that is projected as the perfect, species-typical and therefore essential and fully human. Disability then is cast as a diminished state of being human.
>
> (p. 44)

Like other forms of oppression, ableism dehumanizes children with disabilities by classifying human variations as inferior to typically developing children (Bogart & Dunn, 2019). Additionally, ableism occurs often in schools and community settings when children with disabilities are expected to function identically to non-disabled peers. Ableism takes many forms such as segregating children with disabilities into separate classrooms, failing to incorporate braille on signs in a school building, failing to incorporate accessibility plans, using restraint or exclusion as means for modifying behavior, and talking about a child with a disability rather than talking to the child with a disability.

Social Model

The narrative of the social model of disability emphasizes that the term "disability" is a social construct imposed on children with impairments (Norwich, 2002). Scholars and disability activists that view disability from a social model lens dismantle disability and impairment. In light of this, disability is defined as the "disadvantage or restriction of activity caused by a contemporary social organization which takes little or no account of people who have physical impairments and thus excludes them from participation in the mainstream of social activities" (Shakespeare, 2010, p.1).

On the other hand, impairment is characterized as a long-term biopsychosocial abnormality that impacts functioning (Goodley, 2001). In this framework, disability exists primarily due to societal attitudes and responses to children with variations (Reindal, 2008). Therein, supporting children with disabilities following a social model of disability includes removing institutional barriers, improving inclusion and quality of life, and altering negative stereotypes and attitudes, all of which lead to an increased sense of self within disability culture (Bingham et al., 2013; Brittain, 2004).

Considerations for Children with Disabilities

Disability Rights

Children with disabilities have defined rights under three pieces of legislation: the Individuals with Disabilities Education Act (IDEA), the Americans with Disabilities Act (ADA), and Section 504 of the Rehabilitation Act of 1973 (Section 504). Together, these laws create a foundation for children with disabilities in securing access to educational opportunities and protection from disability discrimination. Specifically, the IDEA mandates that eligible children with disabilities receive a "free appropriate public education" (FAPE) as outlined in an individualized education program (IEP; Raj, 2021). Eligibility requirements for having a disability under IDEA are fairly restrictive. To qualify for services under IDEA, a child must meet criteria for being assigned to at least one of the 13 legal categories of disability (https://sites.ed.gov/idea/regs/b/a/300.8), the disability must create an impairment that adversely impacts academic functioning, and consequently, the child requires individualized education and related services (Raj, 2021).

Contrarily, Section 504 and the ADA provide discrimination protection to all children with disabilities. Broadly, both laws safeguard children with (a) an impairment that is "otherwise qualified, (b) with a physical or mental impairment that substantially limits one or more major life activities, (c) with a record of such an impairment, (d) who is regarded as having such an impairment" (Raj, 2021). Importantly, Section 504 and the ADA aim to ensure that children with disabilities are provided with equitable access to services and programs as well as protection from disability discrimination.

Although disability rights laws have led to some improvements in services provided to children with disabilities, critics argue that the laws are based on the medical model of disability and that enforcement of the statutes is problematic (Bogart & Dunn, 2019) and restrictive in terms of protecting children's universal rights (Raj, 2021). Additionally, because Western society has not fully embraced inclusion and universal design, parent(s)/guardian(s) tend to bear the responsibility in ensuring that their children receive appropriate accommodations and services (Raj, 2021).

Barriers

Children with disabilities experience undue barriers for participation in home, school, and community settings. Often, the existence of barriers faced by children with disabilities results in reduced participation, consequently impacting wellbeing and quality of life (Bedell et al., 2013). The International Classification of Functioning defined participation as "involvement in life situations" (WHO, 2007; p. 7) that encompasses multiple aspects (Granlund, 2013), and is evaluated according to both the rate of participation and level of engagement in life situations (Bedell et al., 2013). Specifically, numerous barriers produce restricted opportunities to engage with peers, use assistive technology, participate in educational programs, sports, hobbies, and leisure activities, and access buildings and environmental spaces (Guichard & Grande, 2018).

According to the Centers for Disease Control and Prevention (CDC, n.d.), children with disabilities experience the following barriers: communication, physical, policy, programmatic, social, and transportation. Communication barriers exist when children with disabilities have difficulty understanding or communicating, hearing, reading, or writing, whereas physical barriers occur when mobility is obstructed or inaccessible. Policy barriers come about when disability laws and regulations are not enforced, whereupon programmatic barriers exist when health and social services are inaccessible. Social barriers occur when discrimination, policies and the distribution of resources affect "the conditions in which people are born, grow, live, work and age" (CDC, n.d.), whereas transportation barriers come about when children are unable to move around independently due to insufficient or inaccessible transportation.

Play Therapy Considerations for Working with Children with Disabilities

Although many play therapists have been trained under the medical model of disability, many within the disability community prefer the social model of disability. In a clinical setting, it is well understood that diagnosis is necessary for utilizing insurance benefits, thus we encourage therapists to work to understand clients using a social model of disability and as a succession, develop humanistic treatment goals rather than cure-focused goals. In this light, play therapists are urged to embrace a worldview that does not seek to "fix" children with disabilities, rather ponder how children can be supported within the cultural and structural disabling environment within which they live. For example, a child who uses a wheelchair is not disabled until they attempt to access a space with stairs and no ramp or elevator. An autistic person, who communicates via AAC, is not disabled if they can communicate using their device.

Disability Identity

Similar to identity research relating to race, disability identity occurs through a developmental process. While forming a disability identity, individuals with variabilities navigate a society that medicalizes disability and idolizes normalcy and as such, assign meaning to their impairments. A negative disability identity occurs when one internalizes oppressive, ableist, discriminatory macro- and micro-level messages about their impairment. For example, I (KLS) worked with an elementary-aged boy with ADHD who often shared his experiences of navigating a society that prizes a neurotypical way of being. Specifically, the child often stated: "My ADHD makes me bad; I make everyone mad because I have ADHD; I wish I didn't have ADHD." In contrast, a positive disability identity comes to fruition when people with disabilities accept and value their unique strengths and limitations. When individuals embrace their impairments, they tend to experience increases in self-esteem, coping skills, and achievement (Arnold-Oatley, 2005). A positive disability identity also leads to a sense of connection with the broader disability community and culture (Dunn & Burcaw, 2013).

Over the last decade, the disability community has advocated for humanizing language regarding disability identification. Historically, scholars believed that person-first language was the most humanizing way to describe individuals with disabilities, as it emphasized the person, not the disability (Dunn & Andrews, 2015). However, many communities prefer identity-first language because "the person-first approach subtly implies that there is something inherently negative about disability and that use of constructions such as 'with a disability' or 'with diabetes' unnecessarily dissociates the disability from the person" (Dunn & Andrews, 2015, p. 257). As an example, the autistic community generally prefers identity-first language (Brown, n.d.). In the autistic community, many consider person-first language as a form of ableism because they consider autism as a central part of their identity, and one of which to be proud, not ashamed (Brown n.d.). Play therapists are encouraged to honor the client and their family with respect to identity. Therefore, play therapists need to discover and keep pace with identification preferences of clients served.

Diagnostic Overshadowing and Masking

Play therapists should also be familiar with two important diagnostic concepts in their work with children with disabilities: diagnostic overshadowing and masking. In *diagnostic overshadowing*, a term originally discussed by Reiss et al. (1982) referencing individuals with "mental retardation" (now referred to as intellectual disability), individuals with disabilities may be overlooked in areas of possible co-occurring mental health diagnoses, such as depression and anxiety, due to difficulty in verbally communicating their areas of needed support (Rush et al., 2004). Because play therapists often gather information from parents and significant others regarding behaviors outside of session, and do not require child verbalizations, appropriate diagnoses and other supports will often be discovered and implemented in the process of working with caregivers. However, play therapists should always be mindful to keep diagnostic overshadowing in mind, thus we encourage further assessment from outside professionals if warranted. For example, I (AAS) worked with a young girl in play therapy who had a family history of autism, but she herself was not diagnosed autistic by medical professionals due to her ability to make good eye contact with them. She was instead diagnosed with speech delay and ADHD by her primary care doctor. However, her play behaviors, as well as the parent report of behaviors outside of session, seemed to point to autism. For example, in session, sensory play was a primary theme (i.e. jumping on couches, trampoline, bop bag, using kinetic and regular sand and painting her hand every session, etc.). In addition, this client had a diagnosed delay in speech, and she did not engage in pragmatic communication in and out of session as might be expected for her age. Her parents also reported struggles in understanding peer relationships, including reporting having no friends, as well as getting in trouble at school for copying inappropriate behaviors of other students but not understanding why they were problematic. Finally, parents reported some other developmental delays, such as continued struggles with using the bathroom appropriately. Because I was aware that autism sometimes presents differently in females, and because of the strong family history of autism, it seemed important to share with parents about the possibility of autism. In one of our regular parent consultation sessions, where I gave feedback about session progress, I shared some literature about the female presentation of autism and shared that a neuropsychology evaluation could help provide more clarity about her diagnosis, if they were interested. The parents chose to complete a neuropsychology evaluation, for which she was diagnosed autistic, and subsequently, the family and school staff were more understanding and accepting of her challenges and more appropriate supports were put in place at school.

Another important concept is *masking*, also known as *camouflaging*. Masking and camouflaging are defined as behaviors that neurodiverse individuals engage in to disguise or hide their true selves to avoid stigma, feel safe, connect socially, and avoid mistreatment and bullying from neurotypical standards of behavior (Hull et al., 2017). Thus, professionals may perceive that neurodiverse children are functioning well, and may not realize the difficulties they experience due to camouflaging (Hull et al., 2017). Girls are thought to be undiagnosed or diagnosed with autism later in adulthood more frequently due to masking (Hull et al., 2017). "Because of the way women are socialized to 'fit in' and pick up on social cues, underlying traits of autism or ADHD or other neurological makeups essentially get missed" (Nerenberg, 2020, p. 10).

Ethics, Training, and Collaboration

Disability is an element of diversity that has been disregarded by most helping professions (Woo et al., 2016). For decades, activists and researchers have declared that professionals in human services, counseling, and social work are not sufficiently trained to work with children with disabilities (Korinek & Prillaman, 1992; Lebsock & DeBlassie, 1975; Smart & Smart, 2006). Research also indicates that mental health training programs are devoid of specialized coursework and clinical training aimed at supporting individuals with disabilities in therapeutic settings (Feather & Carlson, 2019). Because ethically and professionally competent child counselors are obligated to be aware of their own beliefs and to garner the appropriate education and training for working with diverse clients (ACA Code of Ethics, 2014), we propose that play therapists need to participate in additional training and clinical supervision for supporting children with disabilities. Play therapists are also encouraged to seek knowledge from adults with disabilities as they are the most knowledgeable about disability culture, discrimination, and stigma. Finally, because children with impairments often receive an array of services including special education services, speech therapy, physical therapy, and occupational therapy, we believe it is imperative to consult regularly with specialists providing supportive therapies for clients.

Access and Play Materials

The disability-affirming play therapist must provide appropriate building accessibility and appropriate materials. In a study examining the impact on environmental adaptations in play therapy, Eisert et al. (1988) found that children with disabilities demonstrated increased play behaviors following the development of a play environment specifically designed to meet their unique needs and interests. In constructing the environment, Eisert et al. (1988) reduced stimulation, provided areas for self-directed activities, and adapted the space for individuals with physical disabilities. Therefore, play therapists need to provide accessibility for clients with physical disabilities (wheelchair accessibility for entry to building and rooms as well as access to items in the playroom). Research also indicates that children with disabilities including autism and ADHD have increased challenges with processing and integrating sensory experiences. Specifically, Nerenberg (2020) notes that sensory sensitivity "implies a certain heightened reaction to external stimuli – experiences, noise, chatter, others' emotional expression, sound, light, or other environmental changes" (p. 9). Thus, for children with unique sensory channels, it is important for therapists to consider how sensations are experienced in the playroom. For example, some clients may find aromas off-putting and distracting, whereas some children may get overwhelmed by bright visual stimuli and cluttered rooms.

In addition to using traditional play therapy items as recommended by Landreth (2012), we have discovered that children with unique sensory processing benefit from the following items: small trampoline, play tipi, weighted blanket, water beads, kinetic sand, and fidget toys.

Another accommodation for promoting engagement in play therapy is the inclusion of adaptive equipment and materials such as adaptive toys and switches, positioning and pointing devices, and Photovoice. Play therapists also need to be aware of how to support children's communication, thereby including an array of augmentative and alternative communication which may include tactile symbol communicator, picture communication boards, and speech–generative devices. Play therapists specializing in working with children with impairments are also encouraged to be fluent in American Sign Language.

Cultural Opportunities in Working with Children with Disabilities

Our preferred approach for supporting children with variabilities is child-centered play therapy (CCPT). CCPT is regarded as one the of most humanistic approaches in child therapy (Cooper et al., 2007). CCPT is rooted in the belief that all children organically move towards growth and development when provided with the opportunity to experience an empathically attuned relationship. When children with disabilities experience a growth enhancing alliance, it is believed that children with disabilities experience "a form of letting go, merging freely into experience, immersing oneself totally in the moment so that there is no distinction between self and object or self and other" (Moustakas, 1959, p. 2). As a result of experiencing acceptance, unconditional positive regard, and empathy, children develop a positive self-concept, assume increased self-responsibility, become self-directing, self-accepting and sensitive to coping, engage in self-determined decision-making, experience a sense of control, develop an internal source of evaluation, and increase trust in self (Landreth, 2012).

In CCPT, therapists accept children's holistic way of being moment by moment and honor and value their interests and unique ways for communicating and engaging.

Although the mechanisms underlying child growth and movement in CCPT are not known, researchers speculate change occurs due to the child experiencing the core relationship conditions inherent within CCPT (Landreth, 2012). Ray et al. (2013) developed a theory in which empathy and emotional expression are conceptualized as the primary factors of change in CCPT. Similar to their model, we speculate that the therapeutic relationship, characterized by acceptance, empathy, and attunement plays an important role in the creation of an attachment bond that directly influences affect-regulation and promotes positive changes. Figure 6.1 displays our model for enhancing cultural opportunities in supporting children with disabilities in CCPT.

A primary ingredient for promoting growth for children with disabilities involves ensuring that a child experiences an attuned, therapeutic relationship that is expressed as unqualified acceptance of the child's embodied experience. In this way, play therapists honor and follow a child's movement and seek to understand the child's unique and unconventional way of relating and behaving. Thus, play therapists working with children with disabilities do not expect children to emote, behave, or communicate in a neurotypical manner. Additionally, we believe that the therapist's sensitive attunement establishes what neuroscientists refer to as "neuroception of safety," creating a soothed autonomic nervous system and secure attachment for children with children with disabilities. (Porges, 2011). Thus, when a child feels safe in the therapeutic relationship, the child may express sensorimotor needs, affective arousal, and dysregulation through play, gestures, and behaviors. For example, I (KLS) worked with a child who was diagnosed with a global developmental delay, sensory processing disorder, and

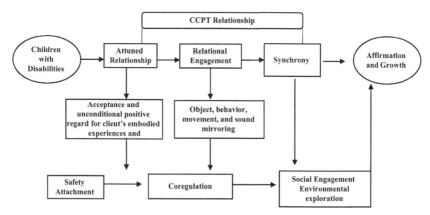

Figure 6.1 Proposed model for supporting children with disabilities in play therapy

speech delay. In one of our sessions together, my client crashed toys together, poured sand on his head, and pushed toys off the shelves. In attuning to embodied communication, I noticed that his sensory inputs and outputs were an expression of emotional distress. In meeting with his guardian, I discovered that the family had experienced several deaths during a seven-day period.

Another important component for supporting children with disabilities in play therapy is to relationally engage with clients in ways that meet their sensory preferences. Specifically, we utilize mirroring as a means for increasing connection, promoting awareness and social engagement, and enhancing communication. In mirroring, we reflect and mirror salient aspects of a child's movement, behavior, or communicative expression. For example, if a child sways back and forth, we will imitate the client's behavior and move back and forth. We may also layer on verbal reflections if appropriate by stating, "You are moving back and forth, I am moving back and forth." If a client looks in the mirror and begins to hum, we will imitate the client's expression by humming. In this approach, we also sensitively utilize verbal reflections and attune to client feedback on use of our verbalizations. For example, in using choices and limit-setting, we utilize picture communication systems as a means for engaging with clients who are unconventional communicators. Thus, in our approach, we acknowledge and respect that verbalization is one of many sensorimotor input systems, and as such, we do not solely rely on verbal reflections for engaging with clients with disabilities.

Through the process of creating safety and relationally engaging through use of multi-sensory inputs, a child with a disability may experience a co-regulating encounter (Porges, 2011; Schore, 2001) which then influences a child's sense of synchrony, that is, a shared experience of being with and alongside another person (Porges & Daniel, 2021). Amid this synchronous relationship, mirror neurons are activated, the pathways to social engagement are strengthened, and affective responses are internalized (Panksepp & Biven, 2012). As a result, we believe that children sense affirmation, which leads to increased environmental exploration, congruence, and ultimately growth (Porges, 2021)

Working with Parents/Guardians

Providing care to a child with a disability may pose unparalleled challenges. Research suggests that caregivers of children with disabilities experience more psychological stress and financial strain (Goudie et al., 2014) as compared to caregivers of children without disabilities. Studies have also shown that parent(s)/guardian(s) of children with disabilities tend to experience increased psychiatric distress, e.g. anxiety, depression, sleep disorders (Pinquart & Sorensen, 2007), and social isolation as well as a decreased quality of life (Evans et al., 1993). Conversely, research indicates that parents who have a positive perception of disability tend to have increased coping and family adjustment (Lustig, 2002). Further, qualitative accounts reveal that caregivers have reported that having a child with a disability has led to an increased sense of meaning and spirituality (Hastings & Taunt, 2002), personal maturation (Scorgie & Sobsey, 2000), and meaningful social relationships (Scorgie & Sobsey, 2000). Because all families respond idiosyncratically to parenting a child with a disability, it is important for play therapists to support caregivers in ways that maximize their own internal and external resources.

To build and maintain therapeutic rapport with parents, play therapists are encouraged to subscribe to a parent consultation model. In our work with caregivers of children with disabilities, we flexibly utilize a child-centered parent consultation model (Schottelkorb et al., 2015). In this particular model, the therapist-parent relationship is just as important as the child-therapist relationship. In this way, play therapists embrace a Thou-I relationship as portrayed by Schmid (2007): "in a nutshell: to understand is to listen, to realize is to appreciate, to become aware of is to follow (and not to direct – hence the 'non-directiveness', to be understood as facilitative responsiveness)" (p. 42). Therefore, therapists working with parents of children with disabilities are encouraged to develop a therapeutic alliance with caregivers by attuning to their needs, values, beliefs, and strengths, while also conveying the core relational conditions of empathy, congruence, and unconditional positive regard (An & Palisano, 2014).

> Through the process of creating and maintaining a trusting relationship, play therapists also regard parents as authority of their own children. Thus, therapists acknowledge that caregivers possess lived experiences that make them the true experts on their children's developmental pathways, needs, and experiences of ableism and discrimination. Consistent with research examining parents' perspectives in professional-caregiver relationships, parents indicate a desire for professionals to actively seek their knowledge and input.
>
> (Cohen & Mosek, 2019)

As the therapist-caregiver relationship evolves, we assert that it is important to share knowledge about disability rights and adaptive supports (www.wrightslaw.com, www.ctdinstitute.org). Play therapists can also teach parents ways to support the development of their children's disability identity. Additionally, we believe it is vital for therapists to engage parents in understanding their children's communications and behaviors. Oftentimes, children with disabilities are referred for therapy due to concerning behaviors. As play therapists, it is essential to understand the child's unique expression and help parents recognize that behaviors are a form of communication. Some children are unconventional communicators and correspondingly, are not able to communicate in ways that are understandable to parents, thus we believe we can help by serving as translators for children that struggle to communicate their intentions and needs.

Working with Systems to Advocate

Children with disabilities are often involved in an array of health, educational, and community systems. Primary obstacles across all settings include lack of accommodations, low quality services, and exclusive practices (Colver et al., 2011). More concerning, children often face participation restrictions in home, school, and community settings (Colver et al., 2011; Coster et al., 2011; Coster et al., 2013). At the heart of all these obstacles is ableism. Alleviation of social problems inherent to ableism will require macro-level societal transformation. Play therapists, however, are in a unique position to engage in advocacy and social justice activities that can lead to micro-level changes. Specifically, play therapists are called to collaborate with individuals and systems that influence a child's wellbeing (Constantine et al., 2007). Play therapists can engage in consultation with professionals with the purpose of facilitating awareness of ableism and prejudice towards children with disabilities. For example, therapists can advocate for inclusive practices that foster children's sense of belonging and disability identity and champion anti-ableist IEP goals. Consequently, because belonging "is so essential to well-being, it is important to examine how social inclusion and belonging might be fostered in school and community settings" (Scorgie & Forlin, 2019, p. 13). In particular, play therapists can work with professionals and educators and advocate for (a) increased prospects to interact with peers, (b) identifying and challenging barriers to inclusion, (c) fostering reciprocity and contribution, (d) promoting socially inclusive values, (e) examining social and cultural structures that impact power and privilege, and (f) attending to the voices of children with disabilities (Scorgie & Forlin, 2019). Ultimately, we believe that play therapists should support children with disabilities and their caregivers by challenging the oppressive societal belief and consequences that children with disabilities need to be fixed. Instead of focusing on a change or a cure, play therapists can critically examine social systems and advocate for the creation of spaces that unconditionally accept all children, those with and without impairments.

Conclusion

Play therapists are in unique positions to combat ableism and discrimination in their places of work and social communities. As such, they may benefit from examining their competencies and beliefs in working with children with disabilities. Play therapists are also encouraged to ponder their identity, experiences, and education and reflect on how their lived experiences impact their sense of competency and self-efficacy in working with children with disabilities. Additionally, we have discovered that the therapeutic alliance has been strengthened when we have shared our own experiences of being part of the neurodiverse population; therefore, therapists with impairments are encouraged to use appropriate self-disclosure for instilling hope and helping families of children with disabilities navigate the various social systems.

In authoring this chapter, our greatest hope was to foster an understanding of the inequities faced by children with disabilities. By increasing cultural competence, play therapists may dismantle the visible and invisible challenges that perpetuate social inequalities among children with impairments. Further, we hope that the knowledge shared about this marginalized population inspires therapists to expand their professional competence in how to best serve children with variabilities. We also want to acknowledge that our work as play therapists in supporting children with variances has been informed by our own unique lived experiences, thus we end this chapter by sharing our positionality statements.

Positionality Statements

Karrie

I identify with multiple intersecting identities. I am an enrolled tribal member, I am neurodiverse (diagnosed with ADHD), and my family of origin was impacted by poverty, thus I view the world through low social class values. Additionally, many of my family members were impacted by various disabilities including autism, intellectual disability, ADHD, and specific learning disorders. In contrast to many of my family members, I have an invisible variation that has largely influenced my sense of feeling that I am not as capable as most of my peer group. To a degree, I have internalized ableism and the notion that my neurodivergent way of being is not acceptable to society. However, I also recognize there is an advantage to having an invisible impairment as compared to my aunts and uncles who had visible disabilities.

At an early age, I witnessed continual discrimination and harmful attitudes toward my family members. Even one of my earliest childhood memories involves a situation wherein my mother was publicly ridiculed because she allowed my autistic aunt to provide childcare for my sister and me. My childhood experiences ultimately inspired me to become a special education teacher. I consider myself deeply fortunate for serving as a humanistic special education teacher and in having relational experiences with children with varying abilities and strengths, but I'd be amiss if I failed to mention that I fought against systemic inequities in the K-12 system every single day. As I reflect on my knowledge and lived experiences, I find it difficult to separate my identity as a play therapist from the sum of all my experiences; however, I acknowledge that my intersecting identities and engagement in various systems have influenced my humanistic worldview and anti-ableist beliefs.

April

I recently recognize myself as a neurodiverse person, similar but different than my two neurodiverse children. The process of delving into the neurodiversity movement has helped me more clearly see myself as a highly sensitive person who is anxious. As a play therapist who has always believed in the child-centered/person-centered philosophy, I feel more accepting of myself, my children, and my clients who are neurodiverse with knowledge about the neurodiversity paradigm. I feel fortunate that I received training from child-centered practitioners, because I do believe that, as we learn more about neurodiversity, humanistic interventions, like CCPT, will be the preferred intervention for neurodiverse children who struggle with anxiety and depression. Neurodiverse individuals process information differently than neurotypical individuals; however, this difference is not a detriment and, in many cases, is a strength. My high sensitivity is an asset as a therapist, as I am highly empathic and connect easily with the children and parents with whom I work. My high sensitivity also means that I am highly affected by my work with clients, and thus I need to limit the number of sessions I have in a day, as that can burn me out quickly.

The biggest growth I have made as a human, parent, and therapist is because of my autistic daughter. Being a parent of a child with high support needs is helpful as a therapist, as I can better understand the discrimination and barriers of navigating in a neurotypical world. I believe that parenting a child with high support needs can be more stressful than parenting a neurotypical child, due to society not understanding or accommodating for different needs. When play therapists work with children and parents who are neurodiverse, I hope they have empathy for the extra amount of stress that can bring to the family.

I am sad to admit that I had my daughter participate in all interventions recommended by medical professionals, even when some of them were against my own beliefs. I am now trusting myself and listening to autistic adults, and we will never again participate in applied behavioral analysis (ABA) or any ABA-like therapies. I also know, as a former school counselor, that ABA and behaviorism are a big part of public schools. Thus, oftentimes ABA is a part of a neurodiverse child's life without perhaps being aware of it. As a mother and play therapist, I hope that play therapists will read the research about behavioral therapies through the lens of autistic adults and recognize the possible harmful effects. I do believe that CCPT is a neurodiversity-affirming practice as we believe that experiencing acceptance within the therapeutic relationship is the healing factor that allows children to be their best selves.

References

American Counseling Association (2014). *ACA code of ethics*. ACA.

An, M., & Palisano, R. J. (2014). Family-professional collaboration in pediatric rehabilitation: A practice model. *Disability and Rehabilitation*, 36(5), 434–440. doi:10.3109/09638288.2013.797510.

Armstrong, T. (2010). *The power of neurodiversity: unleashing the advantages of your differently wired brain*. Da Capo Press.

Arnold-Oatley, A. E. (2005). *Students with physical disabilities adaptation to university.* (Master's thesis). York University, Toronto, Canada.

Bedell, G., Coster, W., Law, M., Liljenquist, K., Kao, Y.-C., Teplicky, R., Anaby, D., & Khetani, M. A. (2013). Community participation, supports, and barriers of school-age children with and without disabilities. *Archives of Physical Medicine and Rehabilitation*, 94(2), 315–323. doi:10.1016/j.apmr.2012.09.024.

Bingham, C., Clarke, L., Michielsens, E., & Van De Meer, M. (2013). Towards a social model approach? British and Dutch disability policies in the health sector compared. *Personnel Review*, 42, 613–637. doi:10.1108/PR-08-2011-0120.

Blustein, J. (2012). Philosophical and ethical issues in disability. *Journal of Moral Philosophy*, 9, 573–587. doi:10.1163/17455243-00904002.

Bogart, K. R., & Dunn, D.S. (2019). Ableism special issue introduction. *Journal of Social Issues*, 75(3), 650–664.

Brittain, I. (2004). Perceptions of disability and their impact upon involvement in sport for people with disabilities at all levels. *Journal of Sport & Social Issues*, 28, 429–452. doi:10.1177/0193723504268729.

Brown, L. (n.d.). Identity-first language. *Autistic Self Advocacy Network.* http://autisticadvocacy.org/home/about-asan/identity-first-language.

Byrne, G. (2018). Prevalence and psychological sequelae of sexual abuse among individuals with an intellectual disability: A review of the recent literature. *Journal of Intellectual Disabilities: JOID*, 22(3), 294–310. doi:10.1177/1744629517698844.

Campbell, F. (2001). Inciting legal fictions: "Disability's" date with ontology and the ableist body of the law. *Griffith Law Review*, 10 (1), 42–62.

Centers for Disease Control and Prevention (CDC) (n.d.). www.cdc.gov/ncbddd/disabilityandhealth/disability-barriers.html.

Cohen, A., & Mosek, A. (2019). "Power together": Professionals and parents of children with disabilities creating productive partnerships. *Child & Family Social Work*, 24(4), 565–573. doi:10.1111/cfs.12637.

Colver, A. F., Dickinson, H. O., Parkinson, K., Arnaud, C., Beckung, E., Fauconnier, J., Thyen, U. (2011). Access of children with cerebral palsy to the physical, social and attitudinal environment they need: A cross-sectional European study. *Disability and Rehabilitation*, 33(1), 28–35. doi:10.3109/09638288.2010.485669.

Constantine, M. G., Hage, S. M., Kindaichi, M.M., & Bryant, R. M. (2007). Social justice and multicultural issues: Implications for the practice and training of counselors and counseling psychologists. *Journal of Counseling & Development*, 85, 24–29.

Cooper, M., O'Hara, M. O., Schmid, P. F., & Wyatt, G. (2007). Preface. In M. Cooper, M. O'Hara, P. Schmid, & G. Wyatt (Eds.), *The handbook of person-centered psychotherapy and counseling* (pp. xxi–xxiv). Palgrave Macmillan.

Coster, W., Bedell, G., Law, M., Khetani, M. A., Teplicky, R., Liljenquist, K., Kao, Y. C. (2011). Psychometric evaluation of the Participation and Environment Measure for Children and Youth. *Developmental Medicine & Child Neurology*, 53 (11), 1030–1037. doi:10.1111/j.1469-8749.2011.04094.x.

Coster, W., Law, M., Bedell, G., Liljenquist, K., Kao, Y. C., Khetani, M., & Teplicky, R. (2013). School participation, supports and barriers of students with and without disabilities. *Child: Care, Health and Development*, 39(4), 535–543. doi:10.1111/cch.12046.

Department for International Development (2000). Disability, poverty and development. Retrieved from https://hpod.law.harvard.edu/pdf/Disability-poverty-and-development.pdf.

Dunn, D. S. & Andrews, E. E. (2015). Person-first and identity-first language: Developing psychologists' cultural competence using disability language. *American Psychologist*, 70(3), 255–264.

Dunn, D. S., & Burcaw, S. (2013). Disability identity: Exploring narrative accounts of disability. *Rehabilitation Psychology*, 58, 148–157. doi:10.1037/a0031691.

Eisert, D., Kulka. L., & Moore. K. (1988). Facilitating play in hospitalized handicapped children: The design of a therapeutic play environment. *CHC*, 3(18), 201–208.

Evans, R. L., Dingus, C. M., & Haselkorn, J. K. (1993). Living with a disability: a synthesis and critique of the literature on quality of life, 1985–1989. *Psychological Reports*, 72(3), 771–777. doi:10.2466/pr0.1993.72.3.771.

Feather, K. A., & Carlson, R. G. (2019). An initial investigation of individual instructors' self perceived competence and incorporation of disability content into CACREP-accredited programs: Rethinking training in counselor education. *Journal of Multicultural Counseling and Development*, 47(1), 19–36. doi:10.1002/jmcd.12118.

Goodley, D. (2001). Learning difficulties, the social model of disability and impairment: Challenging epistemologies. *Disability & Society*, 16, 207–231. doi:10.1080/09687590120035816.

Goudie, A., Nacisse, M., Hall, D. E., & Kuo, D. Z. (2014). Financial and psychological stressors associated with caring for children with disability. *Family, Systems, and Health*, 32, 280–290. doi:10.1037/fsh0000027.

Granlund, M. (2013). Participation: challenges in conceptualization, measurement and intervention. *Child Care Health Development*, 39, 4. doi:10.1111/cch.12080.

Griffin, M. M., Fisher, M. H., Lane, L. A., & Morin, L. (2019). In their own words: Perceptions and experiences of bullying among individuals with intellectual and developmental disabilities. *Intellectual and Developmental Disabilities*, 57(1), 66–74. doi:10.1352/1934-9556-57.1.66.

Guichard, S., & Grande, C. (2018). Differences between pre-school children with and without special educational needs functioning, participation, and environmental barriers at home and in community settings: An international classification of functioning, disability, and health for children and youth approach. *Frontiers in Education*, 3(7). doi:10.3389/feduc.2018.00007.

Hastings, R. P., & Taunt, H. M. (2002). Positive perceptions in families of children with developmental disabilities. *American Journal of Mental Retardation: AJMR*, 107 (2), 116–127. doi:10.1352/0895-8017.

Hull, L., Petrides, K. V., Allison, C., Smith, P., Baron-Cohen, S., Lai, M. C., & Mandy, W. (2017). "Putting on my best normal": Social camouflaging in adults with autism spectrum conditions. *Journal of Autism and Developmental Disorders*, 47 (8), 2519–2534.

Korinek, L., & Prillaman, D. (1992). Counselors and exceptional students: Preparation versus practice. *Counselor Education and Supervision*, 32, 3–11. doi:10.1002/j.1556-6978.1992.tb00168.x.

Kraus, L., Lauer, E., Coleman, R., and Houtenville, A. (2018). *2017 Disability Statistics Annual Report*. University of New Hampshire.

Landreth, G. L. (2012). *Play therapy: The art of the relationship* (3rd ed.). Routledge.

Lebsock, M. S., & DeBlassie, R. R. (1975). The school counselor's role in special education. *Counselor Education and Supervision*, 15, 128–134. doi:10.1002/j.1556-6978.1975.tb00997.x.

Lustig, D. C. (2002). Family coping in families with a child with a disability. *Education and Training in Mental Retardation and Developmental Disabilities*, 37(1), 14–22.

Mitra, S. (2006). The capability approach and disability. *Journal of Disability Policy Studies*, 16, 236–247. doi:10.1177/10442073060160040501.

Matthias, R. E., & Benjamin, A. E. (2003). Abuse and neglect of clients in agency-based and consumer-directed home care. *Health & Social Work*, 28, 174–184. doi:10.1093/hsw/28.3.174.

Moustakas, C. E. (1959). *Psychotherapy with children: The living relationship*. Ballantine Books.

Norwich, B. (2002). Education, inclusion and individual differences: Recognising and resolving dilemmas. *British Journal of Educational Studies*, 50(4), 482–502.

Nerenberg, J. (2020). *Divergent mind: Thriving in a world that wasn't designed for you*. HarperCollins.

Nettelbeck, T., & Wilson, C. (2002). Personal vulnerability to victimization of people with mental retardation. *Trauma, Violence, & Abuse*, 3, 289–306.

Panksepp, J. & Biven, L. (2012). *The archaeology of mind: Neuroevolutionary origins of human emotion*. Norton.

Pinquart, M., & Sorensen, S. (2007). Correlates of physical health of informal caregivers: A meta-analysis. *Journal of Gerontology: Psychological Sciences and Social Sciences*, 62, 126–137.

Porges, S. W. (2021). Play as a neural exercise: Insights from the polyvagal theory. In: Porges, S. W. (Ed), *Polyvagal safety: attachment, communication, self-regulation*. W. W. Norton & Company.

Porges, S.W., & Daniel, S. (2021). Play and the dynamics of treating pediatric medical trauma: Insights from polyvagal theory. In: Porges, S. W. (Ed), *Polyvagal safety: attachment, communication, self-regulation*. W. W. Norton & Company.

Porges, S. W. (2011). *The polyvagal theory: Neurophysiological foundations of emotion, attachment, communication and self-regulation*. W. W. Norton & Company.

Raj, C. (2021). The lost promise of disability rights. *Michigan Law Review*, 119(5), 933. doi:10.36644/mlr.119.5.lost.

Ray, D. C., Stulmaker, H., Lee, K., & Silverman, W. (2013). Child-centered play therapy and impairment: Exploring relationships and constructs. *International Journal of Play Therapy*, 22(1), 13–27.

Rees, K. (2017). Models of disability and the categorisation of children with severe and profound learning difficulties: Informing educational approaches based on an understanding of individual needs. *Educational & Child Psychology*, 34 (4), 30–39.

Reindal, S. M. (2008). A social relational model of disability: A theoretical framework for special needs education? *European Journal of Special Needs Education*, 23(2), 135–146.

Reiss, S., Levitan, G. W., & Szyszko, J. (1982). Emotional disturbance and mental retardation: Diagnostic overshadowing. *American Journal of Mental Deficiency*, 86, 567–574.

Rose, C. A., Monda-Amaya, L. E., & Espelage, D. L. (2011). Bullying perpetration and victimization in special education: A review of the literature. *Remedial and Special Education Research*, 32(2), 114–130. doi:10.1177/0741932510361247.

Roush, S. E., & Sharby, N. (2011). Disability reconsidered: The paradox of physical therapy. *Physical Therapy*, 91, 1715–1727. doi:10.2522/ptj.20100389.

Rush, K. S., Bowman, L. G., Eidman, S. L., Toole, L. M., & Mortenson, B. P. (2004). Assessing psychopathology in individuals with developmental disabilities. *Behavior Modification*, 28(5), 621–637.

Schmid, P. F. (2007). The anthropological and ethical foundations of person-centered therapy. In M. Cooper, M. O'Hara, P. Schmid, & G. Wyatt (Eds.), *The handbook of person-centered psychotherapy and counseling* (pp. 30–46). Palgrave Macmillan.

Schore, A. N. (2001). Effects of a secure attachment relationship on right brain development, affect regulation, and infant mental health. *Infant Mental Health Journal*, 22(1–2), 7–66.

Schottelkorb, A. A., Swan, K. L., & Ogawa, Y. (2015). Parent consultation in child-centered play therapy: A model for research and practice. *International Journal of Play Therapy*, 24(4), 221–233. doi:10.1037/a0039609.

Schottelkorb, A. A., Swan, K. L., & Ogawa, Y. (2020). Intensive child-centered play therapy for children on the autism spectrum: A pilot study. *Journal of Counseling and Development: JCD*, 98(1), 63–73. doi:10.1002/jcad.12300.

Scorgie, K., & Sobsey, D. (2000). Transformational outcomes associated with parenting children who have disabilities. *Mental Retardation*, 38(3), 195–206. doi:10.1352/0047-6765(2000)038<0195:TOAWPC>2.0.CO;2.

Scorgie, K. & Forlin, C. (2019). Social inclusion and belonging: Affirming validation, agency and voice. In C. Forlin & K. Scorgie (Eds.), *Promoting social inclusion* (pp. 3–16). Emerald Publishing.

Shakespeare, T. (2010). The social model of disability. In L. J. Davis (Ed.), *The disability studies reader* (pp. 266–273). Routledge.

Smart, J. F., & Smart, D. W. (2006). Models of disability: Implications for the counseling profession. *Journal of Counseling & Development*, 84, 29–40. doi:10.1002/j.1556-6678.2006.tb00377.x.

Swan, K. L. & Ray, D. C. (2014). Effects of child-centered play therapy on irritability and hyperactivity behaviors of children with intellectual disabilities. *Journal of Humanistic Counseling*, 53(2), 120–133.

U.S. Census Bureau (2019). Childhood disability in the United States: 2019. Retrieved from www.census.gov/content/dam/Census/library/publications/2021/acs/acsbr-006.pdf.

Ware Balch, J., & Ray, D. C. (2015). Emotional assets of children with autism spectrum disorder: A single-case therapeutic outcome experiment. *Journal of Counseling and Development*, 93(4), 429–439.

Woo, H., Goo, M., & Lee, M. (2016). A content analysis of research on disability: American Counseling Association journals between 2003 and 2013. *Journal of Multicultural Counseling and Development*, 44, 228–244. doi:10.1002/jmcd.12051.

World Health Organization (2007). *International classification of functioning, disability and health for children and youth (ICF-CY)*. World Health Organization.

World Health Organization (2011). World report on disability. Retrieved from www.who.int/disabilities/world_report/2011/report.pdf.

7   Cultural Opportunities with Indigenous Populations

Geri Glover

"We do not inherit the Earth from our Ancestors, we borrow it from our Children."

— Tribe Unknown (Weiser-Alexander, 2020)

From *Chinook*, as told by Jessie Marsh (1976).

The old one thought for a while, remembering the stories he had been told long ago. Then he began. When the world was very young, the Creative Spirit gave a small part of it to the Thunderbird. It was the North Crow Creek canyon of the Mission Range. Thunderbird was very happy to have a canyon of her own where her jealous rival Coyote could not enter. Here she could be free to lay her eggs and hatch her young. Coyote could not bother her. So, it was here in the North Crow Creek canyon that she gave birth to three daughters, Bluejay, Magpie, and Crow. All went well for a time. Thunderbird was kind to all that came from the Bitterroot valley to hunt, or fish, or gather huckleberries. If Thunderbird saw a storm coming from the East pass, she would make thundering noises. This would warn the hunters to leave before the storm struck.

Then one day a careless hunter failed to put out his campfire. It started a great fire. The fire spread all through Thunderbird's canyon destroying everything in its path. Angrily, Thunderbird beat her huge wings against her breast. She thundered out her punishment. "You have killed everything that grew in my beautiful valley. Even the elk and deer have fled. So, I will keep all of you away forever." She called the Northeast wind. "Stay in the pass," she told him. "Keep on blowing your icy breath. Keep on blowing until I tell you to stop. For I mean to destroy the people who have destroyed my land."

Shivering with cold, the Indians left their homes. They fled to the Bitterroot country. Even Thunderbird's daughters, Bluejay, Magpie, and Crow left with the others. Thunderbird was alone. Many moons passed before Thunderbird's anger softened. Then an Indian scout came back and reported to his tribal chief. "I heard Thunderbird sobbing. She sounded lonely."

DOI: 10.4324/9781003190073-10

All the Indians and the animals were sorry to hear this except Coyote. "Let the big bird who makes the big noise live alone in the country she has made too cold for us to live in," Coyote said. But Thunderbird's daughter Bluejay went to the Chief and offered her help. "When the right time is here," she said, "I will fly West. I will find Chinook and tell him what has happened. I will ask him to come to our valley and help us."

So Bluejay flew West, found Chinook and told him the story. "You are a good little, bird," Chinook said. "You should always be gay and happy. So, I will follow back to Montana if you will fly ahead of me and lead the way." So Bluejay flew ahead of Chinook until they reached the Mission Range. And there below the Mission Range, Chinook blew his warm breath across the land. The ice melted. New trees and grasses and flowers grew. And the Indians and animals returned.

Once more Thunderbird was happy. Turning to Bluejay she thanked her. "What can I do to show you how happy you have made me?" she asked. "You can keep your temper down, my mother," said Bluejay, "so that the innocent ones need never again suffer for the careless ones because of your anger." And so it was. And to this day Thunderbird's land is one of the prettiest spots in Montana.

Cultural Considerations

To know a people, listen to their stories. Listen to how they teach their children the lessons of life. Native Peoples of the Americas have used the oral transmission of stories, histories, lessons, and other knowledge to sustain their cultures and identities. Coyote stories should only be told in the dark winter months, when the snow is on the ground, and there is time to listen and learn. To share a coyote story here shows just how acculturated I am, but it demonstrates an avenue by which we can reach our clients; whether they are small children or parents. Telling a story puts things into context, making ideas easier to understand. In addition, the lesson is indirect and does not accuse the listener of wrongdoing. It is just a story.

What's in a Name?

When asked to write a chapter for this text, I was immediately confronted with the dilemma of appropriate nomenclature. Language and what a people call themselves is foundational to a culture. Names placed upon a group by others discounts the essence of a people. We all know the story of Columbus's voyage "toward the regions of India," coming to the Americas, and thinking that he had circled the globe to Asia. He used the word Indios to refer to the peoples of the so-called New World that resulted in the misnomer, Indian, that has lasted for centuries (Zimmer, 2009). My father was of the generation who, after many years of cultural decimation and forced assimilation tactics, finally in his later years was proud to call himself Indian. In New Mexico, we have billboards proclaiming that you have entered Indian Country and should be respectful of the land and people who live there.

The U.S. Census Bureau uses the terms American Indian and Alaska Native (AI/AN) to identify persons belonging to the tribal nations of the continental United States (American Indians) and the tribal nations and villages of Alaska (Alaska Natives) (Norris et al., 2012). This is also the language used in federal treaties and laws and in much of academia. In the United States, Native American was popular in the 1970s and 80s, but according to the National Museum of the American Indian (2018), it is falling out of favor with some groups as it perpetuates the continued use of the term Indian which was assigned by the White oppressors.

Five prominent Native voices shared their thoughts about the terms Native American vs. Indian with columnist Amanda Blackhorse (Diné) (2019). White Hawk (Sicangu Lakota) said that naming is important because, "Understanding our names is a base level of understanding of who we are. When people don't respect your request to be identified by your name, by your own definition, it's hurtful and de-validating." Abrahamson (Lemhi, Boise Shoshone, and Interior Salish) stated, "I prefer indigenous, but I am comfortable with 'Native American' or 'American Indian'. The reason I prefer indigenous is because being indigenous means you are of a place, one place on earth, which is unique to you. It identifies our peoples well because we refer to ourselves as from a place or location."

By the end of the 20th century, the preference of tribal peoples from across the world became the term Indigenous and this was recognized by the United Nations when it established the Permanent Forum on Indigenous Issues (2000) and later passed the Declaration of the Rights of Indigenous Peoples (2007). In this chapter, you will see all of these terms as I relate research to the various sections, including the collective terms Native and Native Peoples which are what I choose when speaking of the Indigenous Peoples in the United States.

Demographics

According to the National Congress of American Indians (2020), there are 574 sovereign tribal nations, located across 35 states, which have a formal nation-to-nation relationship with the U.S. government. Estimates of the population of Indigenous people in North America prior to 1890 ranged from 1.5 million to 20 million (Seattle Times, 2016). That number fell below 250,000 between 1890 and 1910. As of 2010, there were an estimated 5.2 million people who were classified as American Indian and Alaska Native alone or American Indian and Alaska Native in combination with one or more other races making up 1.7% of the total U.S. population.

Data from the 2010 U.S. Census (2011) showed that the largest tribal nations in the U.S. by population were Navajo, Cherokee, Choctaw, Sioux, Chippewa, Apache, Blackfeet, Iroquois, and Pueblo. Of the total population of Native Peoples, 33.9% were under the age of 18, while only 5.6% were over the age of 65. The median age of Native Peoples was 31 years, compared to the median age of 37 years for the overall U.S. population. Native Peoples have a life expectancy that is 5.5 years less than the total U.S. population (73.0 years to 78.5 years, respectively); however, this figure can vary significantly in relation to any specific tribal nation. For example, in Oglala Lakota County, South Dakota, the average life expectancy is just 66.81 years, which is 13 years less than for the state as a whole (Institute for Health Metrics and Evaluation, 2016).

Quality of Life

Three of the primary indicators of quality of life include wealth, education, and health (Centers for Disease Control and Prevention, 2000). According to the American Community Survey (Guzman, 2020), the estimated median family income for Native Peoples of the United States during the five-year period from 2015 to 2019 was $43,825 as compared to $68,785 for the non-Hispanic White population. Most reservations have few jobs. Many of those are limited to professionals with college degrees, such as teachers, nurses, doctors, counselors, accountants, and administrators. These professionals are usually not from the reservation, creating a situation of dependence on outsiders for services and less control over their own programs. Only 77% of this population age 25 and over had at least a high school diploma as compared to 90% of non-Hispanic Whites (Office of Minority Health, 2021). 13% had at least a bachelor's degree in comparison to 31% of non-Hispanic Whites and only 4.5% had an advanced graduate degree.

Native Peoples have long experienced lower health status when compared with the general U.S. population (Indian Health Service, 2019). There is a high prevalence of risk factors for mental health concerns and suicide, obesity, substance abuse, sudden infant death syndrome (SIDS), teenage pregnancy, liver disease, and hepatitis (Indian Health Service, 2019). The infant death rate is 60% higher than the rate for non-Hispanic Whites. Native Peoples are twice as likely to have diabetes as non-Hispanic Whites. For example, the Pima Nation of Arizona has one of the highest diabetes rates in the world.

Native Peoples experience higher levels of disease and causes of death including heart disease, cancer, unintentional injuries (accidents), diabetes, and strokes (Office of Minority Health, 2021). In my first six months of working on the Alamo Navajo Reservation, we lost one or two community members each month: two elders; a young woman and her little sister to a car accident; a middle-aged adult to liver failure due to alcoholism; and a young man to an accidental shooting. These deaths resulted in what felt like an endless stream of funerals and grief. The emotional impact was even more intense because of the bonds by blood, marriage, and long friendships that typify Native life. Frequent losses diminish a person's coping capacity. There is often no time to recover from a loss before another occurs.

All of these quality of life issues appear to be rooted in economic adversity and poor social conditions (Norris et al., 2012). Warne et al. (2017) conducted a study of adult residents of South Dakota whose Native population is nearly 10% of the total state population using the Adverse Childhood Experiences (ACEs) survey. The original ACEs study had found a significant relationship between exposure to emotional, physical, or sexual abuse, and household dysfunction during childhood to health risk behavior and disease in adulthood (Felitti et al., 1998). Warne et al. (2017) found that Native respondents to the ACEs survey had a significantly higher prevalence of all categories of childhood abuse, neglect, and household dysfunction compared with non-Native respondents. While the impact of ACEs scores was similar for both Native and non-Native respondents, Native respondents reported significantly higher prevalence of PTSD, depression, and cigarette smoking. Of American Indian respondents, 32.38% reported four or more ACEs compared to 11.27% of non-American Indian respondents. Armed with this information, both play therapy and parent training which is culturally appropriate and responsive would be part of a comprehensive plan to intervene with children and families who are at risk for these adverse experiences and their related outcomes.

Play Therapy Considerations

My training and preferred therapeutic modality is in Child-Centered Play Therapy (CCPT) (Landreth, 2012), which falls under the umbrella of humanistic approaches. Humanistic approaches emphasize that each person has their own way of looking at the world and that each person can make their own choices. These approaches focus on the present and treating the whole person rather than looking at a specific problem or diagnosis. Skills in CCPT include being fully present with a child, responding to the child's behaviors and feelings, and setting limits on behavior only when necessary. The child chooses to play or not to play, to speak or not to speak. The child leads and the therapist follows.

Underpinned by Rogers' (1951) early version of his Client-Centered Approach, CCPT is compatible with Native values, including relationship, striving for balance between the mental, physical, and spiritual aspects in one's environment, a deep respect for individuals, a liberal childrearing ideology, noninterference, and supporting independence. CCPT is based on Carl Rogers' (1951) initial principles of nondirective therapy and was adapted for children by Virginia Axline (1969). The conditions Rogers and Axline identified as necessary for positive change can be linked to the Native values identified above.

Relationship

First, a relationship must exist. Axline (1969) named a warm, caring relationship as the first of eight basic principles of play therapy. The need to establish a trusting relationship between the play therapist and both the child client and the child client's parent(s)/guardian(s) is essential in any therapeutic situation. This relationship takes on additional significance when a lack of trust has been developed over generations with broken promises and poorly administered health care that disregarded the cultural context of Native Peoples.

Incongruent Client and Congruent Therapist

Rogers (1951) identified incongruence or vulnerability in the client as a necessary condition for therapy as the feelings of fear and anxiety are often what bring an individual to therapy. In the case of children, that incongruence is felt and observed by adults. Native Peoples define health as being balanced within the framework of a harmonious and generous life (Cross, 1997). Illness equals imbalance or incongruence (Williams & Ellison, 1999).

As noted by Rogers (1951), the healer must be congruent, healthy, balanced. I remember a story, but not who told it to me, about a village that was suffering because it had not rained for a very long time. The people of the village traveled far to find a shaman (medicine healer) to come and bring the rain back to their village. The shaman went with the people and stayed with them in their village, but the people became angry as the shaman did nothing to bring the rain. The people cried, "Why did we bring you here?" After several days, the clouds started to fill the skies and soon the rain began to fall. The people were grateful and came to thank the shaman. The shaman said, "I did nothing to bring the rain." The people asked, "Then how is it that the rain has returned?" The shaman said, "I have grown old and gained much wisdom from the mountains and rivers, wind and trees. With this, the Great Spirit Creator is pleased. My space and the space around me is balanced, and now all is in order."

Unqualified Acceptance and Permissiveness

Rogers (1951) referred to the necessary condition of unconditional positive regard (UPR) which Axline (1969) addressed in two of her principles as unqualified acceptance and creating a feeling of safety and permissiveness. The child is accepted by the therapist without any conditions or judgment. This would be a familiar style for Native children. Parenting styles affect children differently in different cultures (García & Gracia, 2009). By extension, a play therapist's style could affect clients differently in different cultures. According to García and Gracia (2009), in some collectivist societies where the group is prioritized over the individual, parents motivate children through affection, acceptance, and involvement. They tend to perceive strictness and firm parental control as unnecessary, and perhaps even harmful. Gfellner (1990) found Native parents demonstrated more liberal practices in comparison with White parents. Parental behaviors support self-direction while helping children to learn to balance this with community and family responsibilities. CCPT provides a non-judgmental, understanding, and accepting environment to foster positive development in children.

Empathy

Rogers (1951) identified the requirement of demonstrating empathy by recognizing the emotional experiences of the client, and Axline (1969) stated this simply as being sensitive to the child's feelings. Mesman et al. (2016) measured the universality of responsiveness to infant distress in parents from different cultures. Although Native parents did not display the same degree of smiling, kissing, or cuddling as in Western cultures, there was still evidence of affection for the infant and a demonstration of sensitivity to the child's needs. This mirrors Rogers' recommendation to recognize emotions without getting emotionally involved.

Respect and Understanding

Rogers' (1951) final condition is that the client must perceive to some degree the therapist's unconditional positive regard and empathic understanding. This is covered in Axline's (1969) two principles of respecting the child's ability to solve personal problems and allowing the child to lead. The concept of noninterference supports letting things happen the way they are meant to be (BigFoot & Funderburk, 2011). Briggs (as cited in Sprott, 1994), in his work with Alaska Native families, observed that children were not prevented from making mistakes unless the mistake might be life-threatening. Children grow strong when they are given the opportunity to make choices without coercion (Brendtro et al., 1990). This is similar to a strength-based perspective which honors the power of the self to heal and right itself with the help of the environment (Saleebey, 1997).

Maslow (as cited in Brendtro et al., 1990) described the process of supporting personal autonomy and responsibility by relating the following story. He recalls watching a toddler trying to open a door to a cabin. This was a big, heavy door and he was shoving and shoving. Non-Native adults would probably get up and open the door for him. The Blackfeet (Pikuni) sat for half an hour while the toddler struggled with the door until he was able to get it open himself. Everyone praised him because he was able to do it himself.

Patience

Axline's (1969) final principle is an admonition to not attempt to hurry the process. Traditional Native Peoples have a present-oriented relationship with time. Time is not rigidly structured, it is circular. There is never a lack of time (Glover, 2001). Time is always with us; things happen in their own time (Garrett et al., 2014).

The parallels between Native values and CCPT help Native parents to ally with the play therapist. Being with a child and allowing that child to make their own choices are not foreign practices to Native parents and do not require the same explanations often requested by non-Native parents when they are first introduced to CCPT.

Cultural Opportunities

Access the Native Community

Literature often cites the statistic that 72% of those who identify as Native Peoples live away from their tribal homeland in urban areas (First Nations Development Institute, 2017). This figure is misleading as it uses the Census definition of "urban," as any town with more than 2,500 residents. A town of 2,500 is hardly urban by today's standards. A more accurate description is provided in an analysis of race and ethnicity in America in a 2012 report which found that 54% of the nation's Native population resides in rural or small-town areas. Thirty percent live in suburban areas just outside of a city or exurban areas which are nearly rural, and only 16% live in high population density urban areas. Kingsley et al. (2014) found that 68% of Native Peoples live on or near their tribal homelands.

Berry et al. (2002) noted that individuals living near reservations in surrounding counties are connected to their reservation culturally, socially, and politically. They participate in rituals and traditions, have social ties with friends and families, and vote in tribal elections. Living on or near Native homelands or reservations has a strong effect on an individual's identity and self-esteem because individuals are supported in feeling proud of their racial and ethnic heritage (First Nations Development Institute, 2017). Physical place plays an important part in developing and maintaining an identity as an individual, as a member of a community, and as a member of a racial or ethnic group. Huyser et al. (2018) discovered that individuals who spent the majority of their lives on the reservation had lower odds of psychological distress than individuals who spent some proportion of their lives off the reservation. This was true for both the Northern Plains tribal members and the Southwest tribal members who participated in the study.

With these things in mind, play therapists can expect to have access to tribal communities to learn about the specific cultural aspects of their clients as well as for sources of support for their clients. Neighborhood networks and sharing responsibility for the wellbeing of children are positive features of the extended family concept (Harrison et al., 1990; Red Horse, 1980). A colleague of mine who prefers not to be named presented this advice for becoming involved with Native Peoples.

Try to attend local functions, church services, traditional dances that allow outsiders, community blessings or feedings. Sporting events are huge in Native communities. Attend local high school sporting events. Over time you will become more accepted if you are seen as part of local events. The people that have made the biggest impact among outsiders seem to be those who immerse themselves into the community. I remember a lady. She came to the local clinic over 10 years back. She showed up to community meals and gatherings and followed all customs and traditions like a local native. She brought her offerings/donations, like the rest of us and knew to bring the good stuff like donuts and soda! When there was a death, she brought her offerings for the family. She often pitched in around the cooking fires or food prep in the homes. I noticed she aligned herself with one of the family women she worked with. That was key to her acceptance at these gatherings.

> (Counselor (Jicarilla Apache, Pueblo), personal communication,
> May 1, 2021)

Acknowledge Traditional Parenting Skills

In traditional Native culture, autonomy is highly valued, and children are allowed to make their own decisions and operate semi-independently at an early age with freedom to experience natural consequences (LaFromboise & Low, 1998). Native Peoples have practiced inductive discipline for thousands of years. Warnings about the consequences of bad behavior are presented in community terms and by identifying how others view the behavior. Native parents rarely use physical punishment. Shame, otherwise known as embarrassment, is a common disciplinary tool used to correct unacceptable behaviors (Burgess, 1980). In the playroom, limits are set only when needed for the safety of the child, the therapist or the materials in the room. Autonomy is highly valued and children are allowed to learn from experience. Recognizing and acknowledging this shared perspective about child behavior can help the therapist to align with Native parents.

Disciplining might include disapproving words, ignoring the child, or requiring the child to give restitution for wrongdoing, such as apologizing to members of the family for embarrassing them (LaFromboise & Low, 1998). Discipline may be administered in ways and forms not noticeable to outsiders, including the play therapist, who might be concerned that a parent does not understand the importance of setting limits. The play therapist can ask the parent what they do when their child misbehaves. They might learn that some parents pass information of an indiscretion onto another family member who will then dispense the punishment. This is done to protect the bonds between the parent and child and to reinforce the extended family involvement. Parents generally have a primary responsibility, but uncles and aunts share values, impart wisdom, serve as role models, and enforce tribal teachings.

All parents want their children to be generous, be respectful, get along with others, make responsible choices. Native families actively teach by modeling and storytelling from the earliest moments of a child's life. Through storytelling, children learn about proper relationships, other people in the environment, and moral development. Play therapists can also learn about what is important to a particular Native community by seeking out and listening to the stories they tell their children. In a culturally inclusive playroom, materials are available for children to share their own stories as well as the stories they have been told using dolls, puppets, and other toys.

Native Peoples believe that children are a special gift from the creator (Northwest Indian Child Welfare Institute, 1986). Praise and reassurance are used to encourage a positive loving relationship between parents and children. Naming ceremonies help the child to establish a role and dignity in the tribe. Cradleboards were used to keep newborns close. Cradleboards are not common today; however, infants continue to be held rather than left alone in car seats or strollers. The whole community recognizes the child's growth and development through rites of passage ceremonies. Children are taught to be good observers to understand the meaning of nonverbal communication (Garrett et al., 2014). Play therapy skills mirror traditional Native parenting in a number of ways. Play therapists value and respect children. They encourage a warm relationship through unconditional positive regard, acknowledgment, and non-judgmental encouragement. They support their young clients in their growth and development. Observation and understanding nonverbal communication are key skills for play therapists. These comparable behaviors provide another opportunity for play therapists to recognize and acknowledge a shared perspective about children with Native parents.

All Native Peoples have become acculturated to varying degrees into the dominant culture; however, the level of acculturation depends on the strength of the family support system and the degree of their own conviction about maintaining traditions. Within the extended family, oftentimes children turn not only to their parents and aunts and uncles for support, but also to other significant adults. All elders may be referred to as grandmother or grandfather. Cousins may be referred to as brothers and sisters. Within the extended family environment, traditional values of generosity, respect for elders, respect for all creation, harmony, and individual freedom can be modeled and supported. Knowing this is a common approach to raising children in a traditional Native community, the play therapist can encourage parents to reach out to their immediate and extended family for support, and rather than question the validity of multiple caregivers, commend parents for this communal style.

Utilize the Play Therapy Environment

Although the relationship between child and therapist is probably the single most important tool in CCPT, the environment also plays a significant part in the intervention. Martinez and Valdez (1992) asserted that the play therapy environment should contain items that convey the therapist's openness to the child's cultural background. It is the therapist who has control over the environment in which the therapy occurs. Toys can be selected without cultural responsiveness, assuming that any doll will do as a vehicle for children to express themselves. However, therapists must be on guard not to assume that simply because a Native child plays happily with the toys provided, the playroom is culturally appropriate. Toys are an important part of the therapeutic work, as is noted by Landreth (2012), the toys are a child's words. Dolls with dark skin and hair, cradleboards, drums, traditional foods, utensils and cooking pots, multi-racial, skin-toned crayons, paints and markers, beads and feathers for art projects, horses, dogs, and forest animals will give Native children permission to bring culture into their play; to bring themselves into the play.

In therapy with Native children, actual play behaviors are not unlike those of children from the dominant culture. Both girls and boys enjoy using art materials, easel painting, role playing, playing store, and creating scenes in the sand. Many girls are attracted to doll play and caring for babies. Many boys are attracted to aggressive play with action figures. Some children talk while they play while others are silent. Children may speak in their tribal language rather than English.

Promote Family Participation

Any work with Native children must honor and respect the family. Children learn their culture through their family and community. Native families prefer to include the whole family in any experience and flexibility regarding both time and structure is essential. Child/Parent Relationship Training (CPRT) (Landreth & Bratton, 2020) provides the motivation for incorporating parents and other significant adults in therapy; however, the model must be adjusted to fit Native values and needs (Glover, 2001). Typical CPRT brings parents together to learn basic CCPT skills and child development information. The training is set up as a closed ten-week group. Once the basic skills have been presented and practiced within the group, special play sessions with an identified child begin at home and the training group becomes more of a support group providing a venue for the parents to share their experiences in and outside the special play sessions.

In general, open-ended, drop-in groups are more appealing for Native Peoples who cannot predict their consistent availability for an entire ten-week period (Glover, 2010). Providing childcare and transportation makes the training more accessible. Conducting the training with children available during the group time for practice alleviates the difficulties of doing play sessions at home where there is typically no quiet space. Family groups can be encouraged to attend making it possible to include all children in the practice sessions. Longer training segments with fewer sessions and creating an atmosphere of a social event by providing food for all participants recognizes the holistic nature of Native Peoples where learning and socializing are not separate activities.

The Native style of communication is to listen and learn through observation, especially in the presence of a respected elder or authority (Garrett et al., 2014). Enlisting elders and professionals from the community to participate lends credibility to the group process. Using storytelling to present concepts provides context for the skills that are being taught. Supporting an atmosphere of cooperation, sharing, and harmony with patience and minimal interruption can promote helping processes that are more sustainable and respectful for all individuals.

Working with Families

To understand the Native family, you must look at how history has so negatively impacted this group. Almost from the beginning of European settlement in North America, but especially in the 19th and 20th centuries, various efforts were made to eliminate or change the many tribal cultures. No therapist should underestimate the current impact of historical trauma. It is real and it is pervasive.

The removal policy of 1835 relocated Native Peoples to Indian Territory where the land was often unproductive with few natural resources. The Dawes Severalty Act of 1837 allocated each member of an Indian tribe according to age, a specific portion of land (Monahan, 1995). This contributed to the land base of Native Peoples being reduced from approximately 140,000,000 acres to approximately 50 million. The excess land was made available to settlers (Edmonds, 1981). Proponents of this act assured the public that the Indian would accept individual landholdings, move away from their collectivist lifestyle, and become completely assimilated.

Interference with the Native family generally occurred through the education system. The primary effort of education was on civilizing, and assimilating Native Peoples into White society (Reyhner, 1994). Boarding schools were established in the United States in the 1900s. Schools were highly authoritative and run in a strict military fashion (National Indian Child Abuse and Neglect Resource Center, 1980). Boarding schools effectively destroyed the intergenerational transmission of family and parenting knowledge and also introduced new and dysfunctional behaviors, such as sexual abuse and the use of severe corporal punishment. The general purpose stated of the boarding schools was to "Kill the Indian, save the man" (Pratt, 1973/1892). Those who spent their childhood in boarding schools were deprived of the opportunity to experience family life. They reached adulthood without any clear concept of appropriate parenting. Again, my colleague shares her thoughts.

> We are three generations away from boarding schools, but the effect is still very profound today. I grew up in a home without any kind of

nurturing or affection. That was common for my generation. No one was hugged or told we were loved. We knew we were cared for, and we had homes and general acceptance, but we were not shown affection. We were spanked and disciplined harshly, but it was common practice. I believe these were behaviors learned from boarding school life. We raised our children in the same manner and now come to realize that they need affection and nurturing. It wasn't until I experienced this from my mother-in-law, that I knew I had missed an integral part of my childhood.

(Counselor (Jicarilla Apache, Pueblo), personal communication, May 1, 2021)

In the 1950s, after World War II and the Korean conflict, the GI Bill and the Bureau of Indian Affairs Relocation Program for Job training moved significant numbers of Native Peoples to large urban areas. From 1958 to 1968, The Child Welfare League of America supported the Indian adoption Project (George, 1997). The league's philosophy was that the forgotten child on the reservation could be adopted and placed where there was less prejudice against Indians. In determining the placement, the best interests of the child were to be considered. Poverty was judged a factor leading to neglect and abuse and most Native Peoples living on the reservation were poor. Middle-income European American families were often chosen to be the more the more beneficial placement. In 1978, this unprecedented removal of children from their families was halted by the Indian Child Welfare Act.

It is essential to develop an understanding of the group's cultural makeup, historical and contemporary, and have a sense of the problems that the group is facing. It is impossible to learn essential aspects of history or culture from a young child (Glover, 2001). The therapist needs to learn what is appropriate for a particular child within their culture and this knowledge can only be captured by personal research and high involvement with the adults in the child's life.

Working with Systems

Native Peoples frequently contend with issues that prevent them from receiving quality medical care. These issues include cultural barriers, geographic isolation, inadequate sewage disposal, and low income (National Congress of American Indians, 2020). In a plan for Native American Mental Health Services 1990, the Indian Health Service recognized that the incidence and prevalence of mental health problems and family disruption is high, in part because of the conflicts between traditional and Western practice.

Western helping methods split the person. We give physicians the body. Educators and psychologists, the mind. Social workers, the context and clergy, the spirit. Each looks at the same person and finds different problems and different solutions. Physicians medicate them away. Educators teach them away. Psychologists counsel them away. Social workers advocate them away and clergy pray them away. Each is unable to communicate effectively to the other what the problems are or what to do about them.

(Cross, 1997, p. 30)

Utilization of the professional healers of a Native community shows respect for their powerful knowledge about how to care for an illness of mind, body, or spirit. When this knowledge is not recognized there may be less confidence in any intervention that is attempted. For example, when a physical wound is treated in Western society, it is the wound that receives the treatment. A Native person might assume that the underlying cause of the wound was actually spiritual (Williams & Ellison, 1999). It is important to understand why the wound occurred. An event may have caused a change in body, mind, or spirit that resulted in disharmony significant enough to cause the wound. Tending to the physical aspect of the wound is only part of the treatment. If a Native person does not become invested in the intervention, it is unlikely to be of any help.

Weaver (1999) suggested that the practitioner learn to define both the problem and the solution from a Native perspective. There must be harmony between the treatment and the person being treated. In the case of children, the family must be supportive as well. For example, a child was assessed by a therapist as depressed and in need of medication (Glover, 2001). The educational system supported this plan and advised the family that either the child must be placed on medication, or he should not return to school. The family felt that certain ceremonies needed to be done; however, the grandfather was ill and could not participate at that time. In order to appease the professional, the family accepted the medication compliance requirement, but later chose not to give the medication to the child. Agreeing with authority figures initially, but then not following through with recommendations is not an unusual response for those who feel their objections will be ignored.

A Navajo (Diné) therapist who has worked with many Navajo families cautions that even Native practitioners must always be aware of differences even within an individual tribe (Glover, 2001). Native adults and children are not accustomed to sharing their feelings verbally. The therapist honored this belief and used other forms of expression such as drawing and clay as an avenue for exploring emotional issues. This approach appeared to be more acceptable and useful to the clients.

Researchers have long struggled with conducting rigorous studies with Native Peoples. Tribal governments block studies to protect the privacy of their members. Native Peoples have been naturally resistant to participating in projects conducted by researchers from outside the Native community (Warne et al., 2017). The approaches to increasing participation with research yield helpful insights for working with Native community systems in general. Tribal councils and other key stakeholders take seriously their responsibility to protect the best interests of their community members. They have a great deal of power within the community and want to know about any intervention programs that may be introduced. A collaborative approach will ensure transparency and any program introduced can be modified as needed with input from these experts.

Successful relationships require a long-term process and commitment (Warne et al., 2017). This can be achieved in part through including para-professionals from the community as co-leaders of groups and psychoeducational interventionists. It is not uncommon for community members to lack the resources needed to travel to meetings and appointments, such as no childcare or transportation. A practitioner may need to go to their client or work with the community systems that are likely in place to reach members who need assistance. Therapists can make a practice of providing optional ways of communicating for Native parents and children that expands on the typical verbal style of Western-trained therapists (Hulen et al., 2019). Finally, it is important to be proactive in developing relationships with community members in addition to those who seek out services through unstructured community events.

Conclusion

Native Peoples have survived through significant hardship. They are a resilient group even as each nation has its own language and customs. If parents have lost their connection to traditional parenting, help them find their way back. Values are deeply rooted in a people and I believe that the traditional ways of raising children are more intuitive to Native parents than the parenting style of the dominant culture. It does take a village to raise a child. As a play therapist, you become a member of the village. You are not alone. Seek out the respected elders, acknowledge the strengths of the community, respect traditions, enjoy the humor, grieve the losses, celebrate life, and share your gifts.

Positionality Statement

Geri

My professional experience with Native Peoples is varied. I have practiced CPRT with families on the Flathead reservation in northern Montana as part of my doctoral research. I have worked with children from the Pueblos of New Mexico, displaced urban Natives from several different nations, and children and youth on the Alamo Navajo Reservation, a small community in central New Mexico isolated from the Big Navajo Reservation of western New Mexico and eastern Arizona. I am very aware that I am not an enrolled member of my father's nation. I am an outsider. I did not grow up on the reservation and my mother raised my siblings and I from a Norwegian farming family perspective. However, as noted throughout this chapter, the traumatic events that have impacted Native Peoples throughout history touched my family. I have experienced the consequences of poverty, alcoholism, and dysfunctional parenting. This gives me insight into the challenges many Native families face. Young children who participate in play therapy are not separate entities from their families. In order to work successfully with Native children, a play therapist must develop a partnership with the child's parents and family.

References

Axline, V. M. (1969). *Play therapy*. Ballantine Books.

Berry, K., Henderson A., & Martha, L. (2002). Envisioning the nexus between geography and ethnic and racial identity. In K. Berry & M. Henderson (Eds.), *Geographic identities of ethnic America: Race, space, and place* (pp. 1–14). University of Nevada Press.

BigFoot, D. S., & Funderburk, B. W. (2011). Honoring children, making relatives: The cultural translation of parent–child interaction therapy for American Indian and Alaska Native families. *Journal of Psychoactive Drugs*, 43(4), 309–318.

Blackhorse, A. (2019, November 20). Blackhorse: "Native American" or "American Indian"? 5 more Native voices respond. *Indian Country Today: Digital. Indigenous. News.* https://indiancountrytoday.com/archive/blackhorse-native-american-or-am erican-indian-5-more-native-voices-respond.

Brendtro, L. K., Brokenleg, M., & Van Bockern, S. (1990). *Reclaiming youth at risk? Our hope for the future*. National Education Service.

Burgess, B. J. (1980). Parenting in the Native American community. In M.D. Fantini & R. Cárdenas, *Parenting in a multicultural society* (pp. 63–73). Longman.

Centers for Disease Control and Prevention (2000). *Measuring Healthy Days*. CDC. www.cdc.gov/hrqol/pdfs/mhd.pdf.

Cross, T. L. (1997). The world view of American Indian families. In Child Welfare League of America (Ed.), *Culturally competent practice: A series from Children's Voice magazine* (pp. 23–31). CWLA Press.

Edmonds, R. D. (1995). Native Americans, new voices: American Indian history, 1895–1995. *The American Historical Review*, 100(3), 717–740.

Felitti, V. J., Anda, R. F., Nordenberg, D., Williamson, D. F., Spitz, A.M., Edwards, V., Koss, M. P., & Marks, J. S. (1998). Relationship of childhood abuse and household dysfunction to many of the leading causes of death in adults: The adverse childhood experiences (ACE) study. *American Journal of Preventive Medicine*, 14(4), 245–258. doi:10.1016/S0749-3797(98)00017–00018.

First Nations Development Institute (2017). Research note – Twice invisible: Understanding rural Native America. First Nations Development Institute. www.usetinc.org/wp-content/uploads/bvenuti/WWS/2017/May%202017/May%208/Twice%20Invisible%20-%20Research%20Note.pdf.

García, F., & Gracia, E. (2009). Is always authoritative the optimum parenting style? Evidence from Spanish families. *Adolescence*, 44(173), 101–131.

Garrett, M. T., Parrish, M., Williams, C., Grayshield, L., Portman, T.A.A., Rivera, E.T., & Maynard, E. (2014). Invited commentary: Fostering resilience among

Native American youth through therapeutic intervention. *Journal of Youth and Adolescence*, 43(3), 470–490. doi:10.1007/s10964-013-0020-8.

George, L. J. (1997). Why the need for the Indian Child Welfare Act? In G. R. Anderson, A. Shea Ryan, & B. R. Leashore (Eds.), *The challenge of permanency planning in a multi-cultural society* (pp. 165–175). Haworth Press.

Gfellner, B. M. (1990). Culture and consistency in ideal and actual child-reading practices: A study of Canadian Indian and white parents. *Journal of Comparative Family Studies*, 21(3), 413–423.

Glover, G. (2001). Parenting in Native American Families. In N. Boyd Webb (Ed.), *Culturally diverse parent-child and family relationships: A guide for Social Workers and other practitioners* (pp. 205–234). Columbia University Press.

Glover, G. (2005). Musings on working with Native American children in play therapy. In E. Gil & A. A. Drewes (Eds.), *Cultural Issues in play therapy* (pp. 168–179). Guilford Press.

Glover, G. (2010). Filial therapy with Native Americans on the Flathead Reservation. In J. N. Baggerly, D. C. Ray, & S. C. Bratton (Eds.), *Child-centered play therapy research: The evidence base for effective practice* (pp. 311–321). Wiley.

Guzman, G. (2020). *Household income by race and Hispanic origin: 2005–2009 and 2015–2019*. American Community Survey Briefs, ACSBR-007, U.S. Census Bureau, Washington, DC.

Harrison, A. O., Wilson, M. N., Pine, C. J., Chang, S. Q., & Buriel, R. (1990). Family ecologies of ethnic minority children. *Child Development*, 61, 347–362.

Hulen, E., Hardy, L. J., Teufel-Shone, N., Sanderson, P. R., Schwartz, A. L., & Begay, R. C. (2019). Community based participatory research (CBPR): A dynamic process of health care: Provider perceptions and American Indian patients' resilience. *Journal of Health Care for the Poor and Underserved* 30(1), 221–237.

Huyser, K. R., Angel, R. J., Beals, J., Cox, J. H., Hummer, R. A., Sakamoto, A., & Manson, S. M. (2018). Reservation lands as a protective social factor: An analysis of psychological distress among two American Indian tribes. *Socius: Sociological Research for a Dynamic World*, 4, 1–13. doi:10.1177/2378023118807022.

Indian Health Service. (2019, October). Indian health disparities. www.ihs.gov/newsroom/factsheets/disparities.

Institute for Health Metrics and Evaluation (IHME). (2016). U.S. health map. IHME, University of Washington. http://vizhub.healthdata.org/subnational/usa (Accessed 05/01/2021).

Kingsley, T. G., Pettit, K., Biess, J., Bertumen, K., Budde, A., Narducci, C. & Pindus, N. (2014). *Continuity and change: Demographic, socioeconomic, and housing conditions of American Indians and Alaska Natives*. HUD.

LaFromboise, T. D., & Low, K. G. (1998). American Indian children and adolescents. In J.T. Gibbs, L. N. Huang *et al.* (Eds.), *Children of color: Psychological interventions with culturally diverse youth* (pp. 112–142). Jossey-Bass.

Landreth, G. L. (2012). *Play therapy: The art of the relationship* (3rd ed.). Routledge.

Landreth, G. L., & Bratton, S. C. (2020). *Child parent relationship therapy: (CPRT): a 10-session filial therapy model* (2nd ed.) Routledge.

Marsh, J. (1976). *Indian culture series: Chinook* (H. Gilliland, Ed.). Montana Indian Publication Fund.

Martinez, K. J., & Valdez, D. M. (1992). Cultural consideration in play therapy with Hispanic children. In L. A. Vargas & J. D. Koss-Chioino (Eds.), *Working with culture: Psychotherapeutic interventions with ethnic minority children and adolescents* (pp. 85–102). Jossey-Bass.

Mesman, J., Van IJzendoorn, M. H., & Sagi-Schwartz, A. S. (2016). Cross-cultural patterns of attachment: Universal and contextual dimensions. In J. Cassidy & P. R. Shaver (Eds.), *Handbook of attachment: Theory, research and clinical applications* (pp. 852–877). Guilford Press.

Monahan, T. C. (1981). *An exploratory study of selected characteristics of parent committees associated with projects funded under Title IV, Public Law 92–318, The Indian Education Act, Part A*. Rutgers University.

National Congress of American Indians (2020). Tribal Nations and the United States: An introduction. www.ncai.org/tribalnations/introduction/Indian_Coun try_101_Updated_February_2019.pdf.

National Indian Child Abuse and Neglect Resource Center (1980). *Indian culture and its relationship to child abuse and neglect*. Revised (ERIC Document Reproduction Service No. ED 229 193).

National Museum of the American Indian (2018). *Do all Indians live in tipis? Questions & answers from the National Museum of the American Indian* (2nd ed.). NMAI and Smithsonian Books.

Norris, T., Vines, P. L., & Hoeffel, E. M. (2012). The American Indian and Alaska Native population: 2010. Report Number C2010BR-10. U.S. Census Bureau. www.census.gov/history/pdf/c2010br-10.pdf.

Northwest Indian Child Welfare Institute (1986). *Positive Indian parenting: Honoring our children by honoring our traditions*. Author.

Office of Minority Health (2021). Profile: American Indian/Alaska Native. U.S. Department of Health and Human Services. https://minorityhealth.hhs.gov/om h/browse.aspx?lvl=3&lvlid=62.

Pratt, R. H. (1973). The advantages of mingling Indians with Whites. In F. P. Prucha (Ed.), *Americanizing the American Indians: Writings by the "Friends of the Indian" 1880–1900* (pp. 260–271). Harvard University Press. [Reprinted from Official Report of the Nineteenth Annual Conference of Charities and Correction (1892), 46–59.]

Red Horse, J. G. (1980). Family structure and value orientation in American Indians. *Social Casework: The Journal of Contemporary Social Work*, 61(8), 462–467.

Reyhner, J. (1994). *American Indian/Alaska Native education*. Phi Delta Kappa Educational Foundation (ERIC Document Reproduction Service No. ED 369 585).

Rogers, C. R. (1951). *Client-centered therapy: Its current practice, implications and theory*. Houghton Mifflin.

Saleebey, D. (1997). *The strengths perspective in social work practice*. Longman.

Seattle Times (2016). Washington Indian tribes today: Culture protecting the environment and natural resources, enriching people, building communities. Retrieved from http://nie.seattletimes.com/wp-content/uploads/sites/12/2016/10/WIGA_10-16-16_8PageTab_final.pdf.

Sprott, J. E. (1994). One person's "spoiling" is another's freedom to become: Overcoming ethnocentric views about parental control. *Social Science Medicine*, 38 (8), 1111–1124.

Stiffman, A. R., Brown, E., Freedenthal, S., House, L., Ostmann, E., & Yu, M. A. (2007). American Indian youth: Personal, familial, and environmental strengths. *Journal of Child and Family Studies*, 16(3), 331–346. doi:10.1007/s10826-006-9089-y.

United Nations (2000). *Establishment of a permanent forum on Indigenous issues*. Economic and Social Council (ECOSOC) Resolution 2000/22, 45th plenary meeting (28 July 2000). www.un.org/esa/socdev/unpfii/documents/about-us/E-RES-2000-22.pdf.

United Nations (2007). United Nations Declaration on the Rights of Indigenous Peoples, 61/295, 107th plenary meeting (13 September 2007). www.un.org/development/desa/indigenouspeoples/wp-content/uploads/sites/19/2018/11/UNDRIP_E_web.pdf.

Warne, D., Dulacki, K., Spurlock, M., Meath, T., Davis, M. M., Wright, B., & McConnell, K. J. (2017). Adverse Childhood Experiences (ACE) among American Indians in South Dakota and associations with mental health conditions, alcohol use, and smoking. *Journal of Health Care for the Poor and Underserved*, 28(4), 1559–1577. doi:10.1353/hpu.2017.0133.

Weaver, H. N. (1999). Indigenous people and the social work profession: Defining culturally competent services. *Social Work*, 44(3), 217–225.

Weiser-Alexander, K. (2020). Native American proverbs and wisdom. *Legends of America: Exploring history, destinations, people, & legends of this great country since 2003*. www.legendsofamerica.com/na-proverbs.

Williams, E. E., & Ellison, F. (1999). Indigenous people and the social work profession: Defining culturally competent services. *Social Work*, 44(3), 217–225.

Zimmer, B. (2009). The biggest misnomer of all time? Image or text from the Visual Thesaurus (www.visualthesaurus.com), Copyright © 1998–2021. Thinkmap, Inc. All rights reserved.

8 Cultural Opportunities with African American Populations

LaKaavia Taylor and Krystal K. Turner

The societal portrait of the African American child is often one of inferiority, shame, and discouragement. However, these societal perceptions result in negative labels and pathologizing of African American children (The National Child Traumatic Stress Network, 2018). Instead, it is critical to view their lived experiences as being a Black child in America. If only assessing them externally, emotional and behavioral responses of Black children can be interpreted as threatening or acting out when the behavior is actually their attempt to survive and remain resilient in the presence of continued systemic oppression. In our combined experiences as play therapists who are Black, countless times we have commonly heard statements from African American children and parents such as, "I want my child to know they are smart and beautiful, despite social media messages," "I worry every day if my child will come home alive," "How do I prepare my child for a world that hates them because of their skin?" "I do not like my black skin," and "Will they shoot me too?" These statements evoke an immense sense of empathy as we have had and lived through similar experiences growing up. Furthermore, we know all too well the emotional internalization these statements cause. In our play therapist experiences, we are often confronted with the difficult task of armoring ourselves with the resilience we have developed from overcoming our racial challenges to help normalize the pain of our African American child clients. Therefore, we heavily rely on the therapeutic relationship to affirm our clients' existence in a world that views them as a threat to humanity. We strive to see the gift in their cultural strengths and assets. The relational connection becomes a sacred factor in helping African American children feel that their lives indeed matter.

Cultural Considerations

The State of the Black Child

It is impossible to begin the play therapy process with African American children and families without first examining the role of race, culture, and

DOI: 10.4324/9781003190073-11

socioeconomic factors in their lives. According to recent estimates by the U. S. Census Bureau (2019), 10 million African American children reside in the United States. Population trends indicate the growth of African Americans in the U.S. will continue to rise, reaching a significant increase in the next decade (Harris & Graham, 2014). Currently, African American children account for 14% of the child population. In the last 50 years, African Americans have made progressive strides, particularly in regard to education and wealth (Williams, 2016). However, it is essential to avoid equating progress and resilience with equality. African American children and families continue to face persistent disparities and inequalities educationally, economically, and socially. Specifically, African Americans are disproportionately impacted by poverty, food insecurity, and under-resourced schools (Belgrave & Allison, 2013). These disparities, coupled with historical and current racism, predispose African American children to higher risks for psychological impairments (Philippe, 2014).

Racism and Racial Discrimination

Being a Black child means constantly questioning your visibility and existence. Many African American children grapple with the daily trauma and stressors of racism in their social experiences. Saleem et al. (2016) found that Black children experience at least five racial discriminatory encounters a day. The effect of racism has a lifelong impact on physical and mental health (Trent et al., 2019). Specifically, racism leads to chronic stress and psychological impairment (Shattell & Brown, 2017). For example, Nyborg and Curry (2003) found that perceived experiences of racism in African American children is related to internalized problems such as feelings of inadequacy, somatic complaints, and low self-esteem. In my own experience (LaKaavia), at the young age of seven years old, I was called the "N" word for what I never realized would be one of numerous times. I experienced a rush of mixed emotions, including confusion, anger, and most of all, sadness. The experience was one of my earliest memories of questioning whether who I am and what I looked like was acceptable.

Racism does not just happen at the individual level for African American children but institutionally as well. The public school setting is the biggest culprit of alarming implicit biases and institutional racism (Brooks & Watson, 2019). In public schools across the U.S., the achievement gap is substantially large for African American children in comparison to other groups regarding testing and academic grades (Cokley, 2016; Weir, 2016). This gap is attributed to public schools failing to facilitate learning for African American children. Thus, it is not a competence issue, but the limitation is related to a cultural mismatch with the learning environment (Hale, 2016). For example, most school settings emphasize an analytical learning environment with a significant focus on logic and facts, whereas African Americans tend to have more expressive and harmonious learning styles

(Nieto, 2018). This discrepancy is evident in the overrepresentation of Black students in special education and underrepresentation in gifted and talented programs (Fish, 2017). These factors drastically interfere with academic achievement. As a result, Black children might experience a lack of confidence and powerlessness, feelings of rejection, or identity issues in school settings. To further complicate the academic experiences are suspension and expulsion rates beginning as early as preschool (Gilliam et al., 2016). In the U.S., public school suspensions and expulsion rates are highest for African American children in all 50 states (Teasley et al., 2017). African American children engage in misbehavior at the same rate as other groups but are three times more likely to receive suspension or expulsion (Haight et al., 2016). This racial disparity is a social justice issue considering repeated suspensions are correlated with academic difficulties, early dropout rates, and entry into the criminal justice system (Noltemeyer et al., 2015).

Barriers to Mental Health

African Americans have different perspectives and values about mental health. Mental health challenges in the Black community are viewed as medical, spiritual, or familial, leading to the underutilization of mental healthcare (Belgrave & Allison, 2013). African American parents tend to believe emotional and behavior problems of children are attributed to character flaws, poor parenting, or discipline practices rather than psychological distress. Furthermore, there is still a historical legacy of distrust between the healthcare system and Black populations (Santiago & Miranda, 2014). When treatment is available, it is often inaccessible and incongruent with the cultural values of African Americans. As a result, mental health treatment is frequently sought after problems become severe. We can see this reflected in the overutilization of pediatrics emergency department visits for severe mental health concerns for African American children. Using a five-year institutional study, Abrams et al. (2020) found that in comparison to other groups, African American children had increasingly higher use of emergency departments to address mental health challenges. The results show the critical need to provide early intervention for the problems and concerns of African American children.

Play Therapy Considerations with African American Children

Therapeutic Relationship

Due to the treatment and status of African American children, they are prone to fear and distrust systems in which they interact. Furthermore, African American children could be racially socialized to mistrust others outside of their racial group (Saleem et al., 2016). Therefore, African American children are likely to have a guarded stance for self-protection due to feelings of betrayal and hurt by the devaluing of their culture. These factors convey the importance of building meaningful and trusting relationships with Black children to facilitate credibility and psychological safety. Significant individuals providing services for African American children must "first build relationships that reflect genuine honor, trust, and respect" (Rashid, 2013, p. 35). This suggests a need for relational-based interventions for African American children. In play therapy, the child-therapist relationship is the most fundamental factor of change (Ray, 2011). Specifically, full acceptance of the child and their world is the cornerstone of the child-therapist relationship. When the therapeutic relationship is emphasized in play therapy, not only is the therapist helping Black children, but they are dismantling dehumanization commonly experienced in oppressive environments outside of the playroom. Thus, play therapists from racially similar and dissimilar ethnic groups should ensure their verbal and nonverbal communication conveys safety and acceptance, such as communicating warmth and care through vocal tone, body language, and facial expressions. The play therapist should be careful not to rush the relationship-building process as African American children might be reminded of their own experiences that make them more skeptical of therapeutic relationships with individuals outside of their family systems. Therefore, genuine acceptance and clear communication enhance credibility, trust, and the overall therapeutic relationship.

Enhancing Self-Esteem

Play therapy can help children develop a positive self-concept and become self-accepting, integral to self-esteem development (Ray, 2011). Thus, play therapists have the unique opportunity to help African American children buffer the self-defeating impact of racism and microaggressions through esteem-building. Researchers indicate that negative racial messages can lower self-esteem (Constantine & Blackmon, 2002; Harris-Britt et al., 2007). When African American children have low self-esteem, it prevents them from effectively managing their emotional and behavioral responses to racial and cultural challenges and experiences (American Psychological Association, 2008). Therefore, the more therapeutic opportunities African American children are given in play therapy to feel secure and confident with themselves, the more positively they will feel about confronting tasks, addressing challenges, and overcoming failure. Consider an eight-year-old African American boy presenting with low self-worth due to being left out by racially dissimilar peers at school. In play therapy, the child can be affirmed through esteem-building responses, encouragement, and returning responsibility through play (Landreth, 2012). These experiences would give the child renewed opportunities to feel positive about self-structure and capabilities despite negative messages internalized or received outside of the playroom. The power of play therapy for African American children is that low self-esteem can be mediated through playing away pain from the lack of understanding and rejection they often experience in social contexts.

Facilitation of Racial Identity Development

Racial identity encompasses the attitudes, perceptions, and beliefs that an individual holds about their racial group (Mann & Randolph, 2011). Play therapy lends itself to meet the racial identity needs of African American children because it is through play that children can learn about themselves and engage in self-expression (Bennett & Eberts, 2014). African American children are often grappling with the questions: Who am I? How do I relate to my race and culture? Do I belong? How can I respond when people treat me negatively because I am Black? Facilitating racial identity development allows African American children to engage in daily life experiences without feeling powerless or resentful about racism and discrimination (APA, 2008). Play therapists have the opportunity to help African American children flesh out stereotypes and negative self-perceptions to develop a healthy evaluation of their identity. Specifically, it is through the play therapist understanding the child's unique world communicated through the relationship, empathic responding, and reflections of feelings that African American children can address and reveal feelings about their level of racial and connection. Furthermore, reflecting on themes and meaning about the African American child's identity and self-awareness is critical. Through the African American child's play, they can develop new solutions and perspectives that support appreciation of their racial identity. This is critical considering positive racial identity mitigates the social-emotional effects of being exposed to negative images, discourse, and stereotypes that devalue Blackness and Black identity (Rowley et al., 2008; Shin, 2011).

Cultural Opportunities

Broaching

It is not abnormal that there will be concerns on behalf of the play therapist and the Black family regarding a potential negative racial encounter. Despite fears, addressing race is the core of a healthy and therapeutic relationship. Thus, broaching is the first cultural opportunity. Day-Vines et al. (2007) defined broaching as the invitation for client exploration of race and infusing racial considerations throughout the therapeutic process. Considering the possible racially charged experiences of African American children and families, it is essential that they feel comfortable to share their experiences with the play therapist verbally and nonverbally. This can be especially difficult to do with a racially dissimilar therapist. The African American child and parent need early indicators that this will be accepted and do not need to hold back a piece of their identity. Not only should the parent hear from the therapist that there are cultural and racial differences in the therapist-child relationship, but the child as well. For example, expressing to the child, "There are some differences between me and you [providing examples, e.g. pointing to your skin and hair]. I do not know everything about who you are. When you play with the toys in here, you will help me understand your world and who you are." Although verbal broaching is commonly discussed in the literature, little focus is given to nonverbal broaching. For example, consider the following questions related to nonverbal broaching: (1) Is your staff diverse? (2) Is there diverse artwork in your office or on your website? (3) Do you have any connections to Black-owned businesses or organizations? (4) Are there books that represent Black culture included in your space or recommended to parents? (5) Are race and cultural-related questions on your paperwork? Culture and diversity should be authentically and intentionally embedded in your practices in a way that Black families can receive. Black children and families alike need safety and security in the play therapy process.

Black Racial Identity

According to the Association for Play Therapy (APT) Play Therapy Best Practices (II.3, 2020), "play therapists make every effort to support and respect the culture and cultural identity of clients and their families." The biggest cultural opportunity will come when Black children engage verbally or nonverbally about their racial identification, specifically around physical attributes and experiences of racism. These factors tend to be the most emotionally provoking for the Black child and the play therapist. Racial identity exploration provides play therapists with an understanding of an African American child's view of self and navigation in the world (Gaskin 2015; Harris & Graham, 2014). Through play, the play therapist should assess the child's overt and covert play and verbalizations for rejection of culture, confusion about identity, devaluing of self-expression, and dissatisfaction with physical characteristics (hair texture, skin color, and appearance).

As early as three years of age, children can identify individuals based on physical characteristics (Branch, 1999). Furthermore, during this development period, children begin to show signs of societal messages affecting how they feel about racial identity. Therefore, the child may make comments or engage in play behaviors that reflect stereotypical or negative racial attitudes about being African American. These views might manifest in interpersonal difficulties. For example, imagine eight-year-old Kyla saying, "I wish my skin color were like the other kids in my class. I do not want it to be black." The best way to address this would be to engage in reflections that allow the client to fully explore their feelings, such as "You want me to know that you wish you were not Black" or "You believe things would be better if you were not Black." It is essential to communicate empathy when reflecting rather than rescue the child from their emotions and thoughts. How a play therapist responds will determine how much the child continues in play or verbalization and their future sharing. African American children also need opportunities to process and explore positive feelings about their identity. When they express positive feelings or thoughts, it is essential to affirm and encourage them, such as "You feel proud about being Black" or "You like yourself just the way that you are." These examples also convey the importance of having diverse toys and materials. Diverse dolls, puppets, and figures should be used to help Black children process racial identity, develop a positive self-image, and form a well-rounded view of the world. Society often devalues darker skin colors and natural hair textures. Therefore dolls, puppets, and figures should reflect the Black culture, which will affirm that they belong and are significant. Furthermore, the addition of various toys from other racial backgrounds helps normalize and build empathy for cultural/racial differences. The available dolls and figures must have variations in skin tone, body size, and textures. Furthermore, providing parents with resources for racial exploration outside of therapy such as Black children's books, organizations, and cultural events can be helpful.

Due to current events related to Black/African Americans in society, African American children might show preoccupations with racially charged and sociopolitical events (Gaskin, 2015). The preoccupation is an African American child's attempt to make sense of experiences happening to people who look racially similar. Therefore, validation of their emotions and thoughts is very healing in play therapy. It provides a therapeutic avenue to engage in the self-regulation of emotions and behaviors. I (LaKaavia) recall a second-grade African American boy walking into the playroom after the 2014 national publicized shooting of Mike Brown. The child walked into the playroom and looked at the gun on the shelf. The child looked back at me and gasped. He said, "I cannot play with this," and proceeded to bury the gun in the sandbox. He then moved on to other play activities. A few times through his play, he would go back into the sandbox to recover the gun and play with it briefly and bury it again. He did this about three times in the playroom. The child did not engage with the gun until about three sessions later. When he finally played with the gun again, he pretended to be a police officer keeping robbers from stealing from the store. The way I interpreted it was the child trying to grapple with the idea that the gun can be used to protect and hurt. Black children could use aggressive toys such as non-realistic guns and handcuffs to help them understand and process events related to social injustices of African Americans. However, it should be noted that Black parents might show concerns and worries about their child showing interest in toy guns in that they could be perceived as a threat if playing with one outside of the playroom. In these cases, it would be necessary first to normalize the feelings of parents concerning aggressive items. Furthermore, thoroughly provide a rationale explaining the purpose of having them in the playroom.

In working with African American children, confusion around racial background and features will likely manifest in the playroom. This is one of the biggest cultural opportunities because the target of distress for many African American children is physical attributes, specifically their natural hair. Natural hairstyles for African American children and adults are not always accepted. For African American children, their natural hair can be the basis to how others treat and view them and how they feel about themselves. Black children may need opportunities to play with their own hair or hair of dolls to process their feelings of physical acceptance. In our many experiences working with African American children, there is often mention or a play theme around natural hair for children, specifically for African American girls.

Religion and the African American Community

Traditionally, African American families have looked to religion to serve as a focal point for connection and guidance (Frame & Williams, 1996). The church has become integrated into the African American community and serves as a base where members of the congregation often consider religion when making life choices (Plunkett, 2014). While many African Americans seek guidance from community members, elders, and church leaders, the church may not always provide counseling and therapeutic resources. This extends to families seeking guidance for child rearing. In a phenomen-ological study addressing African American parents' perceptions of play therapy, one participant was quoted saying, "We don't need that, we pray to God and you talk to your pastor or your grandparents or something like that, but you don't need a counselor" (Brumfield & Christensen, 2011, p. 217). This quote provides an illustration of the traditional outlook on the importance and reliance on religious practices over therapeutic services.

Frame and Williams (1996) also suggest that elders within African American communities reinforce the importance of obtaining fulfillment through church which may deem therapeutic services as unnecessary. Furthermore, traditional psychological practices have presented as more secular in nature and are not readily delivered in a way that caters to spiritual and religious clients (see e.g. Plunkett, 2014; Frame & Williams, 1996). These practices in psychotherapy may be limiting for the African American community that places a high premium on religious beliefs. Plunkett (2014) discusses how, over recent years, African American churches have begun to collaborate with outside therapeutic services to better serve its congregation. As the push for psychotherapy to be more multiculturally inclined grows, therapists are attempting to find ways to understand and integrate the importance of religion for the African American community (Plunkett, 2014). As it stands, there is limited research on spirituality and religion in conjunction with play therapy; however, this does not suggest that play therapists ignore the use of spirituality for the African American population. It may suggest that religion in play therapy is a nuanced concept. Having a strong understanding of the child's culture and traditional family values will help illuminate the importance of religious practices for the client. The play therapist that is culturally empathetic can show their respect to the family's religiosity by discussing with the caregivers how their family's religious beliefs may impact the child's behavior. Parent consultation and family involvement serves as a crucial portal into the child's world which can include their religion.

Working with Families

My (Krystal) first experience working with Black families in play therapy began with a single mother, Deanna, and her ten-year-old son, Isaiah whom I was seeing for play therapy. I experienced Isaiah as composed, trusting, and cooperative; however, his teacher described him to me as an angry child, one who often did not work well with others, was disrespectful, and lacked self-control. This opposing description of Isaiah encouraged me to get in contact with his family as soon as possible to get a better understanding of his world. Given that I identify as Black, I was confused about my anxiety for my first consultation with a Black parent. Though Isaiah's mother was open and receptive to me, I now understand my anxiety stemmed from messages I was receiving that Black parents were not invested in therapeutic services.

Deanna shared with me that, as a Black single mother, she wanted to instill in her son the values that she had to adopt in order to persevere in America. She wanted her son to be confident, in control of his emotions and behaviors, and independent. I explained to Deanna that her desires for her son aligned well with the values of the humanistic play therapy intervention I would be providing. By the end of our conversation, Deanna understood that the objectives of child-centered play therapy were to "facilitate the child's efforts to become more adequate as a person, in coping with current and future problems that may affect his life" (Landreth, 2012, p. 84). She shared that she felt validated that she had strong wishes for her son and felt enthused that I shared a lot of her same values and hopes for Isaiah. After our initial meeting, Deanna consulted with me regularly to swap updates. Working as a team with his mother while allowing Isaiah to lead his experiences in the playroom made for a beneficial experience, one where his mother and I were on the same page about attuning to his needs. My interaction with Deanna and Isaiah encouraged my desire to further look into Black parental buy-in as it relates to play therapy.

To date, little research has been conducted on Black children in play therapy, consulting with Black families during the play therapy process, and Black families in play therapy-related interventions such as Filial therapy, an intervention that focuses on the parent–child relationship (Landreth & Bratton, 2020). Despite the lack of relevant literature, humanistic play therapy and play therapy-based interventions seemingly align well with common Black family values and parenting traditions. To understand how the objectives of humanistic play therapy pairs with traditional Black family values, an exploration of these customs is warranted.

Traditional Black Family Values

Glover (2001) asserts that African Americans place a high premium on family and racial identity, and that "no person succeeds for self alone, but for family and race" (p. 34). With an established history of oppression in America, a need to remain family centric and to be aware of one's racial identity helps to ensure safety and security. Furthermore, Glover posits that in the face of adversity, oppression, stereotypes, and negative images, Black families prize perseverance and a strong sense of self-esteem. Parenting styles of Black parents have been described as strong or harsh with the rationale including Black parents' desires for their children to be respectful and behave in socially appropriate manner (Solis et al., 2004). In their collectivistic nature, African American families often use extended family members and their community to help ensure their children are maintaining traditions. Landreth and Bratton (2020) describe experiences where extended and non-traditional family members, such as Godparents or grandparents, were included in therapeutic services for the benefit of the child.

It would behoove the play therapist that works with Black families to be aware of these values and approach consultation with these concepts in mind. However, the culturally sensitive therapist may also be aware that while these values are traditional in the African American community, they do not describe the experiences of all Black families. An interview or intake with the parent can provide background information pertinent to the individual child's world (Landreth, 2012) which would eliminate any false assumptions or preconceived notions about the child or child's family that may be damaging to the relationship.

Involving Parents in the Process

When caregivers feel heard, validated, and emotionally connected with the therapist, a partnership can be formed which can elicit positive reactions to the therapeutic experience (Cates et al., 2006). The intake procedure, or initial interview, can serve as an opportunity for the therapist to broach with the caregiver so as to learn about the family's cultural values and additional background information (Landreth, 2012). The therapist may also use the intake session to begin fostering a relationship with the caregiver wherein discussions on how the objectives of play therapy can align with family values. Explaining to the caregiver the purpose of play therapy is a crucial step towards facilitating cooperation from the family (Cates et al., 2006). As Landreth (2012) explains, caregiver cooperation is vital given that it is ultimately the parent's decision if the child will return. Buy-in from parents can pose additional challenges when working with Black families. Traditionally, therapeutic services have been stigmatized in the African American community (Smith, 1977), and many services that have been accepted are more directive in nature, such as cognitive behavioral therapy or trauma focused cognitive behavioral therapy. The non-directive, child-centered approach of many humanistic play therapy modalities, such as child-centered play therapy (CCPT), may feel foreign or not direct and concrete enough for Black caregivers.

For those parents that may feel skeptical, desire a bit more control in their child's therapy, or struggle to trust the process, a culturally sensitive explanation of play therapy can be beneficial in helping the parent feel more at ease with the therapeutic approach. In CCPT (Landreth, 2012), broad therapeutic objectives are emphasized over goal setting for each child. These objectives fit with Landreth's (2012) and Glover's (2001) assertion that CCPT is ideal for multicultural relationships. CCPT's objectives include helping the child accept self, become more autonomous, and experience control and self-regulation. These objectives coincide with African American traditional values for child rearing such as a desire for their child to develop a sense of independence, strong self-esteem, and socially acceptable behaviors. While CCPT may not encompass all the needs Black families exhibit, the emphasis on following the child and accepting them as they are, which in turn means accepting their cultural background (Landreth, 2012), may appeal to a great number of Black families that prize cultural connection.

It may be to the benefit of the relationship with the therapist and parent if the play therapist shares with the parent how they intend to communicate with the parent (Cates et al., 2006). Cates asserts that involving parents in the therapeutic process as much as possible but within limits can maximize the benefits of play therapy. It is not uncommon for African American caregivers to want to ensure their children are behaving correctly (Glover, 2001), so inquiring about their behavior in the playroom may feel like a natural inclination. An in-depth rationale on maintaining confidentiality, and consulting with parents on a regular basis allows parents to feel empowered in the relational triad while also respecting the relationship between therapist and child.

Working with Systems

Research has shown the positive effects of CCPT objectives when used on a systemic level such as Child-Parent Relationship Therapy (CPRT)/Filial Therapy (FT) and Child-Teacher Relationship Therapy (CTRT; Landreth & Bratton, 2020) within schools (see e.g. Post et al., 2020; Helker & Ray, 2009; Gonzales-Ball & Bratton, 2019) and play therapy within residential care facilities (Donald & Ceballos, 2020). CPRT/FT highlights the parent-child relationship as the most significant relationship in a child's life and engages parents in building relationships with their children through home play sessions (Landreth & Bratton, 2020). With an emphasis on familial systemic change, CPRT may appeal to African American caregivers' values of strong sense of family connection (Solis et al., 2004).

CTRT is an adaptation of the filial model where teachers are trained in CCPT principles to help them build relationship skills with their students which may reduce behavioral problems in the classroom (Post et al., 2020). As previously mentioned, Black children consistently struggle with social engagement, academic achievement, and age-appropriate behavior (Taylor & Ray, 2021) which tends to lead to removal from the classroom as punishment. Interventions that can reduce the amount of time spent outside of the classroom may have an ameliorating effect on Black children's social-emotional engagement. CTRT can serve as such an intervention.

Conclusion

African children are smart, resilient, and possess many cultural strengths. Often when attempting to navigate typical developmental challenges, they must also process the personal impact of their racial experiences as being Black. For some African American children, the lived experiences of being Black can lead to psychological distress. If untreated, the distress can manifest into problems related to anxiety, depression, and psychosomatic complaints. Play therapists have the unique opportunity to walk alongside Black children on their journey to healthy self-identity and expression. However, play therapy is not always the first intervention African American caregivers seek. Traditionally, African American families have strong cultural values that may necessitate adaptations to standard forms of therapeutic services, such as play therapy. Conditioning born from a history of oppression, such as reliance on religion and community elders as the therapeutic agent, may prevent Black families from readily seeking individual or systemic therapeutic services for their youth. A clear explanation of the tenets of humanistic play therapy interventions and how the tenets emphasize encouraging autonomy, confidence, and emotional regulation for children may help Black parents feel seen and understood on their desires for their child's growth in America.

Positionality Statements

Krystal

Foremost, it is of utmost importance for me to state that while I identify as Black and therefore clearly have experienced life as a Black child, I in no way identify as an expert on the Black child experience. My experiences are unique to me and in no way speaks for any others who may share my singular identities or intersectional experiences. During my journey to establish myself as a multiculturally focused mental health professional, I quickly became frustrated with systemic failures to address cultural considerations. This is what led me to focus on addressing Black issues to do my part in enacting change.

I grew up in a Jamaican-American home and then was adopted into an American home in my late teens. While the two nationalities have stark differences in culture, one concept that remains consistent in both cultural customs is a preoccupation with giving 200% in school, work, and my outward appearance at all times. There is a frequently spoken rule in the Black community that we have to always give 1,000% in all things just to be considered in the same league as our White counterparts. In my experience with working with the Black community, I have found similarities in the way parents have tried to convey this message to their children. For example, Kim was a five-year old Black girl client of mine. Kim's perfectly coiffed hair and seemingly perfect outward presentation made it clear that her mother took great pride in Kim's appearance and was adamant that Kim do the same. At age five, Kim struggled with her mom's need for her to be perfect. Each session she would contemplate putting sand in her hair but would change her mind at the last minute. Our sessions always ended with Kim sweeping every single toy off the shelves in an attempt to destroy the playroom. My ability to empathize with Kim as a play therapist stems not just from our shared complexion and experiences of being Black in America, but also from my ability to take a step back and consider her mom's perspective and the cultural climate.

I do not in any way pretend to fully understand all cultures, even those with which I identify, but my path through multicultural exploration has brought me through a priceless journey of empathy, understanding, and acceptance. In the time and space we as a nation hold today where cultural persecution seems to be the norm, encouraging cultural humility and appreciation, in my opinion, seems like a great first step towards basic civil rights for all. As I watch the children close to me grow, whether in my personal life, or a clinical setting, I hope for all of them that they come across multiple people in their lives that value the basic tenets of child-centered play therapy wherein unconditional positive regard, warmth, and empathy are conveyed to them consistently and without reservation.

LaKaavia

As a Black woman, my passion and advocacy with African American children stem from my current and past lived experiences, community activism, and journey as a play therapist. I consider myself a competent play therapist with Black children not solely because I am African American but because I have been intentional about integrating what I have learned in real-world experiences outside of the playroom. I recommend play therapists to become familiar with the issues and presenting concerns of the Black community. Specifically, play therapists are encouraged to support, create, and build positive connections with relevant stakeholders and community leaders.

Considering the experiences Black/African children will face across their lifetime, I consider it an honor and privilege to work with this population. It has become my life's purpose to be a voice for Black/African American children in play therapy.

Black/African American children are resilient and possess many strengths; however, it does not minimize the dehumanization and invisibility they might encounter. Personally, my saving grace and buffer to the racism and racial microaggressions I experienced was the promotion of Black pride and appreciation in my family. I strongly believe if it weren't for those messages of racial pride and high self-value growing up to counter what I heard from societal messages, I would not be the Black play therapist I am today. Although I recognize this is my unique experience, at some point in a Black child's life, they will encounter one or more emotionally charged race-related experiences. This speaks volumes for the need of early play therapy interventions and therapeutic opportunities to feel valued, affirmed, and prized. The nature of play therapy allows for the development of adaptive coping and self-regulation to address race-related struggles children African American children will face.

References

Abrams, A. H., Badolato, G. M., Boyle, M. D., McCarter, R., & Goyal, M. K. (2020). Racial and ethnic disparities in pediatric mental health-related emergency department visits. *Pediatric emergency care*. Advance online publication. doi:10.1097/PEC.0000000000002221.

American Psychological Association (APA) Task Force on Resilience and Strength in Black Children and Adolescents (2008). Resilience in African American children and adolescents: A vision for optimal development. www.apa.org/pi/families/resources/resiliencerpt.pdf.

Annie E. Casey Foundation (2018). Kids of color more likely to live in high-poverty neighborhoods now than during great recession. www.aecf.org/blog/kids-of-color-more-likely-tolive-in-high-poverty-neighborhoods-now.

Association for Play Therapy (2020). Play Therapy Best Practices. Retrieved January 7, 2021, from https://cdn.ymaws.com/www.a4pt.org/resource/resmgr/publications/apt_best_practices_-_june_20.pdf.

Belgrave, F. Z. & Allison, K. W. (2013). *African American psychology: From Africa to America* (3rd ed.). Sage Publications.

Bennett, M. & Eberts, S. (2014). Self-expression. In C. E. Schaefer & A. A. Drewes (Eds), *The therapeutic powers of play: 20 core agents of change* (2nd ed., pp. 11–25). Wiley.

Branch, C. (1999). Race and human development. In R. H. Sheets & E. R. Hollins (Eds.), *Racial and ethnic identity in school practices: Aspects of human development* (pp. 7–28). Taylor & Francis.

Brooks, J. S., & Watson, T. N. (2019). School leadership and racism: an ecological perspective. *Urban Education*, 54(5), 631–655. doi:10.1177/0042085918783821.

Brumfield, K. A., & Christensen, T. M. (2011). Discovering African American parents' perceptions of play therapy: A phenomenological approach. *International Journal of Play Therapy*, 20(4), 208–223. doi:10.1037/a0025748.

Cates, J., Paone, T. R., Packman, J., & Margolis, D. (2006). Effective parent consultation in play therapy. *International Journal of Play Therapy*, 15(1), 87–100. doi:10.1037/h0088909.

Cokley, Kevin (2016). What it means to be black in the American educational system. *The Conversation*. https://theconversation.com/what-it-means-to-be-black-in-the-american-educational-system-63576.

Constantine, M. & Blackmon, S. M. (2002). Black adolescents' racial socialization experiences: Their relations to home, school, and peer self-esteem. *Journal of Black Studies*, 32(3), 325–335.

Day-Vines, N. L., Wood, S. M., Grothaus, T., Craigen, L., Holman, A., Dotson-Blake, K., & Douglass, M. J. (2007). Broaching the subjects of race, ethnicity, and culture during the counseling process. *Journal of Counseling & Development*, 85(4), 401–409. doi:10.1002/j.1556-6678.2007.tb00608.x.

Donald, E. J., & Ceballos, P. (2020). Child-parent relationship therapy with residential care workers. *International Journal of Play Therapy*, 29(3), 163–176. doi:10.1037/pla0000121.

Fish, R. E. (2017). The racialized construction of exceptionality: Experimental evidence of race/ethnicity effects on teachers' interventions. *Social Science Research*, 62, 317–334. doi:10.1016/j.ssresearch.2016.08.007.

Frame, M. W., & Williams, C. B. (1996). Counseling African Americans: integrating spirituality in therapy. *Counseling and Values*, 41(1), 16–28. doi:10.1002/j.2161-007x.1996.tb00859.x.

Gaskin, A. (2015, August). Racial socialization: Ways parents can teach their children about race. *Children, Youth, & Families Newsletter*. www.apa.org/pi/families/resources/newsletter/2015/08/racial-socialization.

Gilliam, W. S., Maupin, A. N., Reyes, C. R., Accavitti, M. & Shic, F. (2016). Do early educators' implicit biases regarding sex and race relate to behavior expectations and recommendations of preschool expulsions and suspensions? Yale University Child Study Center, https://medicine.yale.edu/childstudy/zigler/publications/Preschool%20Implicit%20Bias%20Policy%20Brief_final_9_26_276766_5379_v1.pdf.

Glover, G. J. (2001). Cultural considerations in play therapy. In G. L. Landreth (Ed.), *Innovations in play therapy* (pp. 31–41). Taylor & Francis.

Gonzales-Ball, T., & Bratton, S. (2019). Child-teacher relationship training as a head start early mental health intervention for children exhibiting disruptive behavior. *International Journal of Play Therapy*, 28(1), 44–56. doi:10.1037/pla0000081.

Haight, W., Kayama, M., & Gibson, P. A. (2016). Out-of-school suspensions of Black youths: Culture, ability, disability, gender, and perspective. *Social Work*, 61 (3), 235–243. doi:10.1093/sw/sww021.

Hale, J. E. (2016). Learning styles of African American children: instructional implications. *Journal of Curriculum and Teaching*, 5(2). doi:10.5430/jct.v5n2p109.

Harris-Britt, A., Valrie, C. R., Kurtz-Costes, B., & Rowley, S. J. (2007). Perceived racial discrimination and self-Esteem in African American youth: Racial socialization as a protective factor. *Journal of Research on Adolescence: The Official Journal of the Society for Research on Adolescence*, 17(4), 669–682. doi:10.1111/j.1532-7795.2007.00540.x.

Harris, Y. & Graham, J. (2014). *The African American child, Development and challenges* (2nd ed.). Springer Publishing.

Helker, W., & Ray, D. (2009). Impact of child teacher relationship training on teachers' and aides' use of relationship-building skills and the effects on student classroom behavior. *International Journal of Play Therapy*, 18(2), 70–83. doi:10.1037/a0014456.

Henderson, H., & Bourgeois, J. W. (2021, February 23). Penalizing Black hair in the name of academic success is undeniably racist, unfounded, and against the law. Brookings. www.brookings.edu/blog/how-we-rise/2021/02/23/penalizing-black-hair-in-the-name-of-academic-success-is-undeniably-racist-unfounded-and-against-the-law.

Landreth, G. L. (2012). *Play therapy: The art of the relationship*. Routledge.

Landreth, G. L., & Bratton, S. C. (2020). *Child parent relationship therapy: (CPRT): a 10-session filial therapy model* (2nd ed.). Routledge.

Mann, T. & Randolph, S. (2011). The historical relationship between black identity and black achievement motivation. In N. E. Hill, T. L. Mann, & H. E. Fitzgerald (Eds.), *African American child mental health* (pp.1–31). Prager.

Morin, A. (2020, October 26). Exploring the mental health stigma in black communities. *Verywell Mind*. https://www.verywellmind.com/exploring-the-mental-health-stigma-in-black-communities-5078964.

The National Child Traumatic Stress Network (2018, April 11). Complex trauma: In urban African-American children, youth, and families. https://www.nctsn.org/resources/complex-trauma-urban-african-american-children-youth-and-families.

Nieto, S. (2018). *Language, culture, and teaching critical perspectives*. Routledge.

Noltemeyer, A. L., Ward, R. M., & Mcloughlin, C. (2015). Relationship between school suspension and student outcomes: A meta-analysis. *School Psychology Review*, 44(2), 224–240. doi:10.17105/spr-14-0008.1.

Nyborg, V.M., & Curry, J.F. (2003) The impact of perceived racism: Psychological symptoms among African American boys, *Journal of Clinical Child and Adolescent Psychology*, 32(2), 258–266. doi:10.1207/S15374424JCCP3202_11.

Philippe, C. D. (2014). How might racism impact African American children's thoughts and plans for the future?, *Journal of Adolescent Health*, 54(2). doi:10.1016/j.jadohealth.2013.10.144.

Plunkett, D. P. (2014). The Black church, values, and secular counseling: implications for counselor education and practice. *Counseling and Values*, 59(2), 208–221. doi:10.1002/j.2161-007x.2014.00052.x.

Post, P., Grybush, A., Elmadani, A., & Lockhart, C. (2020). Fostering resilience in classrooms through child-teacher relationship training. *International Journal of Play Therapy*, 29(1), 9–19. doi:10.1037/pla0000107.

Post, P., Grybush, A., Flowers, C., & Elmadani, A. (2020). Impact of child-teacher relationship training on teacher attitudes and classroom behaviors. *International Journal of Play Therapy*, 29(3), 119–130. doi:10.1037/pla0000118.

Rashid, H. M. (2013). Significant – but not sufficient: Quality early childhood education and the development of young African American boys. National Black Child Development Institute. https://www.nbcdi.org/sites/default/files/resource-files/Being%20Black%20Is%20Not%20a%20Risk%20Factor_0.pdf.

Ray, D. C. (2011). *Advanced play therapy essential conditions, knowledge, and skills for child practice*. Routledge.

Rowley, S. J., Burchinal, M., Roberts, J., & Zeisel, S. (2008). Racial identity and race-related social cognition in African Americans during middle childhood. *Developmental Psychology*, 44(6), 1537–1546. doi:10.1037/a0013349.

Saleem, F. T., English, D., Busby, D. R., Lambert, S. F., Harrison, A., Stock, M. L., & Gibbons, F. X. (2016). The impact of African American parents' racial discrimination experiences and perceived neighborhood cohesion on their racial socialization practices. *Journal of youth and adolescence*, 45(7), 1338–1349. doi:10.1007/s10964-016-0499-x.

Santiago, C. D. C., & Miranda, J. (2014). Progress in improving mental health services for racial-ethnic minority groups: A ten-year perspective. *Psychiatric Services*, 65(2), 180–185. doi:10.1176/appi.ps.201200517.

Shattell, M., & Brown, P. J. (2017). Black mental health matters: What nurses need to know about chronic stressors of persons of color. *Journal of Psychosocial Nursing & Mental Health Services*, 55(9), 3–5. doi:10.3928/02793695-20170818-07.

Shin, R. Q. (2011). The influence of Africentric values and neighborhood satisfaction on the academic self-efficacy of African American elementary school children. *Journal of Multicultural Counseling and Development*, 39(4), 218–228. doi:10.1002/j.2161-1912.2011.tb00636.x.

Smith, E. J. (1977). Counseling black individuals: Some stereotypes. *Personnel & Guidance Journal*, 55(7), 390.

Solis, C. M., Meyers, J., & Varjas, K. M. (2004). A qualitative case study of the process and impact of filial therapy with an African American parent. *International Journal of Play Therapy*, 13(2), 99–118. doi:10.1037/h0088892.

Taylor, L., & Ray, D. C. (2021). Child-centered play therapy and social–emotional competencies of African American children: A randomized controlled trial. *International Journal of Play Therapy*, 30(2), 74–85. doi:10.1037/pla0000152.

Teasley, M. L., McRoy, R. G., Joyner, M., Armour, M., Gourdine, R. M., Crewe, S. E., Kelly, M., Franklin, C. G., Payne, M., Jackson Jr., J., & Fong, R. (2017). *Increasing success for African American children and youth* (Grand Challenges for Social Work initiative Working Paper No. 21). Cleveland, OH: American Academy of Social Work and Social Welfare.

Trent, M., Dooley, D.G., and Dougé, J. (2019) The impact of racism on child and adolescent health. *Pediatrics*, 144(2), 1–15. doi:10.1542/peds.2019-1765.

U.S. Census Bureau (2019). Census quick facts. www.census.gov/quickfacts/fact/table/US/PST045219.

Weir, K. (2016, November). Inequality at school: What's behind the racial disparity in our education system? *Monitor on Psychology*, 47(10), 42. www.apa.org/monitor/2016/11/cover-inequality-school.

Williams, J. P. (2016, May 17). Despite progress, Blacks are far from equal with Whites. *U.S. News & World Report*. https://www.usnews.com/news/articles/2016-05-17/despite-progress-blacks-are-far-from-equal-with-whites.

9 Cultural Opportunities with Latinx Populations

Mónica Rodríguez Delgado and Elizabeth V. Aguilar

Nina, a six-year-old Spanish/English speaking child, was happily humming to herself while combing a doll's hair in the corner of the playroom. In the five sessions that Nina had attended, she had never initiated any joint play or even approached me in the playroom. In that instance, I decided to track her play using Spanish. "*Decidiste peinar su cabello*/you decided to comb her hair." Her eyes immediately widened as she turned to me and said, "*Miss, tu sabes Español?*/Miss, you know Spanish?" During the first session, I had introduced the playroom in both English and Spanish. I realized that she had probably forgotten that detail. I replied to her "*Estás sorprendida de que se hablar Español./*You're surprised that I know how to speak Spanish." She stopped what she was doing and began to gather several toys. Once she was done, she grabbed my arm, led me to a section of the floor, and asked me to lie down as she draped a blanket over me. She told me to pretend that I was her sick daughter and said, "*Te voy a untar Vaporub en tu pecho y pies para que te sientas mejor y ahorita te hago un caldo de pollo*/I'm going to spread Vaporub on your chest and feet so you can feel better and in a little bit I'll make you a chicken stew." Nina checked my temperature, pretended to put the medicine on my chest and feet, and spoon-fed me the *caldo de pollo*. This was how my own mother took care of me when I was sick as a child. The same food, the same medicine, and the same fussy comments Nina was expressing. "*Ves, estás enferma porque estabas corriendo sin calcetines*/See, you're sick because you were running around without socks." Nina realized that we had something in common and that realization gave her the opportunity to share her whole genuine experience with me. From that session on, she would always invite me into her play and into her world.

Landreth (2012) stated, "each child possesses a personal perceptual view of self and the world that is reality for the child, and the view of self proves a basis for individual functioning in whatever daily experiences occur in the child's life" (p. 54). It is our job as play therapists to enter into this world and understand the child through their lens, through their eyes, through their cultural context. This is the basis for establishing a healing relationship with the child and a crucial component of play therapy regardless of the play therapist's theoretical approach. I (Mónica) will always remember Nina.

DOI: 10.4324/9781003190073-12

She reminded me of how complex and layered "being with" a child actually is. It was more than just entering a child's world, it was entering a Latinx, bilingual, immigrant child's world with her unique experiences of life, joy, pain, frustration, and beauty. A painful realization later came: Nina had been withholding parts of herself, she altered her behavior, and spoke only English to accommodate me. We do not live in a vacuum; the playroom is a microcosm of what is happening in our society. I asked myself, how many times does this happen in the playroom with children from diverse backgrounds, in this case with Latinx children? What messages are Latinx children receiving both inside and outside of the playroom? How can we as play therapists close that gap to help children like Nina freely express themselves, without hiding, so they can release their own unique way of healing?

Cultural Considerations

Who are We? Latinx Populations in the U.S.

In the United States, the Latinx population is the second largest ethnic group accounting for 18.5% (over 60 million) of the population and is expected to continue to grow (U.S. Census Bureau, 2019a). The Statista Research Department (2021) predicted that by 2060 the Latinx population will comprise 27.5% of the nation's population. School-aged Latinx children (5–17 years old) account for almost a quarter of all children (23%) in the U.S. (Noe-Bustamante & Flores, 2019). While most Latinx children (93%) were born in the U.S., about half have at least one parent born outside of the U.S. (Clarke et al., 2017). Clarke et al. (2017) concluded that about 25–28% of all Latinx children have at least one parent who is considered an undocumented immigrant.

Language is constantly changing and evolving based on our environment and socio-political context (Slemp, 2020). Many individuals under the Latinx/Hispanic umbrella choose to identify in a myriad of ways. Hispanic, Latino, Latin@, Latina/o, Latinx, and Latine are just some of the labels and identities that have been adopted by the community and can create confusion for play therapists. Knowing the history and meaning behind each individual's identity can become a window to a client's internal world and help build a deeper sense of understanding.

Hispanic or Latino (along with the variations of the word) are probably the two labels that are the most familiar for play therapists and have served as umbrella terms to describe individuals with Latin American ancestry. The word "Latino" has seen some major changes as political climates shift. The first variation of the word came with "Latin@" and Latina/o. This change occurred in response to the masculine nature of the world "Latino" and was an attempt to include "Latina" into the narrative. Recently, "Latinx" has been frequently used in academic settings and news/media outlets. The "x" in "Latinx" eliminates gender from the word to be inclusive of gender fluid, gender expansive, and non-binary folx. While some communities have welcomed "Latinx," it is not without controversy. Some scholars argue that using the word "Latinx" is a colonization of the Spanish language given that it enforces U.S. social norms onto other cultures (Guerra & Orbea, 2015). Guerra and Orbea (2015) went as far as calling it a "blatant form of linguistic imperialism." There is not one unifying term to utilize when describing this community, therefore a play therapist will have to pay close attention to how clients choose to self-identify or simply ask a client about their identity. For the purposes of this chapter, we will be using the term "Latinx" to be consistent with existing scholarly literature. However, we also understand that there may be some individuals within this community who do not connect with this term due to the political implications.

Regardless of the identity, one of the most important pieces for play therapists to remember is that while there are many similarities within the Latinx population, there are also great differences. The term Latinx encompasses individuals who have immigrated or have ancestry from more than 20 countries and territories including but not limited to Mexico, Puerto Rico, Cuba, Brazil, Dominican Republic, and El Salvador (Ennis et al., 2011). As colonization and slavery were historically pervasive in many Latin American regions, Black and Indigenous ancestry are also part of the Latinx narrative which include the Afro-Latinx, Indigenous-Latinx, and Mestizo identity.

Each individual culture has their own dialect, cultural meaning, food, celebrations, beliefs, and value systems. It would be important for a play therapist to have knowledge of the country or region to which a family has a connection. Many Latinx individuals have great pride in their own cultural background thus mistakenly calling someone of Puerto Rican ancestry Mexican can be perceived as offensive. The diversity in identities can be daunting for any play therapist, especially a new play therapist. Even as Latinx play therapists ourselves (both authors), it is impossible to know everything about every Latinx culture. We are not the experts of the Latinx experience. Writing a chapter based on any population is a tricky task that could potentially reinforce negative stereotypes. The Latinx community is full of complexities and layers that are impossible to fully cover in a few pages. Therefore, this chapter is a combination of both our personal and professional knowledge of the community and should not be taken as truth of every Latinx child, adult, or family. What helps guide us is a profound curiosity to explore and be in relationship with the person in front of us.

Language

Spanish is the second largest language spoken in the world, only surpassed by Mandarin Chinese (Instituto Cervantes, 2020). The United States ranks fifth in the world in countries with the largest number of native Spanish speakers (Statista, 2020) and Spanish is the second most spoken language in the home (U.S. Census Bureau, 2019b). The Latinx population accounts for 39 million of the Spanish speakers in the U.S. (U.S. Census Bureau, 2019c) and makes up about 16 million English-only speakers. However, Spanish is not the only spoken language within the Latinx community. People within the Latinx population speak over six different languages (Aragones et al., 2014). However, almost 80% of the U.S. population speaks English only (U.S. Bureau Census, 2019b), making it difficult for non-English speakers to feel a sense of belonging and access available resources. I (Eli) remember going to doctors' appointments or receiving letters in the mail and having to translate for my parents and grandparents because they did not know English. Many children of immigrants are placed with the responsibility of communicating between their parents and other adults. This task becomes even harder as children assimilate to the culture and lose or do not learn their parents' native language.

Language is an integral factor for a transfer of cultural values, norms, and identity (Pérez-Rojas et al., 2019). Therefore, for some Latinx individuals, having a limited ability to speak or communicate in Spanish can create a sense of loss in their identity. Many people even incorporate multiple languages (i.e. Spanglish) when they speak in order to effectively communicate their message. For multilingual clients, language has an important impact on the way they express, process, or experience emotions (Pavlenko, 2012). Many of our adult and adolescent bilingual clients who predominantly speak Spanish have mentioned how they could not express their meaning in English and often switch to Spanish. My (Eli) academic experience has been exclusively in English. I have had to navigate and receive extensive supervision in discovering how to provide counseling services in Spanish even though I am a fluent Spanish speaker. Due to my Spanish-speaking abilities, I often place a great responsibility on myself to provide services to Spanish speakers both because it is a passion of mine and due to the limited Spanish-speaking counselors. Many of our Spanish-speaking colleagues experience this same sense of responsibility as well.

Immigration and Assimilation

Almost 45 million people in the U.S. are foreign-born (Budiman et al., 2020) and Latinx individuals account for 44% of the foreign-born population. Individuals migrate to the United States for a myriad of reasons including but not limited to fleeing violence, economic advancement, religious freedom, and hope for a better future for their families. This experience can be traumatic and stressful. As individuals migrate, they are met with anti-immigrant rhetoric leading to discrimination and destructive stereotypes that negatively impact their mental health (Storlie & Jach, 2012). Additionally, youth who migrate experience grief from leaving their friends and family, experience societal and institutional exclusion and rejection due to their immigration status, and experience emotional distress from adjusting to an individualistic culture (Pérez et al., 2009). Furthermore, Latinx immigrant students experience increased isolation, confusion, and fear as they develop (Storlie & Jach, 2012).

Researchers generally conceptualize the Latinx population within separate generations (i.e. first generation, 1.5 generation, second generation; Pew Research Center, 2004). Each generation has their own unique experiences, challenges, and opportunities. Not all Latinx families physically immigrated. For instance, *Tejanos* in the U.S. southern region had their land taken after the 1848 Treaty of Guadalupe-Hidalgo (Cerdeña et al., 2021). Therefore, many Latinx families have lived in the United States for generations. Knowing and understanding the particular generation of clients can provide the play therapist with some context of the client's experience.

Spirituality

For many in the Latinx community, religion and spirituality is a way of maintaining cultural identity (Altarriba & Bauer, 1998). While the Latinx community is represented in many major religions, an estimated 56% of Latinx individuals in the United States identify as Catholic (Gray, 2019) and approximately 17,000 Catholic parishes in the United States (25%) offer religious services in Spanish (Ospino, 2018). Religious leaders may be consulted regarding issues of mental and emotional health. Further, contemporary practices could display influences from Indigenous and African spiritism and folk healing traditions (Andrés-Hyman et al., 2006). Some individuals may seek mental health guidance and support from spiritualism and Santeria. Santeria is a folk religion worshiping saints and combining ritual, magical, and medical beliefs (Altarriba & Bauer, 1998). Spiritualism is "the belief that the world we can see is surrounded by an invisible world. This invisible world is inhabited by good and bad spirits that can enter the visible world and bind themselves to humans" (Altarriba & Bauer, 1998, p. 392). An individual who is knowledgeable about these spirits is referred to as a *curandero* or folk healer and may be sought to provide guidance on emotional/mental, spiritual, and physical health. Additionally, some children or parents may indicate that they see spirits or talk to relatives who died. *Dia De Los Muertos* (Day of the Dead) is a good example of a cultural celebration where Latinx families remember their dead while believing that their spirits visit them on that night.

Discrimination, Racism, and Hate

In recent years the attacks on BIPOC (Black, Indigenous, people of color) have significantly increased (FBI, 2019; Study of Hate and Extremism, 2021). The mass "immigrant round-ups" and deportation of undocumented people have had a direct impact on countless Latinx children. In 2018, many children were separated from their parents (Hegarty, 2018) and by 2019, thousands of them found themselves in child detention centers (BBC, 2019). Latinx children were placed in prison-like conditions. Further traumatic incidents continue to devastate the Latinx community, such as the racially motivated shooting of Latinx persons by a White male in El Paso, Texas in August 2019 which resulted in the murders of 22 Latinx individuals and critical injury of 26 others (Romo, 2019). As I spoke with people within the community both professionally and personally, their reactions varied. Some experienced deep emotional responses (fear, anxiety, sadness, crying episodes) while others, in a flat effect, said, "*cuando te toca, te toca/* when it's your time, it's your time."

Psychological wounding and trauma experienced by adults can be transmitted to children in the form of intergenerational/transgenerational trauma (Cerdeña et al., 2021). Literature on intergenerational trauma suggests that trauma experienced by one generation has a direct impact on the health of children in subsequent generations. Traumas can be personal (i.e. sexual assault) or collective (i.e. wars, genocide, or colonization; Cerdeña et al., 2021). For immigrating families, pre-migration, migration, and post-migration experiences increase the risk of intergenerational trauma (Cerdeña et al., 2021). Financial stress or violence in native countries, the dangers of the journey into the U.S., acculturative stress, discrimination, and anti-immigrant rhetoric exacerbate trauma and negatively affect psychological health for parents/caregivers (Dreyer, 2019). Mass traumas like colonization, hate crimes, and systemic racism also increase the likelihood of intergenerational trauma. After a review of literature, Cerdeña and colleagues (2021) reported that experiencing trauma disrupted a caregiver's capacity to respond to their children, thus altering children's capability to form trusting relationships and regulate their emotional responses. Additionally, Grest et al. (2021) found that second and third generation Latinx youth had a higher level of adverse childhood experiences compared to first generation children, specifically in "household dysfunction." They concluded that these results may be attributed to segregation, low socioeconomic status, discrimination, and political factors like intergenerational racism and criminalizing policies. While trauma can be passed down through generations, so can resilience. Research on intergenerational resilience focuses on the role of positive parenting, strong community narratives, and transfer of knowledge and cultural practices as protective factors for Latinx communities (Budowle et al., 2019; Cerdeña et al., 2021).

The role of discrimination, bias, and trauma for Latinx populations is evident across the practice and supervision of play therapy. In play therapy, I (Mónica) saw an eight-year-old Latinx girl, daughter of undocumented immigrants. She was desperately trying to find something in the "dress-up" area. She found a black dress and put it on. She then said, "Miss, I'm a lawyer. I'm going to make sure that if my parents get deported, I can help them get out of jail. I don't want them to be taken from me." The fear and desperation in the eyes of this eight-year-old child almost had me in tears. There were no words that could make this situation easier for her and I relied on the empathy that I could convey through our relationship. As a play therapist supervisor, I had the opportunity to hold space for another Latinx play therapist (student) who was having an emotional reaction to discriminatory violence against a local Latinx community. She mentioned that no one had asked her how she was doing. She did not realize it was bothering her until I asked her how she was managing the shooting. She processed, we cried, I was authentic with my experience and let her know that I was also impacted and sharing this collective trauma with her. She mentioned feeling understood on a deeper level and eventually we shifted the conversation on how her experience would impact her ability to be with clients. This experience was a good reminder that supervising was more than feedback on essential skills, but an opportunity to really see who was in front of me and how events in society uniquely impact us based on our identities. In both of these examples, I had the opportunity to be with my client and supervisee in a painful yet healing way.

Play Therapy Considerations

The Messages that Latinx Children Receive

Most of us have heard the saying "children are like sponges." They are always absorbing the information around them. What happens when the information they absorb is of hate, "othering," or non-acceptance? Many Latinx children experience internalized oppression, agreeing to the societal belief that White is the preferred race and they are "not as smart, beautiful, resourceful, good, or deserving of success" as their White peers (Monzó, 2016, p. 148). For Latinx children, these beliefs are often linked to their culture, value systems, race, language, and immigration status (Monzó, 2016). Messages of hate can harm children's sense of self; however, messages of acceptance, love, and understanding can also foster resilience. Play therapists are well situated to be able to communicate this unconditional acceptance of Latinx children in order to combat oppressive messages.

I (Mónica) don't have many memories before the age of five, but I remember an experience that has been fundamental to the formation of my identity. In preschool, I changed my name to Jessica. I can actually remember my thought process; I was different and different was not okay. I absolutely hated my name. Now, I'm very particular about correcting people when my name is mispronounced. It's the Spanish pronunciation of Mónica (with accent marks). When I was younger, I would get, "Oh, I can't pronounce that, I'll just call you [insert any Americanized version of my name]." Which can be a testimony on how we invalidate children in our society. We internalize the messages we receive in those younger years. How did the five-year-old me learn to hate my name and by extension hate myself? When my mother heard my classmates call me Jessica she asked, "*Quien es Jessica?*/Who is Jessica?" I replied, "*Me cambié mi nombre, no me gusta Mónica./* I changed my name, I don't like Mónica." My mother knew what was going on. "*Mija, no te sientas avergonzada, ten orgullo en ti misma, en tu familia. Somos humildes pero que nunca se te olvide de donde vienes./*Daughter, don't feel ashamed, have pride in yourself, in your family. We are humble, but never forget where you come from." I have never forgotten those words.

The Relationship

A child-centered play therapist's focus on the relationship (Landreth, 2012) provides an opportunity to work with the Latinx community. An importance of and responsibility to relationships can be seen in Latinx children and their families. Specific values that highlight the significance of relationships include *personalismo, simpatía*, and *familismo* (Ortiz, 2017). *Personalismo* refers to relationships based on mutual respect and trust for people. *Personalismo* is often demonstrated by asking others about their family, engaging in small talk, or sharing meals together. This creates a safe environment that conveys *simpatía*, kind and nonconflicting interactions that create harmony in relationships and in the community. A great value may be placed on being able to collectively interact in a cooperative manner. *Familismo* then refers to the importance of the family which often extends beyond the immediate family system. Individuals often reflect on how they impact and serve others for the greater good of the community through an allocentric lens. Play therapists are invited to build and maintain relationships with Latinx children and their families with these values in mind. For a play therapist, knowing and understanding the importance of and responsibility to relationships within the Latinx population can strengthen the therapeutic relationship and in turn can transcend the playroom.

Self-Actualization

Play therapists aim to empathically understand and accept a child's experience so that the child may feel free to move towards meeting their full potential (Landreth, 2012). Self-actualization is usually understood as an individual experience. However, in the Latinx population, self-actualization includes actualization of the family and the community (Ortiz, 2017). Therefore, a play therapist aims to understand the child's lived experiences rather than make assumptions on what healing may look like based on dominant narratives or personal bias. A play therapist empathically understands and provides unconditional positive regard for the client, their family, and their culture based on their lived experiences and trusts the client will know what they need to move towards self-actualization (Ortiz, 2017). Personally, when I (Eli) am given acceptance and understanding for my experiences, it helps me to better understand myself. Family is very important and major decisions I make are centered around my family. Having a counselor understand this value and how it is one of my strengths rather than have me individuate from my family is conducive to my growth. When I am told to think about what I want and that I am too enmeshed with my family, I feel misunderstood and judged when in fact the relationships in my life play a vital role in who I am.

Rogers (1951) believed the self-actualizing tendency is always present and one's ability to access and fulfill this tendency was influenced by the environment. When specific conditions are met, an individual can move towards the innate self-actualization tendency (Rogers, 1951). Subsequently, an empathic understanding and a prizing of the client can also empower Latinx children who experience oppression because the relational environment of play therapy allows a client to express themselves freely as they become aware of the influence of oppressive factors and the internalized oppression on their self-concept (Swan & Ceballos, 2020). However, Swan and Ceballos (2020) emphasize that this environment cannot be developed if a counselor does not consider that cultural values influence the therapeutic relationship.

Cultural Opportunities in Play Therapy

Procedures

The introduction to the playroom is one of the first opportunities to develop a relationship with Latinx children. Landreth (2012) indicates introducing the playroom with carefully chosen words to communicate the child's freedom, self-direction, and the parameters of the relationship. Typically, one will use a phrase like the following "Eli, this is the playroom and in here you can play with the toys in many of the ways that you would like." As bilingual play therapists (both authors), when working with Spanish-speaking Latinx children, we also introduce the playroom in Spanish and state that they can choose to speak in English, Spanish, or both. Introducing the playroom in this manner allows for an opportunity for a child to choose their language, an experience that may not be conveyed in other settings. Following this introduction, we then follow the child's lead utilizing words or responses in the language the child chooses, sometimes switching between the two throughout the relationship. Bilingual Latinx clients in session are better able to express their thoughts, feelings, and experiences if they speak in their native language (Pérez-Rojas et al., 2019). Although a client may be able to express a message in both English and Spanish, there are times where the use of both languages allows them to accurately articulate their experience. Our assumption is that bilingual children do the same, shift their language according to the linguistic capabilities of the play therapist. To convey acceptance of the child's linguistic capabilities a non-Spanish-speaking play therapist can also introduce a play-room by adding, "In here you can speak English, Spanish, or both. I don't know Spanish, but I will do my best to learn what you say." If a child uses a Spanish word in session with a non-Spanish speaker, we suggest the play therapist learn what the word means outside of session so that in the future the play therapist will know what it means and so that the child can con-tinue to use the word rather than the child having to figure out how to say what they mean in English. We believe this can help the therapeutic relationship.

Toys and Materials

A play therapist must be intentional about incorporating culturally appro-priate toys to allow the child to fully express themselves. Play is a child's language and toys are their words (Landreth, 2012). As play therapists, we want the child to freely express themselves in both their spoken language(s) and through their play language by providing culturally inclusive toys. This goes beyond making generalization of the Latinx population and utilizing stereotypical toys and materials such as Mexican sombreros and sarapes. While, yes, these items may represent some Latinx experiences and could be appropriate for these particular populations, they do not represent the majority and can easily become offensive toys in the playroom. This isn't a "call-out" or judgment for play therapists utilizing these materials; rather, we encourage reflection on selecting culturally inclusive toys and materials. Play therapists are encouraged to take the time to understand and be open to the culture of the subgroups they are working with in order to provide toys, materials, and a space that is representative of the surrounding Latinx community or clients. When choosing toys to use in the playroom, Ray (2011, p. 80) offers three questions for play therapists to ask themselves: "(1) What therapeutic purpose will this serve for children who use this room? (2) How will this help children express themselves? (3) How will this help me build a relationship with children?" We recommend adding a fourth ques-tion when adding culturally specific toys. (4) Is this toy an accurate cultural representation of the diverse children who will enter this room and their surrounding community? Answering these questions while also being aware of both personal bias and the Latinx subgroup's culture including food, clothes, toys, beliefs, and values can help to create a safe space for the child.

Cultural Values in the Playroom

Allowing the child to lead is a hallmark of child-centered play therapy (CCPT; Landreth, 2012) and to a degree infused in many other theoretical orientations. Some Latinx children may experience anxiety from this child-led environment. Due to the value of *Respeto*/respect, many Latinx children are taught to be highly respectful of others. Parents may communicate to the child that they are not allowed to touch other people's belongings unless they have explicit permission. Therefore, some Latinx children may have a hard time initiating play and experience anxiety due to their desire to play while upholding their values of waiting until they are given permission. In an interview, Dr. Peggy Ceballos recommends having a pre-session with Latinx children (Ray, 2019). In this pre-session, a play therapist can take the child to the room for five to ten minutes while touching the toys and stating the typical introductory phrase to indicate that the child is allowed to touch the toys while in the room. Sometimes, this process is done during the first play sessions by giving the child permission to play with the toys. For example, if the play therapist senses a child's desire to play with a dollhouse but the child is hesitant to do so, the play therapist can respond by stating, "It looks like you want to play with that [while pointing to the dollhouse]. In here you can play with that." These actions may seem inconsistent with a traditional approach to CCPT. However, the play therapist is being culturally in tune and responsive to the child and is following the child's lead in their own unique way. Play therapists will have to pay close attention and observe where the child's eyes may go and reflect the client's feelings or desires, rather than wait for the child to initiate verbalization or action. The play therapist does not force a child to play rather allows them to know that it is okay to do so. Typically, these adaptations are only done for the first few sessions. Additionally, from our experience, Latinx children may play with the toys and then clean up after themselves as a sign of respect. Over time this may or may not continue as they learn the "rules" of the room.

Cultural Opportunities with Latinx Children, Families, and Systems

The question is inevitably asked, "Can a non-Latinx play therapist see a Latinx child and it still be a healing experience?" Absolutely! The question that comes after is usually, "Is it more healing for a Latinx play therapist to see a Latinx child?" That answer is more complex and nuanced. A lot may depend on identity/identity development, level of assimilation, language ability, cultural knowledge, and experiences of both the Latinx child and play therapist. Our experiences with Latinx children in the playroom have varied. There have been many sessions where it is clear that our ability to speak a shared language or the child's perception of our sameness or even our insider identity have led to a deeper level of understanding and freedom for the child. Dynamics may shift and change depending on how we are perceived by the child. On other occasions, it did not seem to matter as much. The relationship between the child's family system and play therapist could also influence the child's growth and healing. Either way, to advocate for the children where it does matter means creating safe environments in learning institutions and advocating for more Latinx clinicians, mentors, and supervisors.

Working with Families: The Collective Experience

While many play therapists frequently report working with parents or caregivers as the most difficult part of counseling children (Ray, 2011), working alongside families can provide opportunities to holistically understand the child's system of support. Generally, Latinx families are known to value close knit, loving, supportive, interpersonal relationships that may extend beyond the nuclear family. About 9% of Latinx individuals live in a multigenerational home (Noe-Bustamante & Flores, 2019). Thus, it is not uncommon to have multiple generations living in the same home and finding themselves in the play therapist's office for parent consultations. The caregiver's *comadres* or *compadres* (literal translation is co-mother or co-father but are usually the caregiver's good friends) may become the child's *Tías, Tíos*, or *Padrinos* (aunts, uncles, godparents) and often share an important bond with the child. It would be beneficial for a play therapist to maintain a therapeutic alliance with several important members of the family.

Because *personalismo* relies on trust, it can sometimes be established more easily between people who are perceived as being of the same social/ethnic group (Davis et al., 2019). Additionally, *personalismo* can extend to professional settings including doctors, lawyers, counselors, and their clients. Professional *personalismo* may include interactions such as engaging with clients in small talk about their day, close physical contact (i.e. hugging or sitting in close proximity), gift-giving, or sharing personal information (Davis et al., 2019). Play therapists who are unfamiliar with this cultural value and have been taught to not disclose personal information in a therapeutic setting may feel uncomfortable or believe that these behaviors violate professional boundaries. However, we have found that within the cultural context, they are both appropriate and can lead to positive interactions and a stronger therapeutic alliance between the caregiver(s) and play therapist. Supervision and consultation with a play therapist who has specialized training and knowledge within the cultural framework always encourage discussion of any feelings or experiences that may emerge, as well as mentoring on appropriate boundaries. Each of us (both authors) have had extensive supervision regarding touch, self-disclosure, gift-giving, and other Latinx cultural norms that arise in our caregiver/family consultation.

Rosa, an immigrant mother from Mexico, came into our parent consultation session and immediately moved her chair to sit closer to me (Mónica). *"Doctora, comó está hoy? Y su familia? Oiga, por qué estamos sentadas tan lejos?* [formal Spanish]/Doctor, how are you today? How is your family? Listen, why are we sitting so far away from each other." For six months, I had been telling her that I am not a doctor, I was a doctoral student. She would wave her hand in the air as if to brush off my comment and proceeded to call me *"Doctora."* We engaged in small talk about our families while she shared a batch of cookies with me. We ate the cookies and drank *cafecito* together as we shifted our conversation to her son. This may be a foreign experience for many play therapists; however, I have found that this level of familiarity did not distract from our counseling goals or objectives. These interactions facilitated trust, empathy, and depth in our relationship. Our small talk and sharing of a meal were familiar concepts for her, allowing her to feel comfortable and increase trust. However, her use of formal Spanish and the word "*Doctora*" conveyed a sense of respect for my part in her son's healing journey. When the parent consultation was over, Rosa gave me a big hug and mentioned that next time she was bringing her neighbor because she also had important information to share about her son.

Working with Latinx families may mean working with extended family members or within other systems of support. Rosa felt that her neighbor had a strong enough relationship with her son and trusted her knowledge of his behavior to invite her to the next consultation. Sometimes play therapists will need to re-evaluate their training in order to provide culturally responsive care.

Working Within Systems: Moving from Multicultural Education to Action

Cultural opportunities with Latinx populations transcend the playroom and include working within systems. As previously mentioned, Latinx children make up 23% of the school-aged population. Unfortunately, Latinx children also have the highest school drop-out and suspension rates. They are more likely to experience mental health issues that are often unaddressed and untreated compared to their peers (Ramirez et al., 2017). Research indicates that Latinx children experience increased depression, stress, anxiety, and suicidal behavior due to discrimination, poverty, bullying, violence, acculturation, and immigration status among other familial and community stressors (Ramirez et al., 2017). Rather than receiving mental health care, underrepresented children including those who identify as Latinx receive in-school punishment and incarceration. We recommend working alongside and building relationships with teachers and school-counselors to facilitate safe, protective, and flourishing spaces for children and their families.

Play therapists also indirectly advocate through supporting and encouraging policy changes including but not limited to immigration reform, accessibility to health care, access to education, and economic security. In doing so, we can also affect systems that impact access to higher education so that there may be more Spanish-speaking counselors in the field. Play therapists are encouraged to work alongside Latinx leaders and community advocates who have been at the forefront of addressing issues and systems that impact the Latinx community.

Conclusion

The Latinx population is a diverse group with similar beliefs and values. Play therapists are invited to be open to the cultural opportunities discussed in this chapter and others that may arise when working with the Latinx population to provide culturally inclusive spaces. Understanding the child's world through their lens can strengthen the relationship and the impact of play therapy in the Latinx community.

Positionality Statements

Mónica

I am the daughter of Mexican immigrants. The continued support of my mother, family, extended relatives, friends, and community is the reason for my passion. They motivate me, they make every decision I make crucial, and they help me remember to use my immense privilege to give back to the community that fostered my growth. When I finally add those letters after my name, it will be our moment and not just mine. The colors of my life are often seen as "less than" in environments that were not made for me to flourish. But I am here. This is my lens. My salient identities have profoundly impacted my work and career as a play therapist, researcher, supervisor, and future counselor educator. My personal and professional identities have given me a variety of experiences; some of them were wonderful, some were painful, while others infuriating. So, I was immediately filled with anxiety when I was asked to co-write this chapter. Gloria Anzaldúa (1987) once wrote "I am turtle, wherever I go I carry 'home' on my back" (p. 21). This statement captures both how my culture is interwoven in everything I do and the weight of the responsibility I feel towards my community, my Latinx students/supervisees, Latinx play therapists, and most importantly Latinx children and families. I was afraid that this would become a cookie-cutter approach to working with Latinx children and miss the essence of our community. My hope is that readers were able to see the layers, the colors, and diversity of our people. Each family and child will be unique and will require an individualized relationship. This chapter is only a starting point.

Another realization was that I would have to be vulnerable and re-open old wounds. I'm intimately familiar with racism, trauma, oppression, discrimination, and self-hate. Therefore, writing this chapter was a labor of love, a calling, and an invitation for everyone reading to dive deeper, advocate harder, be uncomfortable, speak out, and step aside when appropriate to hear the stories from the mouths of the community members. Latinx play therapists are already out there doing the work. They are shifting, adapting, advocating, training. They are taking modalities that were meant for White clients and creatively making them work within diverse populations. Each author in this book is using their own experiences of pain or moments of joy as learning opportunities for future play therapists. Honor their stories by entering their world, learning about their perspectives, and paying attention to any defensiveness that is coming up. Right there, that discomfort is a gift, a new opportunity. It was a great honor to write this chapter and an even greater honor to have you read it.

Elizabeth

I am a daughter of Indigenous Mexican immigrants who emigrated from Oaxaca, Mexico. This statement says so much and yet not enough about me. Highlighting the impact of my parents, immediate and extended family, and community is paramount to understanding who I am and how I became. I recognize the privilege I hold in being able to be a part of this chapter and to share my experiences while also feeling a great deal of responsibility in doing so. It is a feeling that other Latinx play therapists in my position may know all too well where we can even begin to question whether we deserve to have this space. We do. Although my Latinx identity and understanding of the culture can facilitate a deeper relationship with the Latinx clients I serve, it is not without its challenges.

As a bilingual Latinx play therapist, I also experience the pain, joy, fear, anger, among other emotions that impact my work. When I initially began working with Spanish-speaking clients, I was worried about my abilities to provide counseling services in Spanish. I felt incompetent as a counselor. How was I now supposed to provide services in Spanish? I had learned all the concepts in English. I now had to figure out how to translate the information. Additionally, I was learning about counseling from an individualistic lens. Integrating what I was learning with who I was, was a complex and fruitful process. As a new play therapist and counselor, I was receiving messages about what to do and what not to do. I was taking information in concretely and then felt ingenuine when attempting to apply these new concepts with my Latinx clients. My relationships with Latinx clients have always felt deeper from the start. However, I wasn't always sure how to integrate my cultural understanding and values within a counseling framework. My confidence has grown since then and the challenges that arise appear through working within systems. As I advocate for my clients, I am also advocating for myself, family, and community. Receiving support from family, friends, colleagues, and supervisors has been an integral component to my development. They help to challenge, encourage, and provide safe spaces for me so that I may be a better play therapist for my clients and to do the same for future Latinx play therapists.

References

Altarriba, J., & Bauer, L. M. (1998). Counseling the Hispanic client: Cuban Americans, Mexican Americans, and Puerto Ricans. *Journal of Counseling & Development*, 76(4), 389–396. doi:10.1002/j.1556-6676.1998.tb02697.x.

Andrés-Hyman, R., Ortiz, J., Anes, L., Paris, M., and Davidson, L. (2006). Culture and clinical practice: Recommendations for working with Puerto Ricans and other Latinas(os) in the United States. *Professional Psychology: Research and Practice*, 37(6), 694–701. doi:10.1037/0735–7028.37.6.694

Anzaldúa, G. (1987). *Borderlands: La frontera: The new mestiza*. Aunt Lute.

Aragones, A., Hayes, S., Hsuan Chen, M., González, J., & Gany, M. F. (2014). Characterization of the hispanic or latino population in health research: A systemic review. *The Journal of Immigrant and Minority Health*, 16(3), 429–439, doi:10.1007/s10903-013-9773-0.

British Broadcasting Corporation (2019). Are US child migrant detainees entitled to soap and beds? *BBC News*. www.bbc.com/news/world-us-canada-48710432.

Budiman, A., Tamir, C., Mora, L. & Noe-Bustamante, L. (2020). Facts on U.S. immigrants, 2018: Statistical portrait of the foreign-born population in the United

States. Pew Research Center. www.pewresearch.org/hispanic/2020/08/20/fa cts-on-u-s-immigrants-current-data.

Budowle, R., Arthur, M., & Porter, C. (2019). Growing intergenerational resilience for Indigenous food sovereignty through home gardening. *Journal of Agriculture, Food Systems, and Community Development*, 1–21. doi:10.5304/jafscd.2019.09b.006.

Cerdeña, J. P., Rivera, L. M., & Spak, J. M. (2021). Intergenerational trauma in Latinxs: A scoping review. *Social Science & Medicine*, 270, 113662. doi:10.1016/j. socscimed.2020.113662.

Clarke, W., Turner, K., & Guzman, L. (2017). One quarter of Hispanic children in the United States have an unauthorized immigrant parent. Hispanic Research Center. www.hispanicresearchcenter.org/research-resources/one-quarter-of-hispa nic-children-in-the-united-states-have-an-unauthorized-immigrant-parent.

Davis, R. E., Lee, S., Johnson, T. P., & Rothschild, S. K. (2019). Measuring the elusive construct of Personalismo among Mexican American, Puerto Rican, and Cuban American adults. *Hispanic Journal of Behavioral Sciences*, 41(1), 103–121. doi:10.1177/0739986318822535.

Dreyer, B. P. (2019). Sustained animus toward Latino immigrants: Deadly con- sequences for children and families. *New England Journal of Medicine*, 381(13), 1196–1198. doi:10.1056/nejmp1908995.

Ennis, S. R., Rios-Vargas, M., & Albert, N. G. (2011). The hispanic population: 2010. US Census Bureau. www.census.gov/prod/cen2010/briefs/c2010br-04. pdf.

Federal Bureau of Investigation (2019). 2019 hate crime statistics. FBI. https://ucr. fbi.gov/hate-crime/2019/topic-pages/incidents-and-offenses.

Gray, M. (2019). U.S. Hispanic Catholic in the pews. *Journal of Prevention & Inter- vention in the Community*, 46(4), 313–323. doi:10.1080/10852352.2018.1507493.

Grest, C. V., Finno-Velasquez, M., Cederbaum, J. A., & Unger, J. B. (2021). Adverse childhood experiences among 3 generations of Latinx youth. *American Journal of Preventive Medicine*, 60(1), 20–28. doi:10.1016/j.amepre.2020.07.007.

Guerra, G., & Orbea, G. (2015). The argument against the use of the term "Latinx". *The Phoenix*. https://swarthmorephoenix.com/2015/11/19/the-argument-against- the-use-of-the-term-latinx.

Hegarty, A. (2018). Timeline: Immigrant children separated from families at the border. *USA TODAY*. https://www.usatoday.com/story/news/2018/06/27/ immigrant-children-family-separation-border-timeline/734014002/.

Instituto Cervantes (2020). El Español: Una Lengua Viva Informe 2020. Centro Virtual Cervantes. https://cvc.cervantes.es/lengua/espanol_lengua_viva/pdf/espa nol_lengua_viva_2020.pdf.

Landreth, G.L. (2012). *Play therapy: The art of the relationship* (3rd ed.). Routledge.

Mensah, M., Ogbu-Nwobodo, L., & Shim, R. S. (2021). Racism and mental health equity: History repeating itself. *Psychiatric Services*. doi:10.1176/appi.ps.202000755.

Monzó, L. D. (2016). "They don't know anything!": Latinx immigrant students appropriating the oppressor's voice. *Anthropology & Education Quarterly*, 47(2), 148–166. doi:10.1111/aeq.12146.

Noe-Bustamante, L., & Flores, A. (2019). Facts on Latinos in the U.S. Pew Research Center. www.pewresearch.org/hispanic/fact-sheet/latinos-in-the-u-s-fa ct-sheet/#length-of-time-in-the-u-s-for-hispanic-immigrants-2000-2017.

Ortiz, F. A. (2017). Self-actualization in the latino/hispanic culture. *Journal of Humanistic Psychology*, 60(3), 418–435. doi:10.1177/0022167817741785.

Ospino, H. (2018). The value and need for new research on the U.S Hispanic Catholic experience to build a stronger sense of communal belonging. *Journal of Prevention & Intervention in the Community*, 46(4), 309–312. doi:10.1080/10852352.2018.1507492.

Pavlenko, A. (2012). Affective processing in bilingual speakers: Disembodied cognition? *International Journal of Psychology*, 47(6), 405–428. doi:10.1080/00207594.2012.743665.

Pérez-Rojas, A. E., Brown, R., Cervantes, A., Valente, T., & Pereira, S. R. (2019). "Alguien abrió la puerta": The phenomenology of bilingual Latinx clients' use of Spanish and English in psychotherapy. *Society for Advancement of Psychotherapy*, 56 (2), 241–253. doi:10.1037/pst0000224.

Pérez, W., Espinoza, R., Ramos, K., Coronado, H. M., & Cortes, R. (2009). Academic resilience among undocumented Latino students. *Hispanic Journal of Behavioral Sciences*, 31(2), 149–181. doi:10.1177/0739986309333020.

Pew Research Center (2004). Generational differences: Fact sheet. www.pewresearch.org/hispanic/2004/03/19/generational-differences.

Ramirez, A. G., Gallion, K. J., Aguilar, R., & Surette Dembeck, E. (2017). Mental health and Latino kids: A research review. Robert Wood Johnson Foundation. https://salud-america.org/wp-content/uploads/2017/09/FINAL-mental-health-research-review-9-12-17.pdf.

Ray, D. C. (2011). *Advanced play therapy: Essential conditions, knowledge, and skills for child practice.* Routledge.

Ray, D. C. (Director). (2019). *Terapia de juego centrada en el niño con niños de cultura latina: Una sesión clínica* [film]. The Center for Play Therapy.

Rogers, C. (1951). *Client-centered therapy.* Houghton Mifflin.

Rogers, C. R. (1959). A theory of therapy, personality, and interpersonal relationships: As developed in the client-centered framework. In S. Koch (Ed.), *Psychology: A study of a science. Formulations of the Person and the Social Context* (Vol. 3, pp. 184–256). McGraw Hill.

Rogers, C. R. (2007). The necessary and sufficient conditions of therapeutic personality change. *Psychotherapy: Theory, Research, Practice, Training*, 44(3), 240–248. doi:10.1037/0033–3204.44.3.240. (Reprinted from "The necessary and sufficient conditions of therapeutic personality change," 1957, *Journal of Consulting Psychology*, 21(2), 95–103.)

Romo, V. (2019). El Paso Walmart shooting suspect pleads not guilty. *NPR.org.* www.npr.org/2019/10/10/769013051/el-paso-walmart-shooting-suspect-pleads-not-guilty.

Slemp, K. (2020). Latino, Latina, Latin@, Latine, and Latinx: Gender inclusive oral expression in Spanish. *Electronic Thesis and Dissertation Repository*, 7297. https://ir.lib.uwo.ca/etd/7297.

Statista Research Department. (2020). Countries with most Spanish speakers 2020. *Statista.* www.statista.com/statistics/991020/number-native-spanish-speakers-country-worldwide.

Statista Research Department. (2021). U.S. population: Ethnic groups in America 2016 and 2060. *Statista.* www.statista.com/statistics/270272/percentage-of-us-population-by-ethnicities.

Storlie, C. A. & Jach, E.A. (2012). Social justice collaborations in schools: A model for working with undocumented Latino students. *Journal for Social Action in Counseling and Psychology*, 4(2), 99–116. doi:10.33043/JSACP.4.2.99-116.

Study of Hate and Extremism (2021). Report to the nation: Anti-Asian prejudice & hate crime. California State University, San Bernardino | CSUSB. https://www. csusb.edu/sites/default/files/Report%20to%20the%20Nation%20-%20Anti-Asian% 20Hate%202020%20Final%20Draft%20-%20As%20of%20Apr%2030%202021% 206%20PM%20corrected.pdf.

Swan, A. M. & Ceballos, P. (2020). Person-centered conceptualization of multiculturalism and social justice in counseling. *Person-Centered & Existential Psychotherapies*, 19(2), 154–167. doi:10.1080/14779757.2020.1717981.

U.S. Census Bureau (2019a). American community survey: ACS demographic and housing estimates. https://data.census.gov/cedsci/table?q=United%20States&tid= ACSDP1Y2019.DP05&hidePreview=true.

U.S. Census Bureau (2019b). American community survey: Language spoken at home. https://data.census.gov/cedsci/table?q=language&tid=ACSST1Y2019.S1601.

U.S. Census Bureau (2019c). American Community Survey: Language spoken at home by ability to speak English for the population 5 years and over (Hispanic or Latino). https://data.census.gov/cedsci/table?q=language&tid=ACSDT1Y2019.B160.

10 Cultural Opportunities with Asian Populations

Yi-Ju Cheng, Regine K. Chung and Yumiko Ogawa

When we (Yi, Regine, and Yumi) gathered to discuss the focus of this chapter, we began our discussion by sharing our feelings about the difficulty and complexity of appropriately presenting the Asian population, a racial group encompassing a wide range of ethnicities, nationalities, and identities. We agreed that it would be important to begin by asking the question, "Who is considered Asian?" before talking about working with Asian children and families in the context of play therapy. Moreover, we would like to note that we use the term Asian populations throughout this chapter to be inclusive of those who identify as Asian or Asian Americans. It is important to respect the identity of each individual by following the person's self-identification of race or ethnicity.

The single-race Asian population, individuals who identify with only the Asian race and not in combination with other races, is the fastest-growing racial demographic in the U.S., with an estimated growth from 10.5 million to 18.9 million between 2000 and 2019. It is projected that Asians will account for 9.3% of the U.S. total population by 2060 (Colby & Ortman, 2015; Pew Research Center, 2021a). According to the U.S. Census Bureau (2020), which adheres to the race and ethnicity standards set in 1997 by the Office of Management and Budget (OMB), the term "Asian" refers to individuals having heritages in the Far East, Southeast Asia, or the Indian subcontinent. As of 2019, 85% of the Asian population is comprised of the ethnic groups by descending order: Chinese, Indians, Filipinos, Vietnamese, Koreans, and Japanese. The remaining 15% are made of nearly 20 groups that are growing more rapidly than the six larger groups over the last two decades. These smaller groups include residents who identify as Pakistanis, Cambodians, Thais, Hmong, Laotians, Taiwanese, Bangladeshis, Burmese, Indonesians, Sri Lankans, Malaysians, Bhutanese, Mongolian, Okinawan, "Two or more Asian ethnicities" and "Other Asians" (U.S. Census Bureau, 2019). We intentionally listed the above ethnic groups to promote the understanding of the myriad groups that encompass the definition of Asian.

Despite how the U.S. government classifies Asians, most people of different races in the U.S. – and even Asians themselves – tend to think of East Asians when they think of what type of person the word "Asian" connotes

DOI: 10.4324/9781003190073-13

(Lee & Ramakrishnan, 2020). Also, East and Southeast Asians along with Whites, Blacks, and Latinx are less likely to see South Asians (e.g. Bangladeshis, Indians, and Pakistanis) as Asian. The disconnect between the official racial assignment of the word "Asian" and the public's understanding of the term has created a pattern of South Asian exclusion (Lee & Ramakrishnan, 2020). The discrepancy between who actually counts as Asian and who people think of as being considered Asian is a reflection of the rapidly changing U.S. demographic profile as well as the phenomenon that the Asian racial group assignment has been neither firmly understood nor well-established. Because different Asian identities have been lumped together and East Asians are perceived as representatives of all Asians, the narratives and images portrayed in public can often be biased and counterproductive to promoting a nuanced understanding of Asians and a racially equitable society. Therefore, it is imperative that play therapists work to be mindful of the vast variability within the Asian population, each of which have their own unique cultural beliefs, language, spiritual and religious practices, socioeconomic circumstances, immigration history, and level of acculturation. The interplay of the multitude of cultural and social components associated with Asian identity has had a profound influence on the mental health needs of the Asian children, Asian parents' attitudes toward mental health services, and the symbolic meanings and expressions of their children's play.

Due to the diversity within Asian populations, our discussion centers on East and Southeast Asian clients; please refer to Chapter 11 on populations of the Middle East, a region that reaches Southwest Asian and North Africa (Marvasti & McKinney, 2004). We also acknowledge that the lack of discussion on the South Asian population is a limitation of this book.

Mental Health of Asian Children

Research on the mental health of young children and families within the U.S. Asian population is scarce. In the U.S., the general public may have the misconception that Asians are less likely to develop mental health issues because Asian populations (specifically Indian Americans and Filipino Americans) are doing well economically, as indicated by statistical figures (Pew Research Center, 2021b). However, the significant differences in income levels and poverty rates among Asian subgroups and the issues regarding racism, acculturation, enculturation, model minority myth, and tendency to internalize experiences highlight that treatment modalities with high sensitivity to assessing and treating internalized symptoms, such as play therapy, seem especially needed for this population. A limited number of studies have shown that Asian American youth tend to have a higher risk of suffering from depression and anxiety and having interpersonal relationship struggles as compared to their White counterparts (Brice et al., 2015; Huang et al., 2012; Huang et al., 2014). Several factors are thought to contribute to the mental health issues of Asian children, especially those whose parents have recently immigrated. These factors include limited English proficiency; low levels of social, human, and financial capital; poor living standards; and inequities associated with social status and access to social services (Huang et al., 2014; Huang et al., 2017; Rhee, 2009). Parent-child acculturation gaps, intergenerational conflict, and experiences of racial discrimination have also been thought to impede the development and psychological adjustment of Asian children (Huang et al., 2014; Wu & Lee, 2015; Zhou et al., 2012). Moreover, previous studies have demonstrated how parenting behaviors and the cultural adaptation of parents can contribute to the development of problematic or adaptive behaviors in children (e.g. Calzada et al., 2009; Capps et al., 2010; Dinh & Nguyen, 2006; Ho, 2014; Huang et al., 2017).

Cultural values have an influence on how parents interpret and respond to the behavior of their children and parent-child interactions. For instance, Asian parents whose parenting style focuses on instrumental support may spend more time providing academic assistance to their children than playing with them. In addition, Asian parents who were raised to control their own emotional expressions may demonstrate less explicit verbal and non-verbal affection towards their children. Cultural values, acculturation, and other societal determinants are factors that can often serve to either strengthen or stress the mental health of Asian children (Zhou et al., 2012).

It is important to note that the mental health risks, concerns, and needs of Asian children differ significantly among the various Asian subcultures (Leong & Lau, 2001). For example, a study showed that Chinese American youth have higher levels of social phobia than Filipino American youth, and Filipino American youth are more likely to have panic disorders, agoraphobia, and obsessive-compulsive disorder than Japanese American youth (Austin & Chorpita, 2004). In addition, while much research has focused on youth from East Asia or Southeast Asia, significantly less attention has been paid to children from South Asia (Huang et al., 2012). This research trend corresponds to the South Asia exclusion discussed above.

Cultural Considerations for Asian Populations

Given the aforementioned complexity and heterogeneity among this group, making universal cultural considerations for *all* Asian populations will be counterproductive. Therefore, in this section, we will focus on a few common threads among some Asian origin groups and their impacts on the mental health of Asian children and their families as part of cultural considerations for play therapists. Those include the model minority myth, immigration experiences, generational gaps, and misconceptions of Asian parenting.

Model Minority Myth and Its Impact on Asian Populations

I (YO) first learned the term, "model minority" in the multicultural counseling class in my graduate program. I vividly remember the mixed feelings that I bore toward this word; "model" sounded good and frankly speaking I felt even a little proud to belong to the minority group that was labeled as "model." In the meantime, it did not feel quite "right" in reflecting back my own as well as other Asian friends' struggles with life in the United States. While I was feeling puzzled with this image of Asian Americans, the Asian Americans chapter in the textbook was relatively quickly covered and we were off to the next chapter. Much later, I learned the complexity of this concept; the reason for its birth, its significantly complicated impacts on Asian population, and the fact that this seemingly positive label and stereotype awarded to this population does not give any protection from hate crimes, prejudice, and discrimination, rather it can bring harm and discrimination to them.

Model minority is a term used to describe the belief that Asians and Asian Americans have achieved economic and academic success through hard work, persistence, patience, and law-abiding attitudes; and therefore they overcame barriers of racism, oppression, and discrimination (Hartlep & Nguyen, 2017; Shih et al., 2019). Chou and Feagin (2015) noted that although the model minority term appears positive, there is a politically motivated racial framing that perpetuates the myth that because Asians and Asian Americans have transcended decades of racism by their work ethic and efforts, other minority groups must be unsuccessful based on lack of diligence rather than systemic injustice. Another issue of the model minority concept is the propagation of a monolithic picture of all Asians being successful despite the diversity within the Asian diaspora which includes vastly different hardships within this population. This politically manipulated and inaccurate image has created indelible difficulties to Asians and Asian American children and their families. One such difficulty is expectation and assumption of success which results in adverse pressure to achieve. Academic pressure and shame for not being able to preserve and perpetuate collective honor to family, community, ethnicity, etc. by failing to meet expectations is often cited as a leading contributing factor for the alarming rate of suicide among young Asian Americans.

In addition, research studies have indicated the negative systemic impact of the model minority myth on Asian children including failure of teachers to identify Asian students who are struggling (Lee, 1994), lack of referrals for Asian students to mental health services by school staff (Guo et al., 2014), and reports by Asian students of discrimination by peers based on teacher favoritism possibly motivated by the model minority myth (Benner & Graham, 2013; Qin et al., 2008; Rosenbloom & Way, 2004; Zang, 2010). The flip side of the model minority myth is an image and perception of Asian and Asian American children as "nerds," "geeks," "weak," "socially awkward," and "not good with sports," which is often exaggerated by media and leads to bullying and discrimination by peers (Qin et al., 2008; Zang, 2010).

Immigration Experience and Generational Gaps

Each Asian ethnic group has its unique origin and complex immigration history in the United States, with the earliest group beginning to arrive in the mid-1800s (Uba, 1994). Over the past 180 years, movements of Asian immigration were dependent upon the political situation in each country as well as the changes in U.S. immigration policies. While a noticeable number of Asian citizens are multiple generations removed from immigration, it is estimated that more than 85% of current U.S. Asians are either first- or second-generation Americans (Frey, 2018). Because of the differences in the history of immigration, pre-and post-migration factors, and acculturation, the psychological characteristics of children within the Asian ethnic communities may vary (Yoshikawa et al., 2016). For example, the experience of stress and anxiety experienced by children of families that immigrate as refugees or asylum-seekers may deviate from the experience of children whose parents immigrated voluntarily to seek higher education and professional mobility. Therefore, understanding the impacts of migration circumstances is a critical element in the play therapy process.

Acculturation and Enculturation

In addition to the discrimination experience, such as the model minority stereotype, Asian children who grow up in the United States encounter other cultural challenges. Asian American children are continually learning to adapt their cultural orientation to feel accepted in two or more cultures. This ongoing cultural experience can be conceptualized as a balance between *acculturation* and *enculturation*. *Acculturation* refers to Asian American children's process of assimilating to the dominant U.S. cultural norms, while the process of retaining their Asian cultural values, behaviors, knowledge, and identity can be described as *enculturation*, a term coined by Herskovitz (1948). When the adherence to one culture conflicts with the other, Asian American children and adolescents may experience a sense of confusion and incongruence (Cheung & Swank, 2019; Fuligni, 2012). The terms *intergenerational cultural dissonance* and *acculturation dissonance* are used interchangeably in the literature to describe the conflicts that arise from cultural inconsistencies between parents and children.

Intergenerational cultural dissonance was found to be a risk factor for Asian American adolescents' behavioral problems and increased adjustment problems (Choi et al., 2008; Uba, 1994; Wu & Chao, 2005). However, other researchers proposed intergenerational cultural dissonance is a normative aspect of acculturation for immigrant families (Fuligni, 2012), and it should not be generalized as an automatic cause of psychological and behavioral maladjustment. Such assumption may cause an oversight of individual differences, parent-child relationships, and acculturation process within immigrant families (Fuligni, 2012; Zhou et al., 2017). Furthermore,

Zhou and colleagues (2017) eschewed the framing of the intergenerational acculturation gap as "the conflict between individualistic and collectivistic values." They suggested this largely generalized narrative of individualistic-collectivistic dichotomy tends to reduce the diversity among various Asian cultures and value systems to a single cultural stereotype. It may even symptomize culture and the acculturation process (Zhou et al., 2017).

Misconceptions of Asian Parenting

Asian American parenting style is often conceived as a monolithic parenting approach, bearing the stereotypical notions that Asian American parents are highly controlling and less expressive in communicating warmth and affection when compared to their European American counterparts (Juang et al., 2013). Scholars and researchers challenged such stereotypical conceptions as a result of comparative research between European American samples and Asian American samples (predominantly Chinese) as one group, with limited studies that focused on capturing within-group differences (Kim et al., 2017). Additionally, the surge of media attention to the portrayal of "tiger parenting" after the publication of the memoir *Battle Hymn of the Tiger Mother* by Amy Chua (2011) further reinforced the myth that all Asian parents are extremely controlling, demanding unquestioning obedience, and value academic excellence over social-emotional wellbeing (Choi et al., 2013; Juang et al., 2013; Kim et al., 2013; Kim et al., 2017). Over the last decade, empirical researchers invested effort attempting to debunk the myth of tiger parenting through examining parenting goals and practices among various Asian groups including Chinese American parents (Cheah et al., 2013; Kim et al., 2013), Korean American parents (Choi et al., 2013), and Hmong American parents (Lamborn et al., 2013). In reviewing the findings from these studies, Juang et al. (2013) synthesized that among various Asian communities, parenting practices deviate from the tiger mother image. Although harsh, demanding, and emotionally unsupportive parenting practice exists among Asian families, it is rather uncommon. A majority of Chinese American parents were found to have high levels of parental warmth, inductive reasoning, parental monitoring, and democratic parenting, while presenting with low levels of parental hostility, psychological control, shaming, and punitive parenting. These parenting qualities are associated with the best developmental outcomes of low academic pressure, high academic achievement and attainment, and a high level of psychological adjustment (Kim et al., 2013). In Korean American families, parents value traditional Korean virtues that are positively associated with Western positive parenting constructs of warmth, acceptance, monitoring, and communication (Choi et al., 2013). Interestingly, Korean American parenting practices can be both authoritative and authoritarian. For example, Choi et al. (2013) suggested that a Korean parent might teach certain culturally appropriate behaviors and give very strict rules (therefore considered authoritarian), but at the same time, the parent might provide the rationale for their expectation in the context of parental acceptance, which eventually strengthens the parent-child relationship. Moreover, studies on Hmong American families offered new understandings of the understudied Southeast Asian population, that Hmong American adolescents perceive their parents to be supportive, loving, openly communicative, and showing warmth (Lamborn et al., 2013). Altogether, empirical inquiries among different Asian ethnic groups illustrated the nuanced conceptualizations of myriad Asian parenting practices. We encourage play therapists to respect cultural values behind Asian parenting approaches and to explore aspects that influence parenting behaviors instead of adopting a blanket definition of "Asian parenting style."

Play Therapy Considerations for Asian Populations

From a child-centered perspective, we believe play therapy offers an authentic multicultural encounter, whereby the child can play out and explore their cultural values through a relationship with the play therapist. The play therapist sees each child as a unique person who is capable and worthy and does not wish the child were different than who they are (Landreth, 2012). This fundamental philosophy offers great opportunities for Asian children to explore, express, respect, and be who they truly are.

Philosophy and Goals of Play Therapy

Child-centered play therapists hold the belief that the relationship between the play therapist and the child is the essential healing factor for children in therapy (Ray, 2011). The child-centered play therapy relationship is characterized by the play therapist's core conditions of genuineness, empathy, and unconditional positive regard for the child. When working with Asian children, the play therapist continues to trust the child's innate ability to move towards a self-enhancing being; at the same time, the therapist remains attuned and sensitive to the cultural nuances or barriers that may hinder the therapist's communication of the core conditions within the therapeutic relationship. When exploring the therapist's unconditional positive regard for an Asian client, the play therapist reflects on their own assumptions toward the definition of wellness, and checks for any biases or expectations of the child's behaviors in session.

Given the holistic nature of the child-centered approach, the therapist conceptualizes the integration of multiple aspects of an Asian child's world and considers the intersection of the child's identities. Asian children's experience of their environment and the impact of oppressive experiences on their growth and development should also be considered. Essentially, play therapists reflect on their understanding of what it is like to be the child client, who is a member of the Asian cultural community today. In addition, sensitivity to cultural barriers is seen in the play therapist's efforts to facilitate Asian children's movement toward congruence as the child struggles with acculturation and enculturation experiences. The play therapist provides a safe space for the child to experience and process inner tensions, such as feelings of anxiety, ambivalence, confusion, anger, shame, or frustration. The play therapist trusts the child's direction in resolving and integrating the experiences without the attempt to rescue. Ultimately, the play therapist's goal is to empower the child within the relationship and release the child's potential for change.

Selection of Toys and Materials

Landreth (2012) suggested that toys are selected instead of collected. The playroom provides opportunities to establish relationships; explore real-life experiences; express feelings, thoughts, and needs; test the limits of reality; enhance self-control; and develop self-understanding (Landreth 2012; Ray, 2011). When setting up a playroom, we recommend that therapists reflect on whether the materials and toys displayed in the playroom reflect the lived experiences of Asian children to such a degree that they feel a certain level of connection and the freedom to express and explore themselves. Asian children develop their identities while navigating the influences of two cultures: the Asian ethnic-specific culture preserved and practiced at home, and the American culture they are exposed to outside of the home environment. Play therapists must, therefore, consider whether the materials they present in the playroom are centered on a specific culture in such a way that they implicitly suggest that one culture is preferred over another. To intentionally create a culturally inclusive and sensitive playroom, play therapists are encouraged to explore their own expectations and assumptions regarding how children interact with toys that appear either relevant or irrelevant to their own culture. For example, should play therapists expect East Asian children to know what dumplings, chopsticks, and buns are? Should play therapists expect East Asian children to play with these specific food toys more often than with hotdogs and burgers? To what degree does the therapist allow the child to make their own meaning on the toys and how do the therapist's assumptions and own internal curiosities influence their understanding of the child's experience of play? The process of selecting toys for a culturally and ethnically diverse range of clients is not merely about the toys themselves – it involves the therapist's continued self-exploration. Moreover, when the play therapist intends to create a playroom that is culturally inclusive, it would be imperative to reflect on the therapist's rationale of the selections to avoid stereotyping. For example, is a Ninja outfit spontaneously relatable for a Japanese child client or is this selection a byproduct of the commercialization of Japanese culture in the U. S. which leads to more stereotypes and biases? We encourage the therapist to be transparent when they are not sure how to include culturally specific toys in the room or whether a specific toy is appropriate and helpful, and to be open to initiating a genuine conversation in parent consultation to learn from parents/caregivers' perspectives. For a thorough discussion of how to create a culturally sensitive playroom for children from diverse cultural backgrounds, please refer to Chapter 15.

Cultural Opportunities

It is impossible to list exactly how and when cultural opportunities emerge in play therapy with Asian children because it depends on many factors such as depth of the relationship between a child and a play therapist, a child's and a therapist's cultural identity development, and sociopolitical issues of the time. We list some of the examples of cultural opportunities that we have experienced working with Asian children in the hope of providing moments to play therapists to hone their awareness of cultural opportunities in play therapy.

Language

One of the first cultural opportunities that may arise in play therapy is a child's selection of language. For Asian children who are English Language Learners (ELL) and/or speak a language other than English at home, their limited English fluency or speaking English with a non-standard American accent may possess a risk of perpetuating a "forever foreigner" status. In addition, their lack of English or English proficiency can be seen as a sign of failure or unwillingness to acculturate and it may result in a source of harassment, mockery, and bullying (Qin et al., 2008). When I (YO) first met a Japanese child client who was internationally adopted by White parents in the U.S., I remembered the adoptive mother had shared during the intake session that the language barrier had been difficult for both of them and the mother wished him to maintain his Japanese roots and heritage. Based on this conversation, I introduced myself to him in Japanese when I met him for the first time at the waiting room, "Hazimemashite. Watashi no namae ha Yumi desu. (Nice meeting you. My name is Yumi)." I remember his face filled with stifled anger, and he said, "English, please!" although his English proficiency was close to none at that point. I felt the sense of urgency in him and quickly switched to English. We left the waiting room which was filled with many other children and their families, and when we turned the corner on the hallway, he stopped and looked at me saying, "Nihongo de hanasite… (Japanese, please…)." This was a learning experience which brought some realization and awareness to me. I failed to tame my excitement to work with a Japanese child, I made a premature assumption that being able to speak in his native language would bring some relief to him, and I was ignorant to the fact that for some bicultural children, which language to speak in at what situation can be a survival decision.

Oftentimes, bicultural children maintain the tendency to switch between cultural frames depending on the setting and employ decisions that fit with the environment they are in. Instead of amalgamating two distinctive cultural frames, they keep them separated and shift between to situationally assimilate. This tendency can be accentuated in Asian children who live in a household where family members communicate in their native language, who go to "Saturday school" which focuses on children's maintenance or acquisition of native language and cultural heritage, and who adhere to cultural practices in the house and in the community. This shift may occur even during a play therapy session, especially when a play therapist and a child have different cultural backgrounds. And yet, the shift is a cultural opportunity that a play therapist should be aware of and possibly reflect upon. I wish I could go back to the moment and respond to him, "It is very important for you to decide when and where to speak Japanese or English… I will follow what you decide."

Action Speaks Louder

In our discussion of Asian cultures, phrases such as "不言実行" (Japanese) and "盡在不言中" (Cantonese) came up. These phrases convey a similar message to "actions speak louder than words" and this idea is sometimes infused into Asian parenting. Some Asian parents may show their love through actions such as cooking and creating or purchasing what their children want or need rather than explicitly and verbally expressing their love by saying, "I love you." This action is based on parents' keen attunement to children's needs, and it is simply one form of expressing their love. Asian children growing up as recipients of such forms of affection may display their fondness toward a play therapist and play therapy in more play or action-oriented ways, such as pretending to cook the therapist's favorite meal or creating art and craft as a gift for a play therapist instead of saying "I like you" and "I love you." Play therapists are adept with listening to and understanding the language of play. Instead of seeing this gesture as shyness or a lack of connection, play therapists should be attuned to the intention and the message behind such play and respond to it accordingly.

Returning Responsibility

Returning responsibility is a therapeutic response that aims to facilitate a child's decision-making ability. It allows the child to take the lead, be independent, and be responsible for the decisions they make in the moment (Landreth, 2012). However, the empowering processes associated with the returning responsibility response may create discomfort and stress for Asian children. Demonstrating obedience and respect to authority figures is a cultural practice that has been adopted by many Asian groups (e.g. Kim & Choi, 1994; Tajima & Harachi, 2010). As members of this hierarchical structure, Asian children are expected to conform and be polite. Consequently, during play therapy, an Asian child new to the therapeutic relationship may wait for the therapist to show them what to play and how to play.

I (YC) had an opportunity to work with a seven-year-old Chinese American child. During the first session, I began by saying, "This is our playroom, and you can play with the toys in a lot of ways you would like" (Landreth, 2012). She stood there, twisted her hands, and looked at me without initiating any movements. I attended to her feelings and reflected, "You seem nervous because it is a new place for you." I stayed silent and observed keenly, hoping that giving her some space and time would help her figure out how to play. A few minutes passed, and she still stood there. She looked at me and appeared to be lost. I said, "It seems like you are not sure what to do and wish I can give you some ideas. In here, you can decide what you want to do, in a lot of different ways you want." She looked at me and responded in a polite and firm tone of voice: "Can you tell me what to play?" I replied, "You are really not sure how to start playing by yourself, and it is important for you that I tell you what to do." Not surprisingly, it took this child a few sessions to realize and adjust to the structure of a playroom that consistently conveys the following message: "In here, it is something you can decide."

The child's expressions of uncertainty could be attributed to the new environment and struggles with autonomy and decision-making. However, settling only for such an interpretation of the scenario risks missing an opportunity to advance cultural sensitivity and understanding. I understood the child's reluctance to play as more than just an instance of discomfort due to unfamiliarity, a common occurrence across all play therapy. It was a cultural moment in which the child genuinely showed her respect for me, a professional and authoritative figure. I also sensed the internal conflict taking place within the child, whose cultural teachings appeared to clash with how I operated, from a CCPT orientation. As I worked to acclimate the child to the playroom, I strived to understand and appreciate the message that the child was sharing with me: "I don't feel comfortable taking the lead right now because it is more important for me to show my respect by following your direction."

It was not an example demonstrating how a child is incapable of self-direction. Rather, it was a moment where the child was adhering to learned cultural values by choosing to be compliant and be her genuine self when embarking on a new relationship. Acknowledging and reflecting this cultural part of the child is essential in conveying acceptance. Instead of making suggestions and being directive, which might be more comfortable for the child and myself, returning responsibility back to the child could be more empowering and facilitative of her experience that I, the therapist, am not an authority figure that she needs to obey. Sometimes it may also be helpful if the play therapist modifies the wording of returning responsibility to meet where the child is culturally by incorporating encouragement or collaboration. For example, "In here, it is something you can *try* to decide," or "In here, you can let me know how we can figure it out together."

Working with Families

Play therapists recognize the importance of including parents and caregivers as significant partners in the therapy process. We believe that increased understanding of the roles and involvement of parents and caregivers may enhance positive therapeutic support for the client (Landreth, 2012; Ray, 2011). Therefore, we focus on the considerations to establish and maintain a collaborative relationship with Asian families.

Recognizing Diversity of Asian Families

Landreth (2012) emphasized the importance for play therapists to remain aware and sensitive to the complexity of family dynamics in current society. This is no exception when working with Asian families. As a matter of fact, the demographic of the Asian population is rapidly changing and diversifying. The family structure and role of parents/caregivers vary within and between Asian ethnic groups of different immigration history and social economic status. Although the majority of Asian American families were shown to be "traditional" households of two parents in the census data, disaggregated data indicated that children from some Asian groups were more likely to grow up in single-parent families when compared to non-Hispanic White children (Asian American Foundation, 2014). The heterogeneity among Asian groups calls for the play therapist's attention to the underrepresentation among some Asian groups and seeks to understand the personal experience of each Asian child client within the home environment. Additionally, grandparents' care is the most common childcare option among Asian preschoolers with a working mother (AAF, 2014). Multigenerational households are also more common among some Asian groups such as Bhutanese and Cambodians (Pew Research Center, 2021b). Therefore, understanding the perspective of significant caregivers other than biological parents, such as grandparents, can enhance the play therapy process for Asian children.

Nevertheless, the therapeutic needs for Asian children growing up in adoptive families cannot be overstated. Currently, in the U.S., the majority of Asian adoptions are interracial adoptions where neither parent was the same ethnic group as the adoptee, exceptions were found among Filipino and Indian groups, where adoptees were adopted by families with at least one parent of the same ethnicity (AAF, 2014). When working with Asian transracial adoptive families, play therapists seek competency training in understanding the unique family processes and parent-child relationships as well as acquiring advanced skills required to promote wellness within the family.

Building Rapport with Asian Parents and Caregivers

Landreth (2012) proposed that "Any effort by the play therapist to be helpful to children must begin with consideration for parameters of the relationship to be established with the parent" (p. 125). Research also suggested the association between the perception of working alliance and positive counseling experiences among Asian clients in the U.S. (Kim et al., 2009). When working with Asian parents and caregivers, play therapists operate with cultural sensitivity and humility, and strive to maintain therapeutic rapport that is signified by empathic understanding and unconditional positive regard.

The Initial Contact

Generally, the very first thing we learn about our client is their name. Naming is of astonishing importance in any culture and naming conventions vary across different cultures. Among Asian communities in the U.S., some parents pick a Westernized first name for their children while some choose to adhere to their Asian heritage when it comes to naming. Because of the linguistic, religious, and other cultural differences, the meaning of Asian names can be abstruse to the people who do not share the same cultural origin and language. Sadly, names in Asian languages often lose their significance when being phonetically transcribed to English. In working with families coming from various Asian cultures, I (RC) found that inviting parents to share the naming process of their children often provided wonderful opportunities to increase my empathic understanding of parents' love and wishes for their children. The creation of the child's name, be it Western or Asian, may involve respect for family members, community leaders, or the name may carry spiritual or cultural meanings. Many parents naturally unfold significant events related to the child's developmental history or some early parenting experiences as they recount the decision-making of their child's name. These recollections provide play therapists with a glimpse of the family dynamics and their cultural expectations. By making the effort to learn the child's name and the story behind it, play therapists show respect to the parent's and child's culture, prize the uniqueness of the child, and establish a more personalized relationship with the child and the parent.

Play therapists may feel nervous about the articulation of a client's name not in their native tongue. Myself being trilingual (RC), I worry about it too, when I come across a client's name that is unfamiliar to me. Usually, I approach my clients with honesty by admitting that "I'm not sure how to pronounce your name" and ask for clarification. I also find it helpful to consult a colleague who is familiar with the specific ethnic group I work with, or to look up name pronunciations on the internet. For children who have both Asian and Western names, I ask for their preference of how to be called. Unless my client invited me to, I do not shorten their name or use a nickname in play therapy sessions.

The Dynamic of Parent–Therapist Relationship

I (YC) have worked with and supervised students working with parents from East Asian countries and have observed how families embrace Asian cultural values and adapt to Western culture to varying degrees. In some Asian ethnic groups, therapists are viewed as professionals with authority who are shown respect by parents (Kao, 2005; Sue & Sue, 2016). For example, in China, play therapists are often called teachers by the child client and the parents/caregivers. Given the dynamic nature of the relationship between parents/caregivers and therapists, play therapists need to be careful about how they approach and maintain their relationships with parents/caregivers. They should do so in a way that facilitates mutual respect and stresses the importance of sharing responsibilities. Play therapists must also be considerate when it comes to delivering information in parent consultation. In particular, they must keep in mind that they are likely to be highly regarded by Asian parents, so their evaluations, suggestions, and feedback need to be carefully supported by comprehensive observation, sound clinical judgment, and appropriate evidence to ensure their credibility.

Due to the high level of respect Asian parents may have for the play therapist and the therapist's expertise, some Asian parents may be less likely to directly express their own opinions or may assume a less active role in the therapy process. They may operate from the following mindset: "I trust the therapist, and they can decide for me and my child." The therapist may mistakenly interpret this as an attitude of indifference or an unwillingness to put effort into the situation. Therefore, having an open conversation about this in parent consultation to discuss parents' roles in play therapy, to convey how their opinions are valuable, and to help them understand the importance of collaboration is essential.

Alignment of Parents' Expectations in Play Therapy

The emphasis on education and strict discipline as the means to achieve optimal child development is prevalent among Asian cultures. Parents/caregivers who share this belief may hold some level of reservation in play therapy – a therapeutic modality that encourages children to express and explore self through play. Some of the Asian parents I (YC) worked with have expected play therapy to be more educational. Some parents expressed worries about their child's academic performance after continuing play therapy for a period of time, despite the fact that none of their initial concerns were related to their child's academic performance. Therefore, it is paramount that the play therapist continues to explore parents' perception of their child's problems, identify parental concerns and treatment goals, and discuss how play therapy can be supportive of the specific issues throughout ongoing parent consultations.

It may be particularly helpful to discuss the connection between social and emotional wellness and academic engagement when working with Asian parents. By emphasizing that meeting children's emotional needs helps them fully engage with academic instruction and the learning environment, many concerns can be assuaged (e.g. Blanco et al., 2012; Blanco et al., 2017; Perryman et al., 2020). In addition, helping Asian parents become familiar with the purpose and processes of play therapy through communicating the anticipated length of play therapy and method of progress evaluation are other ways to align parent expectations in therapy.

Ongoing Parent Support

Play therapists continue to collaborate with Asian parents in parent consultations to help them develop more positive parenting skills and enhance the parent–child relationship. Play therapists may refer to Ray's (2011) parent consultation model for the steps of moving parent consultation into parent education (p. 155–166). Moreover, in recognizing the cultural value of *Filial Piety*, a virtue that emphasizes family coherence as seen in a child's devotion and care for their parents, and the parent's obligation to love and educate the child, play therapists may consider utilizing filial therapy models, such as Child-Parent Relationship Therapy (CPRT; Landreth & Bratton, 2020) with Asian families. CPRT empowers the parents/caregivers' contribution to their children's wellbeing by teaching them therapeutic skills during special play times in the home environment. The emphasis of parental involvement in CPRT appears to be responsive to the Asian cultural values which honors the importance of kinship and child-parent bond (Sheely-Moore et al., 2020).

Working with Systems

When finding ways to provide play therapy to Asian children, it is critically important to recognize the stigma associated with seeking mental health services in many Asian communities. Studies have shown that Asians tend to perceive individuals with psychological struggles as being sick, weak, crazy, or even dangerous (Hwang, 2016). Seeking mental health care can bring about embarrassment or loss of face to the family. These harsh consequences have caused mental health services to be underutilized by many Asian communities (Hwang, 2016; Spencer et al., 2010). Research studies also revealed that internalized model minority myth and the Asian cultural value of emotional self-control are uniquely associated with a poor help-seeking attitude among Asian American college students (Kim & Lee, 2014; Shahid, et al., 2021). If discouraging help-seeking behavior toward emotional support is common among Asian American college students, one can easily imagine that Asian American parents may exhibit hesitancy toward seeking mental health services for their own children. Furthermore, disparities in insurance coverage may serve as an additional barrier to mental health services for the Asian population. Despite the fact that overall Asian Americans were found to have the lowest uninsured rate (7.9%) among all racial groups in 2017–2018 after the implementation of the Affordable Care Act (ACA), an inconsistency existed within this diverse group may continue to create challenges to accessing mental health services across all Asian ethnic groups.

Advocacy in Schools

Within school systems, Asian children were found to encounter vulnerabilities such as disparities in discipline and suspension (Nguyen et al., 2019), overrepresentation in speech and language impairments, and underrepresentation in special education (Coalition for Asian American Children and Families [CACF], 2021). In a state-wide study, Asian students were found to be about half as likely to be disciplined as their White peers when all Asian samples were aggregated. However, Southeast Asian subgroups (e. g. Cambodian, Laotian) were found to be three to five times more likely to be disciplined than the East Asian subgroups (e.g. Chinese, Taiwanese). The disparity among Asian students further supports that some Asian subgroups face significant structural barriers in educational settings and their needs are likely to be overlooked or disregarded when Asian children are seen as a monolithic ethnic group (Nguyen et al., 2019). Based on the review of educational data in New York, Asian Pacific American students are found to be more likely to be diagnosed with speech or language impairments than their peers, even though they are consistently underrepresented of those receiving special education services.

Play therapists uphold the professional and ethical standards of advocacy and seek to remove barriers and obstacles that inhibit clients' access, growth, and development (ACA, 2014, Section A.7.a.). Whether in school settings or private practice, play therapists identify Asian children's barriers to growth, such as lack of academic resources, limited language proficiency, and recognize that academic achievement and mental health are interconnected. Play therapists also need to be aware of the unrealistic expectations of perfectionism or internalized model minority myth among Asian students, which may manifest as internalizing symptoms. Inspired by the recommendations made by CACF (2021), play therapists can advocate for Asian children to promote equity in the school system at different levels. On a microlevel, play therapists can advocate for individual Asian child clients through making referrals for psycho-educational assessment and speech assessment to ensure their educational needs are properly identified and met. Moreover, with the professional knowledge in child development, play therapists work with teachers and administrators to: (a) help them distinguish between language acquisition and special education needs, (b) connect

Asian students to relevant service providers or resources, such as language tutoring, ESL programs, or speech therapy, (c) identify students who present with internalizing or externalizing problems, and (d) provide timely social-emotional support through play therapy. On a meso level, advocacy within the school system may involve removing the barriers to accessing mental health concerns. First of all, play therapists should survey parents' attitudes regarding mental health services and the mental health needs of Asian children within specific communities to avoid overgeneralization. Play therapists are encouraged to collaborate with school counselors and school psychologists in order to educate teachers, parents, and families about the factors influencing the mental health of children. These factors include developmental stages, contextual barriers and resources, cultural adaptation levels, and parenting styles. It can also be helpful to reach out to the principals of local schools and the directors of childcare providers in order to build relationships and discuss ways to promote mental health awareness within Asian families.

Advocacy in the Community

Educating the community about the benefits of play therapy in improving social, emotional, behavioral, and academic concerns of children is vital. When introducing the idea of play therapy to the community, it can be helpful to highlight the theoretical orientations that are evidence-based, and to emphasize that play therapy is empirically supported by multiple studies to be beneficial for Asian children who struggle with a variety of concerns. At the same time, it is imperative for play therapists to validate community members' concerns about mental health services and provide support for parents to work through their own struggles related to acculturation and managing the parental stress. In addition, involving local Asian community centers in the process of de-stigmatizing therapy can be useful. One way to do this is by providing workshops and information sessions aimed at supporting the mental health of children and improving parenting practices. Such workshops and sessions will allow play therapists to engage Asian families and build trust. Given that some Asians tend to communicate mental distress by expressing somatic symptoms (Hwang, 2016), partnering with local pediatricians to enhance parents' understandings of childhood mental health may be another potential avenue for bringing mental health services to the Asian population.

Chang et al. (2014) suggested that one of the factors that hindered Asian clients to seek out mental health services was due to cultural issues such as lack of bicultural and bilingual providers. This posits the need for more Asian play therapists, as well as translators or interpreters in clinical settings. To overcome language barriers, play therapy clinics may consider providing bilingual flyers and clinical documents for Asian parents and caregivers, which may mitigate their hesitancy to seek play therapy services within an unfamiliar clinical setting.

Above all, we encourage all play therapists and mental health professionals who identify as Asian or have served the Asian population to professionally and meaningfully share your experiences or reflections on your professional website or blog (without breaking confidentiality, of course), with the goal to de-stigmatize mental health issues within the Asian community, and to facilitate more dialogues related to the mental health strengths and struggles of different Asian ethnic groups. We would also like to encourage play therapists to intentionally facilitate those conversations by presenting at a national or state conferences on Asian children and families; attend workshops or webinars on serving Asians; or initiate small group discussion focusing on this population within your state branch of the Association for Play therapy or at your workplace. Speaking up for the Asian community and helping each other challenge our own biases, attitudes, and stereotypes towards Asian population are the most crucial tasks that necessitate continued attention and work within the system. Such ongoing advocacy also serves as the foundation to facilitating changes for the overall wellbeing of the Asian population.

Conclusion

We (Yi, Regine, and Yumi) have recognized that our individual cultural identities, levels of acculturation, and lived experiences as Asians both consciously and unconsciously impact the messages we convey in this chapter. As has been previously emphasized, "Asian" is an umbrella term for a racial group that includes heterogenous and distinct subgroups. It should never be seen or understood as a single category or race. Similarly, it is not our goal to present a fixed framework or guideline for working with all Asian children and families in play therapy. Rather, it is our hope that our narratives can inspire more curiosity, questions, and dialogue between play therapists and the clients they serve. We also hope that this chapter will motivate the mental health community to pay more attention to the mental health needs of South Asian children and families as well as continue to advocate for equitable mental health services for the Asian community.

We would like to present Regine's positionality in the following section and please refer to the introduction of this book for Yi and Yumi's positionality.

Positionality Statement

Regine

As an Asian play therapist from Hong Kong, my cultural status changed from being a part of the dominant culture (native-born, ethnic Chinese, and permanent resident) to a member of the minority culture (foreign-born, non-White, and non-citizen). Being a foreigner, a cultural barrier I often encounter is the lack of cultural references. A colleague once shared with me an exciting play therapy breakthrough with her client who was nonverbal in sessions. Through painting a fictional character, the Grinch, this client was able to relate and process their feelings of loneliness and insecurity that they had never spoken about. At first, I was not sure how my colleague made the connection; it was through understanding the backstory of the Grinch's upbringing that I discovered the abandonment and bullying that the Grinch experienced was something that the client identified with. This missing puzzle of cultural reference has become a reminder for me since then. By recognizing my limited understanding, I became more motivated to learn about my clients' unique cultural background and I am more attentive to the nonverbal communications and my client's present being. Over time, my limitations in "not-knowing" made me more sensitive to nuanced growth as well as disruptions within play sessions.

Reflecting on my development, I feel grateful for my clients who allowed me to enter their world and shared their vulnerabilities with me. I am especially thankful for the authentic cultural interactions that occurred in our relationships. After a play session, on the way back to the classroom, my nine-year-old White client took me to a multicultural mural by the school entrance and asked me to identify any landmark I recognize from home. My heart is warmed by this client's desire to connect with me because of who I am, and the opportunity for a genuine multicultural relationship. When my five-year-old biracial client spent sessions combing my brown straight hair, she began to tell me about the differences between her dark curly hair and her mother's blonde straight hair, her brother's white skin, and her grandmother's dark skin. Brushing my hair, that is somewhat "in-between," seemed to facilitate her processes of confusion related to her cultural identity. These clients not only affirmed my trust in the healing power of a relationship but they also taught me that racial differences are not disadvantageous. In the beginning, I saw my ethnic minority status as a shortcoming to my professional therapeutic work. Now, I recognize it as a privilege that I am able to offer a cultural exchange experience to my clients.

I really appreciate the opportunity to contribute to this chapter with Yi and Yumi. I genuinely hope this chapter helps readers adopt a new perspective in learning about Asian cultural identities; and finally, I hope to share some encouragement to my fellow Asian play therapists. Embrace the unique dimensions we bring into the relationship with each and every client we serve.

References

American Counseling Association (2014). 2014 ACA code of ethics. www.counsel ing.org/docs/default-source/default-document-library/2014-code-of-ethics-finala ddress.pdf.

Aratani, Y., & Liu, C. H. (2015). English proficiency, threshold language policy and mental health service utilization among Asian-American children. *Archives of Psychiatric Nursing*, 29, 326–332. doi:10.1016/j.apnu.2015.06.006.

Asian American Foundation (2014). The State of Asian American Children. www.aa federation.org/doc/AAF_StateofAsianAmericanChildren.pdf.

Austin, A. A., & Chorpita, B. F. (2004). Temperament, anxiety, and depression: Comparisons across five ethnic groups of children. *Journal of Clinical Child and Adolescent Psychology*, 33(2), 216–226. doi:10.1207/s15374424jccp3302_2.

Benner, A. D., & Graham, S. (2013). The antecedent and consequences of racial/ethnic discrimination during adolescence: Does the source of discrimination matter? *Developmental Psychology*, 49, 1602–1613. doi:10.1037/a0030557.

Blanco, P. J., Ray, D. C., & Holliman, R. (2012). Long-term child centered play therapy and academic achievement of children: A follow-up study. *International Journal of Play Therapy*, 21, 1–13. doi:10.1037/a0026932.

Blanco, P. J., Holliman, R. P., Muro, J. H., Toland, S., & Farnam, J. L. (2017). Long term child-centered play therapy effects on academic achievement with normal functioning children. *Journal of Child and Family Studies*, 26(7), 1915–1922. doi:10.1007/s10826-017-0701-0.

Brice, C., Warner, C. M., Okazaki, S., Ma, P. W., Sanchez, A., Esseling, P., & Lynch, C. (2015). Social anxiety and mental health service use among Asian American high school students. *Child Psychiatry Hum Dev*, 46, 693–701. doi:10.1007/s10578-014-0511-1.

Calzada, E. J., Brotman, L. M., Huang, K., Bat-Chava, Y., & Kingston, S. (2009). Parent cultural adaptation and child functioning in culturally diverse, urban families of preschoolers. *Journal of Applied Developmental Psychology*, 30(4), 515–524. doi:10.1016/j.appdev.2008.12.033.

Capps, R. C., Bronte-Tinkew, J., & Horowitz, A. (2010). Acculturation and father engagement with infants among Chinese and Mexican-origin immigrant fathers. *Fathering*, 8(1), 61–92. doi:10.3149/fth.0801.61.

Chang, C. Y., McDonald, C. P., & O' Hara, C., *et al.* (2014). Counseling clients from Asian and Pacific Island Heritages. In M. J. Ratts & P. B. Pedersen, (Eds.), *Counseling for multiculturalism and social justice: integration, theory, and application* (4th ed., pp. 127–142). Wiley.

Cheah, C. S. L., Leung, C. Y. Y., & Zhou, N. (2013). Understanding "tiger parenting" through the perceptions of Chinese immigrant mothers: Can Chinese and U.S. parenting coexist? *Asian American Journal of Psychology*, 4(1), 30–40. doi:10.1037/a0031217.

Cheung, C. W. & Swank, J. M. (2019). Asian American identity development: A bicultural model for youth. *Journal of Child and Adolescent Counseling*, 5(1), 89–101. doi:10.1080/23727810.2018.1556985.

Choi, Y., He, M., & Harachi, T. W. (2008). Intergenerational cultural dissonance, parent-child conflict and bonding, and youth problem behaviors among Vietnamese and Cambodian immigrant families. *Journal of Youth and Adolescence*, 37(1), 85–96. doi:10.1007/s10964-007-9217-z.

Choi, Y., Kim, Y. S., Kim, S. Y., & Park, I. J. K. (2013). Is Asian American parenting controlling and harsh? Empirical testing of relationships between Korean American and Western parenting measures. *Asian American Journal of Psychology*, 4(1), 19–29. doi:10.1037/a0031220.

Chou, R. S., & Feagin, J. R. (2015). *Myth of the model minority: Asian Americans facing racism* (2nd ed.). Routledge.

Chua, A. (2011). *Battle hymn of the tiger mother*. Penguin Books.

Coalition for Asian American Children and Families (2021). Asian Pacific Americans for educational equity: Values and policy recommendations. https://static1.squarespace.com/static/5f36d65bb133d41b244bc521/t/607f4aa5be884b677dacb3e0/1618954920729/Education+Equity.pdf.

Colby, S. L., & Ortman, J. M. (2015). Projections of the size and composition of the U.S. population: 2014 to 2060. U.S. Census Bureau. www.census.gov/content/dam/Census/library/publications/2015/demo/p25-1143.pdf.

Department of Labor (1965). *Moynihan Report: The Negro family: The Case for national action.* Office of Policy Planning and Research.

Dinh, K. T., & Nguyen, H. H. (2006). The effects of acculturative variables on Asian American parent–child relationships. *Journal of Social and Personal Relationships,* 23(3), 407–426. doi:10.1177/0265407506064207.

Frey, W. H. (2018). *Diversity explosion: How new racial demographics are remaking America.* Brookings Institution Press.

Fuligni, A. J. (2012). Gaps, conflicts, and arguments between adolescents and their parents. *U.S. New Directions for Child and Adolescent Development,* 135, 105–110. https://doi.org/10.1002/cd.20006.

Gourney, L. (2001). Child-centered play therapy. *International Journal of Play Therapy,* 10(2), 13–31.

Guo, S., Kataoka, S. H., Bear, L., & Lau, A. S. (2014). Differences in school-based referrals for mental health care: Understanding racial/ethnic disparities between Asian American and Latino youth. *School Mental Health,* 6, 27–39. doi:10.1007/s12310-013-9108-2.

Gunha, M. Z., Baumgartner, J. C.., Shah, A., Radley, D. C., & Collins, S. R. (2020). Gap closed: The Affordable Care Act's impact on Asian Americans' health coverage. The Commonwealth Fund. www.commonwealthfund.org/publications/issue-briefs/2020/jul/gap-closed-aca-impact-asian-american-coverage.

Hartlep, N. D., & Nguyen, K. T. (2017). How the model minority stereotype creates moments of (in)visibility. In D. Ball & N. D. Hartlep (Eds.), *Asian/Americans, education and crime: The model minority as victim and perpetrator* (pp. 101–117). Lexington Books.

Herskovitz, M. J. (1948). *Man and his works: The science of cultural anthropology.* Knopf.

Ho, G. W. K. (2014). Acculturation and its implications on parenting for Chinese immigrants: A systematic review. *Journal of Transcultural Nursing,* 25(2), 145–158. doi:10.1177/1043659613515720.

Huang, K.-Y., Calzada, E., Cheng, S., & Brotman, L. M. (2012). Physical and mental health disparities among young children of Asian immigrants. *The Journal of Pediatrics,* 160, 331–336. doi:10.1016/j.jpeds.2011.08.005.

Huang, K.-Y., Calzada, E., Kamboukos, D., Rhule, D., Sharma, K. C., Cheng, S., & Brotman, L. M. (2014). Applying public health frameworks to advance the promotion of mental health among Asian American children. *Asian American Journal of Psychology,* 5(2), 145–152. doi:10.1037/a0036185.

Huang, K.-Y., Calzada, E., Cheng, S., Barajas-Gonzalez, R., & Brotman, L. M. (2017). Cultural adaptation, parenting and child mental health among English speaking Asian American immigrant families. *Child Psychiatry and Human Development,* 48(4), 572–583. doi:10.1007/s10578-016-0683-y.

Hwang, W. (2016). *Culturally adapting psychotherapy for Asian heritage populations: An evidence-based approach.* Academic Press.

Juang, L. P., Qin, D. B., & Park, I. J. K. (2013). Deconstructing the myth of the "tiger mother": An introduction to the special issue on tiger parenting, Asian-heritage families, and child/adolescent well-being. *Asian American Journal of Psychology,* 4(1), 1–6. doi:10.1037/a0032136.

Kao, S. (2005). Play therapy with Asian children. In E. Gil & A. A. Drewes (Eds.), *Cultural issues in play therapy* (pp. 180–193). Guilford Press.

Kawabata, Y., Crick, N. R. (2013). Relational and physical aggression, peer victimization, and adjustment problems in Asian American and European American children. *Asian American Journal of Psychology*, 4(3), 211–216. doi:10.1037/a0031205.

Kim, B. S. K., Ng, G. F., & Ahn, A. J. (2009). Client adherence to Asian cultural values, common factors in counseling, and session outcome with Asian American Clients at a university counseling center. *Journal of Counseling & Development*, 87(2) 131–142. doi:10.1002/j.1556-6678.2009.tb00560.x.

Kim, B. S. K., Yang, P. H., Atkinson, D. R., Wolfe, M. M., & Hong, S. (2001). Cultural value similarities and differences among Asian American ethnic groups. *Cultural Diversity and Ethnic Minority Psychology*, 7(4), 343–361, doi:10.1037/1099-9809.7.4.343.

Kim, P. Y., & Lee, D. (2014). Internalized model minority myth, Asian values, and help-seeking attitudes among Asian American students. *Cultural Diversity and Ethnic Minority Psychology* 20(1), 98–106. doi:10.1037/a0033351.

Kim, S. Y., Wang, Y., Orozco-Lapray, D., Shen, Y., & Murtuza, M. (2013). Does "tiger parenting" exist? Parenting profiles of Chinese Americans and adolescent developmental outcomes. *Asian American journal of psychology*, 4(1), 7–18. doi:10.1037/a0030612.

Kim, S. Y., Chen, S., Sim, L., & Hou, Y. (2017). Stability and change in parenting and adjustment profiles across early, middle and late adolescence in Chinese American families. In Y. Choi & H. C. Hahm (Eds.), *Asian American parenting: Family process and intervention* (pp. 69–88). Springer.

Kim, U., & Choi, S. (1994). Individualism, collectivism, and child development: A Korean perspective. In P. M. Greenfield and R. R. Cocking (Eds.), *Cross-cultural roots of minority child development* (pp. 227–257). Lawrence Erlbaum.

Lamborn, S. D., Nguyen, J., & Bocanegra, J. O. (2013). Hmong American adolescents' perceptions of mothers' parenting practices: Support, authority, and intergenerational agreement. *Asian American Journal of Psychology*, 4(1), 50–60. doi:10.1037/a0031045.

Landreth, G. L. (2012). *Play therapy: The art of the relationship* (3rd ed.). Routledge.

Landreth, G., & Bratton, S. (2020). *Child-Parent Relationship Therapy: An evidence-based 10-session filial therapy model* (2nd ed.). Routledge.

Lee, J., & Ramakrishnan, K. (2020). Who counts as Asian. *Ethnic and Racial Studies*, 43(10), 1733–1756. doi:10/1080/01419870.2019.1671600.

Lee, S. J. (1994). Behind the model-minority stereotype: Voices of high- and low-achieving Asian American students. *Anthropology & Education Quarterly*, 25, 413–429.

Leong, F. T., & Lau, A. S. (2001). Barriers to providing effective mental health services to Asian Americans. *Ment Health Serv Res*, 3(4), 201–214. doi:10.1023/a:1013177014788.

Marvasti, A. & McKinney, K. D. (2004). *Middle Eastern lives in America*. Rowman & Littlefield.

Nguyen, B. M. D., Noguera, P., Adkins, N., & Teranishi, R. T. (2019). Ethnic discipline gap: Unseen dimensions of racial disproportionality in school discipline. *American Education Research Journal*, 56(5), 1973–2003.

Perryman, K. L., Robinson, S., Bowers, L., & Massengale, B. (2020). Child-centered play therapy and academic achievement: A prevention-based model. *International Journal of Play Therapy*, 29(2), 104–117. doi:10.1037/pla0000117.

Pew Research Center (2021a). Asian Americans are the fastest growing racial or ethnic group in the U.S. www.pewresearch.org/fact-tank/2021/04/09/asian-americans-are-the-fastest-growing-racial-or-ethnic-group-in-the-u-s.

Pew Research Center (2021b). Key facts about Asian origin groups in the U.S. www.pewresearch.org/fact-tank/2021/04/29/key-facts-about-asian-origin-groups-in-the-u-s.

Qin, D. B., Way, N., & Rana, M. (2008). The "model minority" and their discontent: Examining peer discrimination and harassment of Chinese American immigrant youth. *New Directions for Child and Adolescent Development, 2008*(121), 27–42. doi:10.1002/cd.221.

Ray, D. C. (2011). *Advanced play therapy: Essential conditions, knowledge, and skills for child practice*. Routledge.

Rhee, S. (2009) The impact of immigration and acculturation on the mental health of Asian Americans: Overview of epidemiology and clinical implications. In N. H. Trinh, Y. C. Rho, F. G. Lu, & K. M. Sanders (Eds.), *Handbook of mental health and acculturation in Asian American families* (pp. 81–98). Humana Press. doi:10.1007/978-1-60327-437-1_5.

Rosenbloom, S. R., & Way, N. (2004). Experiences of discrimination among African American, Asian American, and Latino adolescents in an urban high school. *Youth & Society*, 35, 420–451. doi:10.1177/0044118X03261479.

Shahid, M., Weiss, N. H., Stoner, G., Dewsbury, B. (2021). Asian Americans' mental health help-seeking attitudes: The relative and unique roles of cultural values and ethnic identity. *Asian American Journal of Psychology*, 12(2), 138–146. doi:10.1037/aap0000230.

Sheely-Moore, A. I., Ceballos, P., Lin, W-W. D., & Ogawa, Y. (2020). Culturally responsive CPRT. In G. L. Landreth & S. C. Bratton, *Child-Parent Relationship Therapy (CPRT): An evidence-based 10-session filial therapy model* (2nd ed., pp. 431–443). Routledge.

Shih, K. Y., Chang, T., & Chen, S. (2019). Model minority myth on Asian American individuals and families: Social justice and critical race feminist perspectives. *Journal of Family Theory & Review*, 11, 412–428. doi:10.1111/jftr.12342.

Spencer, M. S., Chen, J., Gee, G. C., Fabian, C. G., & Takeuchi, D. T. (2010). Discrimination and mental health-related service use in a national study of Asian Americans. *American Journal of Public Health*, 100(12), 2410–2417. doi:10.2105/AJPH.2009.176321.

Substance Abuse and Mental Health Services Administration (2015). Racial/ethnic differences in mental health service use among adults. https://store.samhsa.gov/sites/default/files/d7/priv/sma15-4906.pdf.

Sue, D. W., & Sue, D. (2016). *Counseling the culturally diverse: Theory and practice* (7th ed.). Wiley.

Tajima, E. A., & Harachi, T. W. (2010). Parenting beliefs and physical discipline practices among Southeast Asian immigrants: Parenting in the context of cultural adaptation to the United States. *Journal of Cross-Cultural Psychology*, 41(2), 212–235. doi:10.1177/0022022109354469.

Turner, E. A., & Mohan, S. (2016). Child mental health services and psychotherapy attitudes among Asian Indian parents: An exploratory study. *Community Mental Health Journal*, 52, 989–997. doi:10.1007/s10597-015-9976-z.

Uba, L. (1994). *Asian Americans: Personality patterns, identity and mental health*. Guilford Press.

U.S. Census Bureau (2019). Asian alone or in any combination by selected groups (Table ID B02015) [Data set]. 2015–2019. *American Community Survey 5-year Estimates*. https://data.census.gov/cedsci/table?q=ASIAN&tid=ACSDT5Y2019. B02018.

U.S. Census Bureau (2020). About. www.census.gov/topics/population/race/about. html.

U.S. Census Bureau (2021). Asian American and Pacific Islander Heritage Month: May 2021. www.census.gov/newsroom/facts-for-features/2021/asian-american-pacific-islander.html.

Wu, C. & Chao, R. (2005). Intergenerational cultural conflicts in norms of parental warmth among Chinese American immigrants. *International Journal of Behavioral Development*, 29, 516–523. doi:10.1177/01650250500147444.

Wu, T., & Lee, J. (2015). A pilot program to promote mental health among Asian-American immigrant children and their parents: A community-based participatory approach. *International Journal of Child, Youth & Family Studies*, 6, 730–745. doi:10.18357/ijcyfs.641201515055.

Yoshikawa, H., Mistry, R. & Wang, Y. (2016), Advancing methods in research on Asian American children and youth. *Child Development*, 87, 1033–1050. doi:10.1111/cdev.12576.

Zang, Q. (2010). Asian Americans beyond the model minority stereotype: The nerdy and the left out. *Journal of International and Intercultural Communication*, 3(1), 20–37. doi:10.1080/17513050903428109.

Zhou, Q., Tao, A., Chen, S. H., Main, A., Lee, E., Ly, J., Hua, M., & Li, X. (2012). Asset and protective factors for Asian American children's mental health adjustment. *Child Development Perspectives*, 6(3), 312–319. doi:10.1111/j.1750-8606.2012.00251.x.

Zhou, X., Wu, C. S., Juan, M. J. D. & Lee, R. M. (2017). Understanding and addressing parent-adolescent conflict in Asian American families. In Y. Choi & H. C. Hahm (Eds.), *Asian American parenting: Family process and intervention* (pp. 143–163). Springer.

11 Cultural Opportunities with Middle Eastern Populations

Ahou Vaziri Line

In my master's internship at a counseling clinic, I had the opportunity to serve in a supervisory role with incoming interns, and as a Type A, high achieving individual, wanted to complete the requirement with praise-worthy accolades. One evening, as I complained about how much work needed to be completed before I could revel in the completion of my degree, I heard a door slam. A client had run out of a session into the lobby, tears filling her eyes, and a finger pointed at my White colleague. In a thick accent, she yelled, "You don't understand me, and you never even tried!" I gripped my chest as any such outbursts were usually a cue to call our supervisor; however, I hesitated and quietly observed before taking action. The woman was actually a parent of a play therapy client seeking services at our clinic; her son quickly ran after her. She wore a floor-length floral skirt embellished with paisley print and a matching hijab covering her hair and neck. As tears streamed down her face, I noticed her dark complexion, her espresso-colored eyes, and her beautiful thick eyelashes as they were soaked with tears. Before she left the main clinic doors, she stared at me with a look that can only be described as a plea for help and an expression that read, "You look like me. You must understand what I am going through." As I jumped up out of my seat, eager to support the student and commendably serve in my role, I felt an overwhelming feeling of guilt and remorse. Why was I tending to my White colleague rather than chasing after the client to implore what pain had caused her such an outcry of tears?

I learned that my colleague had been providing play therapy services for her son for over seven months and felt as though she was at a standstill. She shared that she believed cultural differences impeded her judgment as a counselor and, in this most recent parent consultation, provided the client's mother with three referrals to Middle Eastern counselors she believed could better serve her family. The counselor shook her head as she described the discrepancy between her observations of the child and his mother's presenting concerns. What came next was a slew of misconceptions about Middle Eastern women, their role as parents, considerations of men in "their culture," and a blank stare when I asked from which country

DOI: 10.4324/9781003190073-14

specifically they immigrated. In this moment, the brief eye contact I shared with the mother who fled our clinic made sense. Though our counselors were well-trained in the art of unconditional positive regard, empathy, and congruence when working with children, working with parents, and specifically Middle Eastern families, appeared to be a growing opportunity.

I share this story not to vilify my colleague. In fact, her ability to empathize and build relationships with her child clients is unmatched. However, her confusion about Middle Eastern culture and failure to connect with this client's mother provided much needed insight into my own cognitive dissonance. As an Iranian American play therapist myself, the expression in that mother's eyes haunted me and plagued me with questions for months after the incident. How are we as play therapists trained to understand Middle Eastern culture? Through our diversity courses, are we exposed to enough of an understanding to know which questions to ask? How are our implicit biases about the culture impacting our work with children and their families? Lastly, where do I, as a Middle Eastern therapist, fit into the equation?

Cultural Considerations

Throughout my life, after my initial introduction of my "unique" name, I often brace myself for the onslaught of questions which usually include something along the lines of, "What are you?" Though I often reply with humor, "I am a human," defining my cultural identity appears to be important to others. It allows individuals to quickly conceptualize me, a person they view as different from them, though often with misconceptions. When I reply that I am Persian, or Iranian, I steady myself again for the questions and assumptions. The Middle Eastern culture is so misunderstood that even defining who "counts" becomes an arduous task. In researching and writing this chapter, I found myself questioning the verbiage to use. Some texts reference Middle Eastern Americans, whereas other texts specifically discuss Arab Americans. In this chapter, I defaulted to the term used by the scholars in their texts. Even the name used to define this population is so nuanced, therefore a clear understanding becomes even more critical.

Who is Considered "Middle Eastern?"

Middle Eastern culture is often pigeonholed into only considering Arab Americans and those who identity as Muslim. However, this narrow definition ignores many individuals who identify themselves as Middle Eastern (myself included) such as those from Pakistan, Iran, and those who identity as Turks. For the purposes of this chapter, I will borrow from Marvasti and McKinney's (2004) conceptualization of Middle Eastern Americans which considered the viewpoint of anyone who "identifies him- or herself as being from or having ancestral ties to the predominantly Islamic region of the world in Southwest Asia and North Africa" (p. xx). The authors noted that, "Middle Eastern Americans, like Hispanic Americans, come from multiple racial, linguistic, religious, and geographical backgrounds [and] constitute a distinct ethnic category in the United States" (Marvasti & McKinney, 2004, pp. xx–xxi).

Americans often lump Arabs, Turks, and Iranians into one category; however, the numbers of Middle Easterners living in the U.S. may be severely underrepresented due to methods used in measuring the population (Marvasti & McKinney, 2004). The census categories only include Black, Hispanic, Asian or Pacific Islander, and American Indian or Alaskan Native, and instructs Middle Eastern Americans to report their race as "White"; therefore, an accurate count of Middle Eastern individuals in the U.S. is not possible (Tehranian, 2009; Marvasti & McKinney, 2004). Furthermore, with a 2018 decision not to include Middle Eastern and Northern African (MENA) as an option on the 2020 census, Middle Eastern Americans must wait at least another decade before they are represented (Measher, 2020). Arab Americans are the largest group of Middle Eastern Americans with over 20 countries represented and most Arab Americans identifying as Christian (Marvasti & McKinney, 2004). With such a large portion of the world encompassed in this label, it is surprising that such a heterogeneous population is typically lumped into narrow stereotypes. In fact, Middle Eastern Americans are often stereotyped as Muslim and Arabic, though Iranians and Pakistanis do not consider themselves Arabic, and only 23% of present-day Arab Americans identify as Muslim (Tehranian, 2009). Middle Eastern children have been referred to as "the lost sheep in the school system" due to their tendency to fall through the cracks (Wingfield & Karaman, 1995), and are often described as being one of the most misunderstood ethnic groups in the United States (Erickson & Al-Timimi, 2001). Furthermore, because Arab American children do not often face failures in school, they are not commonly targeted by research and policy (Khouri, 2016) further subjecting them to misunderstanding and invisibility. The National Center for Education Statistics does not consider Arab or Middle Eastern Americans their own ethnic minority group, further erasing data that could prove useful when studying this population (Goforth et al., 2017).

Discrimination Middle Eastern Children May Face

Not only do Middle Eastern children become lost within a school system; they are also often targets of discrimination. It begs the question, which is worse: being passively forgotten or actively mistreated? My own experience was a blend of both. In the first grade, my parents worked five jobs to move us across the country from a Title I school in California to an affluent district in Texas. When I arrived in my class midyear, I was far behind my peers academically. My teacher quickly alerted the school that I should be placed in English as a Second Language (ESL). As a shy six-year-old whose culture taught me to respect authority, I was too afraid to tell her that I spoke English well but struggled with reading because my previous school was at least a grade level behind. I spent hours in a special education classroom with a bilingual teacher who worked to remediate me by translating Spanish words into English. In 1996, my brown hair, brown eyes, and systems of educational inequity meant that I was stereotyped as a Latinx student who recently immigrated to the U.S. The discrimination became more overt when my teacher sent home additional reading for extra practice. I brought home the books and begged my siblings to help so I could avoid returning to the ESL classroom. Two days later, I brought the books back to my teacher in a clear plastic bag, but my proud smile turned to shame when I was publicly scolded in front of my entire class for lying to her about finishing them. When my mother took a day off work to explain to my teacher that I had in fact read the books, my mother's thick accent was further proof that I must have been lying. Almost three decades later, I still get emotional considering my mother's poor treatment in that classroom and consider how easily it could have been avoided. Unfortunately, I believed my teacher's authority was confounded with superiority, so I took the books home, laid them on my counter until enough time had passed that she might believe me, and took them back two weeks later.

The Role of the 9/11 Terrorist Attacks

September 11, 2001 marked a drastic shift in the roles and lives of many Middle Eastern Americans in the U.S. Many Middle Eastern Americans can describe the dramatic moment where they were stripped of any semblance of belonging in the U.S., and their identity became a national threat (Erickson & Al-Timimi, 2004; Goforth et al., 2017; Khouri, 2016). Following the attacks, the Arab Anti-Discrimination Committee (ADC) confirmed 520 violent crimes impacting Middle Eastern Americans, and over 1,400 hate crimes were reported as of November of that year (Erickson & Al-Timimi, 2004; Tehranian, 2009; Marvasti & McKinney, 2004). Terrorist attacks and media portrayals lead to common stereotypes that Middle Easterners are terrorists, dangerous, greedy, have conservative religious views, and have oppressive families with controlling husbands (Marvasti & McKinney, 2004; Erickson & Al-Timimi, 2004).

Unfortunately, recent spikes in hate crimes against Muslims following immigration bans further alienate Middle Eastern Americans today (Lichtblau, 2016). In 2015, hate crimes against American Muslims increased by 78%, with scholars citing negative rhetoric in the media leading to the increase (Lichtblau, 2016). This was the biggest annual rise since the terrorist attacks in 2001 and was especially pertinent as hate crimes against almost all other groups either only slightly increased or declined (Lichtblau, 2016). Kumar et al. (2015) posit that though many marginalized groups face discrimination, Arab Americans are the only group who face questions related to their allegiance as citizens. It is no surprise that following 9/11, many Middle Eastern Americans displayed American flags or symbols of patriotism to avoid discrimination (Marvasti & McKinney, 2004).

Middle Eastern children feel the impact of this increase in discrimination. Tabbah et al. (2016) found over half of the Arab Americans in their study had experienced discrimination, citing experiences of being called derogatory names including "towel head" or "terrorist." Albdour et al. (2019) found Arab American adolescents reported a "significantly higher prevalence of cyberbullying and victimization while in school (42%) relative to Whites (33%), African Americans (13%), and Hispanics (12%)" (p. 711). Albdour et al. (2019) speculate this may be due to "perceived immigrant status, religious beliefs, and the negative portrayal of Arabs and Muslims in the media" (p. 707). Consider the difficulty Middle Eastern children face by simultaneously having their identity erased by educational statistics and actively persecuted as undesirable and dangerous.

Important Factors for Play Therapists to Consider: The Mitigating Factors of Different Identities

Though discrimination is rampant among Middle Eastern communities, not all children may experience discrimination in the same way. Many texts provide categorical information about Middle Eastern children to help educators better work with them such as "boys and girls are treated differently in Arab cultures" (Manning & Baruth, 2004, p. 119) or "asking Arab American children to look someone in the eyes while talking is in direct opposition to the concept of saving face" and should be avoided (Vang, 2010, p. 150). Though these texts provide valuable information to educators regarding Middle Eastern children, I believe such recommendations may risk further stereotyping such a heterogenous population. Rather, it would be more useful to provide mitigating factors to consider when working with Middle Eastern identifying clients so that play therapists are asking better questions rather than assuming the answers.

Whiteness and Assimilation

Though the census definition of Middle Eastern Americans considers this population as "White," the individual considerations of whiteness within Middle Eastern children is paramount. Many older Middle Eastern Americans merit the ability to "pass" as White and actually insist on avoiding the consideration as a person of color (Tehranian, 2009). Such preference can be understood when considering the role of White privilege in the U.S. However, the preference to be viewed in one way and the reality of how others view Middle Eastern Americans are two very different things. Marvasti and McKinney (2004) consider how factors such as foreign sounding names and skin tone impact how others respond to this population. For example, individuals with darker skin tones are often considered "despised and dangerous" (Marvasti & McKinney, 2004). This phenomenon is especially impactful for Middle Eastern children who have not yet considered how their identities are viewed by others and may feel compounded confusion and fear each time they share their name or have their identities questioned (Marvasti & McKinney, 2004). Tabbah et al. (2016) found that Arab American children's perceptions of discrimination were inversely correlated with their perceptions of their physical appearance. The authors postulate it is possible that children who express their ethnicity more outwardly or have more visible stereotypical features would experience more discrimination (Tabbah et al., 2016).

Furthermore, in conceptualizing Middle Eastern child clients, it would behoove the play therapist to consider the client's perception of acculturation as well as how others may view the child. In considering the following factors of religion, immigration, and language, they may best be understood in their proximity to whiteness especially as many of these factors provide protection from oppression and stereotyping. Abdulrahim et al. (2012) hypothesized proximity to whiteness included an individual's racial identification, ethnic centrality, religion, skin color, and whether or not an individual lived in an ethnic enclave where Arab Americans are the majority. The authors found three of the five variables were statistically significantly associated with discrimination meaning that study participants that identified as Muslim, non-White, and resided in an ethnic enclave reported higher levels of discrimination.

Religion

Confounding ethnicity, race, and religion is a common error related to Middle Eastern Americans. Muslims are predominantly non-Arab (Diller, 1991), and most Arab Americans are not Muslim (Marvasti & McKinney, 2004). Furthermore, confusing words such as Arab and Muslim, as well as avoiding other Middle Eastern countries within this sub context may lead to mistrust between client and play therapist. Perceptions and stereotypes of Islamic individuals include the fear that Muslims are dangerous, the religion breeds oppressive and ritualistic ideals, and that Muslims are violent (Said, 1997). Further, Muslim woman donning head coverings are more likely to become targets for hostility (Marvasti & McKinney, 2004). Following 9/11, Christian Arab Americans reported significantly greater perceptions of assimilation into U.S. culture as compared to Muslim Arab Americans (Amer & Hovey, 2005). Ikizler and Szymanski (2017) found that when compared to non-Muslims, Muslims reported more experiences with ethnic discrimination and that high and average levels of religiosity were correlated with more ethnic discrimination than Muslims reporting lower levels. In recognizing religion as a mitigating factor for discrimination, understanding how a client was taught religion and the family's religious beliefs provides a more comprehensive image of how Middle Eastern identity may impact a child. Furthermore, this understanding allows for a better conceptualization of how religion may impact presenting concerns (Erickson & Al-Timimi, 2004).

Immigration and Language

Citizenship status and reasons for immigration are also important considerations when working with Middle Eastern children. Al-Hawdrawi (2017) found that Middle Eastern immigrants reported higher emotional distress if their immigration was involuntary as opposed to voluntary. Taking the time to understand the process of immigration for families receiving therapy services can help play therapists build rapport with parents and caregivers. Furthermore, recognizing an involuntary immigration helps provide context about presenting concerns specifically if trauma was experienced as a result of the family's refugee experience (Haboush, 2007).

The majority of Middle Eastern families immigrating to the United States did so in hopes for better opportunities or freedom (Awad, Martinez, & Amer, 2013). Many texts coin the term "the American Dream" to describe the promise of equal opportunity and prosperity that lures many immigrants to the U.S. (Marvasti & McKinney, 2004) which can explain why education is important to many Middle Eastern Americans. One Iranian author describes the process of assimilation and the role of education:

> The options may be limited when it comes to skin color, but it is possible to improve one's status in other ways. I think of it as race laundering: the right clothes, the right car, the right neighborhood can help compensate for that fundamental imperfection: nonwhiteness.
>
> (Asayesh, 2006)

Marvasti and McKinney's (2004) interviews with Middle Eastern Americans were laden with considerations of the promises of prosperity with the caveat that if they move their children to the U.S. and they study hard, they can achieve success they may not ever have attained in their home country.

Among the issues related to immigration, Erickson and Al-Timimi (2001) suggest therapists consider, "length of time in the United States, reasons for emigration, whether they have family still living abroad, their ability to return to or visit their home country, and their long-term plans to stay in the United States" (p. 312). Furthermore, the authors consider the disparity between a family's socioeconomic status in their home country as related to their financial means in the U.S. as such a dramatic shift may be an additional source of stress for families (Erickson & Al-Timimi, 2001). Play therapists may consider the role of education and the perception of the American Dream among the family and recognize how parent expectations of the child may be impacted.

In line with the idea of "whiteness" and assimilation, Middle Eastern Americans' ability to communicate effectively in the English language may bring about additional concerns. Middle Eastern Americans may speak a multitude of languages including Arabic, Farsi, Armenian, French, or English, and a child's experience with the English language prior to immigrating differs depending on country of origin (Haboush, 2007). Accents are also important to consider. In Paige et al.'s (2015) study with Iranian Americans, a thicker accent was correlated with perceived prejudice. My own perceptions of my mother's thick Persian accent in contrast to my mother-in-law's thick South African accent provides firsthand insight that all accents are not viewed with the same stigma. In working with parents, play therapists consider their own stereotypes related to accents and recognize that Middle Eastern parents charged with caring for their children may fear that they may not be able to successfully fulfill their role due to struggles with communicating with outside entities such as teachers, school officials, and counselors (Awad, Martinez, & Amer, 2013; Erickson & Al-Timimi, 2001).

Opportunities When Working with Middle Eastern Children

Recognizing Middle Eastern Americans as a heterogenous ethnic group with varying identities, play therapists have a rare opportunity in working with this population because they are uniquely situated to consider the needs of their child client, the family system, and additional systems such as the school and community. With this privileged viewpoint, play therapists have an opportunity not only to impact the child to whom they are providing play therapy services, but the greater community that interacts with this child. Recognizing the confusion and disparity that comes with the Middle Eastern identity, a play therapist has the tools to forge pathways within the systems the child interacts with to help diminish identity concerns and promote advocacy.

Overcoming Stereotypes and Reducing Practitioner Bias

First and foremost, the play therapist has the opportunity to overcome stereotypes and reduce personal bias within this population. Play therapists may critically consider diversity texts that provide a one-size-fits-all approach to working with this population, especially given the vast differentiation among its members. Careful consideration of one's own attitudes and beliefs as well as a clear audit of consumption of media portrayals of Middle Eastern Americans allows play therapists to reduce their own implicit biases (Erickson & Al-Timimi, 2004). Play therapists would benefit from considering their own experiences of September 11, 2001, and how their own perceptions of Middle Eastern Americans may have shifted as a result. Many Muslim Americans, already sensitive to biases within the larger culture, may view non-Muslim play therapists as representative of prejudiced views of society, thus, the more play therapists can understand about cultural practices as well as their own limits and biases, the more likely they will be to avoid further alienating their clients (Altareb, 1996).

Views of Mental Health

The greatest opportunity that play therapists working with this population experience is the fact that they even brought their children to counseling at all. Middle Eastern Americans are less likely to pursue mental health services due to a perceived lack of understanding of mental health, stigma related to mental health symptoms and subsequent treatment including criticism of therapy, shame, and fear of asking for help outside of the family (Mechammil et al., 2019). Mechammil et al. (2019) found that religion also plays a large part in Middle Eastern Americans avoiding counseling services with individuals citing the expectation that religion and God should be leaned upon to resolve mental illness. Furthermore, Mechammil et al. noted that participants in their qualitative study belonged to many different religious backgrounds, indicating that one main religion did not deter individuals from seeking services, but rather, it could be assumed that the intersectionality of culture and religion as well as family concerns led to this hesitation. Perhaps the most pertinent to play therapists is that participants in this study shared the perspective that mental illness was rarely discussed with children, and though family members may have history of struggling with mental illness, participants reported their families would often ensure secrecy in order to avoid further stigmatization (Mechammil et al., 2019). These perceptions of mental illness provide ample opportunity for play therapists to recognize the sheer courage it requires to arrive at an intake appointment.

Among Arab Americans, attitudes toward mental health were impacted by mitigating factors such as education, family values and beliefs regarding mental health, and accessibility of services (Al-Darmaki, 2003). Al-Darmaki (2003) postulated that seeking help from a physician is more acceptable than considering a psychological help provider such as a therapist, therefore play therapists may be the last consideration when families are pursuing services for their children. Historically, Arab American patients often resisted referrals to mental health services when hospitals or clinics recommended them (Lipson, Reizian, & Meleis, 1987). Self-disclosure is often unacceptable and reserved for conversations among family members, thus, sharing difficulties within an intake appointment may stir up cognitive dissonance for parents that are seeking services for their children (Al-Darmaki, 2003).

In considering the specific perspectives of Arab-Muslim Americans, Aloud and Rathur (2009) found that individuals were likely to underutilize mental health services due to the tendency to exhaust all informal resources prior to contacting professional counseling services, and often tended to have less favorable attitudes toward formal mental health services. One opportunity for play therapists is to empathize with parents and caregivers who are experiencing often negative messaging regarding mental health services but chose to arrive to their intake appointment anyway.

Play Therapy Considerations for Middle Eastern Children

Person-Centered Approach to Culture

The child-centered play therapist has ample opportunities in working with Middle Eastern children. Though many texts include distinct accommodations for working with multicultural clients, Patterson (1996) posited such techniques have "overshadowed attention to the nature of the relationship between the counselor and the client" (p. 229). Patterson acknowledged Roger's Person-Centered Counseling may be the best modality for multicultural counseling, and true empathic understanding includes the counselor's ability to convey empathy in a culturally consistent manner. The belief that empathic understanding toward the client is essential supports caution in adopting generalized tips on working with Middle Eastern children. Such a broad approach may reinforce the homogenous stereotypes they have experienced in many other facets of their lives. The best course of action for play therapists would be to consider the individual child with true demonstration of core conditions. However, the play therapist's effectiveness in providing the core conditions is limited unless the child can perceive them. Moreover, if play therapists provide the core conditions in the playroom but avoid providing conditions of empathy and unconditional positive regard with caregivers, multicultural counseling perspectives may not be fully realized.

Self-Discovery of Identity

Middle Eastern children have a unique perspective in multicultural identity development. Middle Eastern Americans are privileged in their ability to more easily "opt out" of their racial categorization due to their racial ambiguity (Tehranian, 2009). Consider a six-year-old Iranian child with a traditional name, light brown hair, fair complexion, and green eyes. Her identity as a Middle Eastern female, or her connection with multiculturalism, may fluctuate depending on who knows her name, what names she chooses to call herself, her family's perception of whiteness, language, and proximity to immigration status. Thus, the issue of cultural identity in Middle Eastern children may not be linear. When considering the Sue and Sue (2003) Racial/Cultural Identity Development model, I would argue that Middle Eastern individuals would not experience a linear development through the stages. For example, children may move to introspection where they are working to differentiate their own personal views from their group views but may experience a set-back to the Dissonance stage when others identify them as Middle Eastern rather than passing as White (Sue & Sue, 2003).

Play therapists have a unique opportunity to promote development through these stages through their use of unconditional positive regard. Play therapists are keenly aware of moments in which cultural identity are apparent through a child's play. For example, a vacillating selection in dolls of different skin complexions to represent a client's sister may lead the play therapist to reflect meaning related to the client's ambivalent identification. Play therapists well-versed in understanding the particular client's world-view may recognize when self-identification of religious preferences or language usage is present in the playroom. These opportunities allow an environment of unconditional acceptance with which a child may journey toward identity development and empathic understanding that respects individual cultural values.

Toys in the Playroom

Landreth (2012) describes the importance of including toys that allow expression of a wide range of feelings, exploration of real-life experiences, and the development of self-understanding. As such, play therapists working with Middle Eastern children would benefit from considering how their current toy selection allows for these specific goals. I recommend the inclusion of dolls of various skin tones (including more than just Black and White dolls) in order to avoid inadvertently attributing to the messaging of Middle Eastern children as the "invisible race" (Erickson & Al-Timimi, 2004) and to promote identity development. Though not all Middle Eastern children may identify this way, familial considerations are paramount to many Arab American children (Erickson & Al-Timimi, 2004), thus, play therapists may consider adding to the doll collection with more options for parents, grandparents, and community members.

Play therapists may recognize how their typical inclusion of American food may prohibit feelings of safety within the room. Middle Eastern children can often cite the feeling of impending doom when they sit at a cafeteria table and take out their "weird smelling lunch" and immediately feel othered by their classmates. As a child still determining my own racial identity, if I was limited in my choice between making a pretend peanut butter and jelly sandwich or a bowl of cereal, I may immediately consider that parts of my cultural identity may not be safe to express in the playroom. Therefore, including more ambiguous items in the kitchen may benefit all clients of color. Consider including items such as rice, unmarked spices, empty and unmarked jars, and boxes that may not have a denoted meaning to allow for greater expression.

As is often the case, though it may not benefit all Middle Eastern children, religion may play an integral role for clients (Erickson & Al-Timimi, 2004). Thus, consider adding religious symbols into the playroom. Children considering their own views on religion may benefit from figures depicting various religions including Christianity, Islam, Judaism, Druze, Bahai, and

Buddhism. Selection of toys may not only benefit Middle Eastern children but may create a more inclusive environment for various multicultural identities. Furthermore, exposing children identifying as White to a variety of food, skin tones, and religions may further play therapists' advocacy efforts.

Working with Parents/Family

Beginning to Build a Relationship

The single-most important consideration in working with Middle Eastern children includes the clear understanding of their worldview. Parents and caregivers are the window to this opportunity, and much like with any child in play therapy, a relationship with parents and caregivers is instrumental in a play therapist's work (Ray, 2011). The intake appointment allows the play therapist an opportunity to understand the child's specific Middle Eastern worldview, develop a relationship with parents and caregivers, and develop clear expectations of counseling. In addition to a play therapist's role in understanding the developmental background of a child at intake, play therapists working with Middle Eastern children may consider taking time to ask parents and caregivers about specific aspects of their experiences with acculturation, their ethnic identity, family relationships, religious beliefs, and cultural beliefs (Erickson & Al-Timimi, 2001). Furthermore, play therapists working with children may consider how the child's acculturation, ethnic identity, religious beliefs, and cultural beliefs may diverge from the family system. In assessing acculturation, play therapists consider parents' assessment of Western values in alignment with their own parenting practices. For example, do parents want their children to "fit in" with American peers or would they prefer that they maintain their culture? This valuation provides play therapists valuable insight in assessing how parenting skills often discussed in consultation may be accepted as Middle Eastern parents may not view the traditional American values in child-rearing in a favorable light (Erickson & Al-Timimi, 2004). Goforth et al. (2015) found discrepancies between parent and child acculturation correlated with more behavioral concerns for Arab American adolescent girls. Muslim Arab Americans who identified the maintenance of their Arab culture reported fewer psychological problems (Goforth et al., 2014). Though not studied with Middle Eastern children specifically, Kim et al. (2013) found that an acculturation gap, defined as a discrepancy between parent and child levels of acculturation, may be correlated with children's mental health concerns. These studies shed light on how questions regarding acculturation allow play therapists the ability to identify concerns that may be present for a child client without a parent discussing them directly.

Play therapists may allow parents to educate them without making assumptions, questioning parenting choices, or offering alternatives. Within a first appointment, play therapists continue to consider the courage parents have demonstrated by moving against cultural norms of mental health counseling. Beginning the counseling process may be difficult for parents, and counselors would benefit from regarding this first interaction as an honor. That being said, an intake appointment should prioritize relationship and trust building. Erickson and Al-Timimi (2001) caution that when working with Arab Americans, play therapists should recognize that "trust may develop slowly, but intense connections are possible" (p. 246), and developing rapport becomes extremely important. Haboush (2007) recommends that mental health professionals do not acknowledge political events as a means of rapport building, but rather, initiate conversations regarding cultural traditions and religion. I recommend approaching the intake appointment with a sense of discovery, allowing the therapist to develop an understanding of the family's phenomenological perspectives of culture and parenting.

Identifying Presenting Problems and Goals of Counseling

Within the intake appointment with the parent or caregiver, demonstrating unconditional positive regard and empathy are paramount. When discussing presenting problems, play therapists clarify goals and provide clear expectations for counseling procedures. Dwairy and Van Sickle (1996) recommend short-term, concrete, and goal-oriented therapy for Arab American clients; however, due to the nature of person-centered counseling, this may not be possible. One such study recommended Arab Americans tend to prefer more directive approaches to counseling; however, this research was related to adults and did not consider the perspectives of children (Nassar-McMillan & Hakim-Larson, 2003). Depending on parent preference, play therapists may prefer to be more direct within the parent consultations and avoid non-directive language when discussing progress and treatment.

Play therapists are empathetic to parent concerns, but also recognize that their perceptions of the child may differ from the parents' perceptions. Erickson and Al-Timimi (2004) suggest that Arab American parents may have strong expectations for their children to practice the family's cultural customs which children may reject (Erickson & Al-Timimi, 2004). Parents may hold strong expectations for their children's behavior and career choices, the effects of which may be seen in a discrepancy between parent goals for counseling and the play therapist's perception of the child. That being said, parent perceptions are still of value in helping contextualize difficulties the child may be experiencing. Through CCPT, children may be given the opportunity to process the discrepancy between their strict lives at home and the childhoods of many of their American friends. Rather than disregarding the parents' concerns, a play therapist would be well suited to empathize with the child's experience and recognize that the play therapist and parent perspectives do not need to align in order for counseling to be effective. Furthermore, the therapist would benefit from recognizing personal biases toward Western child-rearing practices. I recognize that my own parents were considered "strict"; however, their parenting practices were not harmful. Rather, they were grounded in our own cultural ideals where parents were dominant, and children were considered subservient.

Building Upon the Relationship and Communicating Progress

Continued communication with parents and caregivers is paramount to counseling all children (Ray, 2011); however, it specifically allows Middle Eastern parents space to develop trust and confidence in the play therapist's role. In subsequent parent consultations, play therapists should continue to explore aspects of the child's worldview. Consider that parents may not be forthcoming in the initial intake appointment as family secrets are not to be shared among strangers, and a deeper connection and trust with the play therapist may be required (Erickson & Al-Timimi, 2004). As play therapists begin to understand children through their own perceptions, they can begin to explore how levels of acculturation between parent and child may differ. This serves as an opportunity for play therapists to connect parent and child in order to avoid mental health concerns related to acculturation gaps (Kim et al., 2013).

As play therapists begin to measure progress, they consider the discrepancy between the goals of CCPT and many Middle Eastern cultures. The goal of CCPT includes a child's ability to move toward self-actualization. However, this process may challenge many Middle Eastern parents' perceptions of collectivism as a goal for their children (Dwairy & Van Sickle, 1996). Thus, goal formation and communication of progress rely on parents' perceptions of healthy functioning. In my opinion, the most difficult part of working with Middle Eastern children and families is the process of aligning on what healthy functioning may look like in a child and how CCPT's non-directive nature may help a child get there. Psychoeducation regarding normal development at each age may be beneficial to share with parents. Clear communication and a strong relationship allow therapists to understand parenting strategies that are currently being employed. This allows the therapist to tweak existing parenting strategies rather than asking parents to overhaul their entire approach. Play therapists may benefit from engaging in conversations with caregivers about their role as parents and their perception of judgment from others within their broader community in relation to their child's behavior. This may also shed light on perceptions of the role of parenting and caregivers' own experiences as Middle Eastern children. These conversations allow for therapists to meet parents where they are rather than imposing their own biases of Western child-rearing practices on Middle Eastern parents.

Working with the System and Advocacy

Teacher Perspectives of Middle Eastern Children

Research suggests Arab American children perform well academically (Tabbah et al., 2012), Arab Americans have higher average level of education than White Americans, and the median family income of Middle Eastern Americans is substantially higher than the United States median (Marvasti & McKinney, 2004). That being said, though Middle Eastern families may prove their successes through high performance in schools and in careers, they are not immune to negative stereotypes within the school environment. In a study of Arab American adolescents, half of the children included had either experienced discrimination firsthand or had known a peer who had (Tabbah et al., 2012). In measures of scholastic competence, Arab American children were academically high achieving; however, teacher support was not related to this variable or the variable of self-concept (Tabbah et al., 2012).

Teacher perceptions of Middle Eastern children are fraught with misconceptions, so it is no surprise that they are often considered the "lost sheep" of the school system (Wingfield & Karaman, 1995). Alnawar (2015) found that when teachers were asked about their familiarity with Middle Eastern culture and asked to name a country in the Middle East, most teachers in the study fell short. Alnawar (2015) concluded that many teachers had little to no information regarding Middle Eastern culture which may lead to misunderstandings and miscommunication in the classroom.

In considering the perspectives of Middle Eastern parents when viewing elementary education, first-generation Arab American mothers reported a lack of involvement in their children's schooling (Moosa et al., 2001). In comparing survey results from both parents and teachers, Moosa et al. (2001) found parent factors that impacted involvement included cultural and language barriers as well as the assumption that the school is the sole authority on their child's education. In direct contrast, Badiee (2004) explored both Middle Eastern mothers' and teachers' perspectives of the American early childhood system, finding that teachers perceived that it was the parent and child's responsibility to advocate for their own cultural needs (Badiee, 2004).

Play therapists are uniquely positioned to build empathy and understanding with Middle Eastern families and support them in this advocacy. In recognizing the role the system plays within a child client's phenomenological perspective, it is a unique opportunity for play therapists to advocate and help navigate these social systems, especially when they appear to be working against child clients. I recommend play therapists communicate the fruitful conversations from parent consultations to educators in order to help develop empathy and understanding. Play therapists may advocate for more inclusive experiences both at the classroom and district level in order to help alleviate the potential for the child client to be "lost" within the school system (i.e. recognizing how Middle Eastern children are "counted" within testing data and how support services may benefit them). Lastly, play therapists well-versed in school systems may support Middle Eastern families in navigating systems that may benefit their child such as special education services.

Identifying as a Middle Eastern Play Therapist

It is challenging to separate my identity as a Middle Eastern woman, my role as a play therapist, and the need for advocacy into three distinct categories. As such, they meld together and form a passionate plea to play therapists in the field working with Middle Eastern families. I consider my own childhood and the plausibility that one of my colleagues may have worked with me as an anxious, confused six-year-old. I consider my mother's perspectives on mental health and the smile and nod approach she may have taken before returning home and vowing to never return when a play therapist questioned her parenting methods or made incorrect assumptions about our culture. I consider my own covert experiences with discrimination in elementary school with teachers who hesitated to say my name and the overt experiences of discrimination I faced after September 11, 2001.

Middle Eastern play therapists may recognize the great challenges they face in the field. Though not tied to the Middle Eastern culture directly, a study of foreign-born counselors found that immigrant counselors who reported feeling more connected to U.S. culture reported higher levels of clinical self-efficacy (Kissil, Davey, & Davey, 2013). Furthermore, counselors' clinical self-efficacy was not only correlated with their level of acculturation, but appeared to be more strongly correlated to their perception of prejudice from their environment. Kissil et al. (2013) stated, "it is not how much immigrant therapists feel they belong and are accepting of the U.S. culture that is significantly associated with their clinical self-efficacy, but how much they feel accepted in the U.S." (p. 227).

In authoring this chapter, I recognize my distinct privilege as well as the burden I hold. As a Middle Eastern play therapist, I recognize the need for advocacy, training, and practitioner support. However, I also recognize I am one voice, with a narrow understanding of Middle Eastern culture due to my perspective as a first-generation citizen, with advanced education, and limited experience of Arab American customs (as I identify as Iranian). I may be an expert on my own singular experience as a Middle Eastern American but have much room to grow in understanding other perspectives. Middle Eastern play therapists will benefit from considering their unique perspectives related to the intersectionality of their identities. Before supporting our clients, a clear understanding of our own identity is paramount. Furthermore, our processes may be motivating to colleagues.

Rather than condemning my White colleague during my master's program, I empathized with her confusion and powerlessness and discussed my own childhood dissension regarding my parents' views of child-rearing and my desire to assimilate to the culture of my American peers.

It is my hope that this chapter served to illuminate further questions rather than offering a paint-by-numbers approach to working with Middle Eastern children. Among such a differentiated culture, questions of where we all fit become highlighted. One thing is certain, however, in that the views covered in this chapter may not just benefit Middle Eastern clients but may become a blueprint for how to interact with all children and their families. It is an honor to be invited into our child clients' lives and to have their parents and families trust us, and demonstrating empathy for their human experience, especially in regard to multicultural issues, is the ultimate way to repay that honor.

Positionality Statement

Ahou

As the sole author of this chapter, I recognize my distinct privilege in creating this resource, therefore I must share that I unequivocally do not consider myself an expert in Middle Eastern children. As a Middle Eastern American who would have likely benefited from play therapy as a child, I would be remiss not to point out how the intersectionality of my identities provide a unique perspective on this topic.

My family immigrated from Iran to the United States when I was three years old, therefore my perspective as an immigrant is as much of a part of my identity as being a Middle Eastern female. My racial identity development was steeped in memories of being different than my peers, as compared to my older siblings who were able to experience larger portions of their life as part of the majority in Iran. I always wondered if my name was not foreign, if we celebrated Christmas, and if my parents did not have accents, if others would recognize my "otherness" as much as they did. I imagine many Middle Eastern children also grapple with their racial identity as I did because it always felt ambiguous to me.

The sacrifice my parents made in order to raise their three children in the United States also informs my clinical practice. I watched my parents work five jobs to afford the rent for a house zoned for a high-performing school district to ensure their children could live out the American Dream for which they sacrificed so much. I often consider how many children of immigrants consider success a non-negotiable as a means of repaying their parents' sacrifices just as I do. I imagine these experiences rear their heads in my writing as I recognize the role parents play in their children's lives. This has also made me an advocate for clinical practice in working with children and parents who identify as immigrants. It is important to me to honor and encourage parents and caregivers who often feel torn between their home and the world in which they are raising their children. This is an experience many of us will never truly understand which is why empathy and compassion are at the forefront of our work.

I have learned so much in authoring this chapter and feel indebted to the editors for developing this text. As a result, I have learned that to fully advocate for clients, I must first unapologetically explore my own identity. Throughout this chapter, I often considered which perspectives would be beneficial to consider if I was writing this as a child working to advocate for my own needs with those with power and privilege. I imagined myself communicating these messages clearly and passionately to allow others to best understand me and my family which is why so many of my personal stories run through the text.

Though my experience is unique to my own identities, it is my hope that my voice can be one of many dedicated to recognizing opportunities in working with Middle Eastern Americans. As play therapists develop in their cultural humility, I hope that one day, my own daughter will have the privilege of growing up in a world where individuals consider empathy first, value the beauty in our differences, and honor those differences with acceptance and compassion.

References

Abdulrahim, S., James, S. A., Yamout, R., & Baker, W. (2012). Discrimination and psychological distress: Does whiteness matter for Arab Americans? *Social Science and Medicine*, 75(12), 2116–2123. https://doi.org/10.1016/j.socscimed.2012.07.030.

Albdour, M., Sung Hong, J., Lewin, L., & Yarandi, H. (2019). The impact of cyberbullying on physical and psychological health of Arab American adolescents. *Journal of Immigrant and Minority Health*, 21, 706–715. doi:10.1007/s10903.

Al-Darmaki, F. R. (2003). Attitudes towards seeking professional psychological help: What really counts for United Arab Emirates University students? *Social Behavior and Personality*, 31(5), 497–508. doi:10.2224/sbp.2003.31.5.497.

Al-Hawdrawi, H. (2017). The effect of immigration on the mental well-being of Middle Eastern immigrants in the United States. *Research Journal of Pharmacy and Technology*, 10(7), 2069–2074. doi:10.5958/0974-360X.2017.00361.4.

Alnawar, H. J. (2015). *Raising teachers' cultural knowledge of Middle Eastern students in the classroom*. [Unpublished master's thesis]. California State University, Monterey Bay.

Aloud, N. & Rathur, A. (2009). Factors affecting attitudes toward seeking and using formal mental health and psychological services among Arab Muslim populations. *Journal of Muslim Mental Health*, 4(2), 79–103. doi:10.1080/15564900802487675.

Altareb, B. Y. (1996). Islamic spirituality in America: A middle path to unity. *Counseling and Values*, 41, 29–38.

Amer, M. M & Hovey, J. D. (2005). Examination of the impact of acculturation, stress, and religiosity on mental health variables for second-generation Arab Americans. *Ethnicity and Disease*, 15(1), 111–112.

Asayesh, G. (2006). I grew up thinking I was white. In Azam Zanganeh, L. (Ed.), *My sister guard your veil, my brother guard your eyes: Uncensored Iranian voices*. Beacon Press.

Awad, G. H., Martinez, M. S., & Amer, M. M. (2013). Considerations for psychotherapy with immigrant women of Arab/Middle Eastern descent. *Women and Therapy*, 36(3), 163–175. doi:10.1080/02703149.2013.797761.

Badiee, S. (2004). *Middle Eastern mothers' perspectives of U.S. early childhood schools* [Unpublished master's thesis]. Oregon State University.

Camarota, S. A. (2002, August 1). Immigrants from the Middle East. *Center for Immigration Studies*. https://cis.org/Report/Immigrants-Middle-East.

Diller, C. D. (1991). *The Middle East* (7th ed.). Congressional Quarterly.

Dwairy, M. & Van Sickle, T. (1996). Western psychotherapy in traditional Arabic societies. *Clinical Psychology Review*, 16(3), 231–249.

Erickson, C. D. & Al-Timimi, N.R. (2001). Providing mental health services to Arab Americans: Recommendations and considerations. *Cultural Diversity and Ethnic Minority Psychology*, 7(4), 308–327. doi:10.1037//1099-9809.7.4.308.

Erickson, C. D. & Al-Timimi, N. R. (2004). Counseling and psychotherapy with Arab American clients. In T. Smith (Ed.), *Practicing multiculturalism: Affirming diversity in counseling and psychology* (pp. 234–253). Pearson.

Goforth, A. N., Oka, E. R., Leong, F. T., & Dennis, D. (2014). Acculturation, acculturative stress, religiosity, and psychological adjustment among Muslim Arab Americans adolescents. *Journal of Muslim Mental Health*, 8, 3–19.

Goforth, A. N., Pham, A. V., & Oka, E. R. (2015). Parent-child conflict, acculturation gap, acculturative stress, and behavior problems in Arab American adolescents. *Journal of Cross-Cultural Psychology*, 46(6), 821–836. doi:10.1177/0022022115585140.

Goforth, A. N., Michols, L. M., Stanick, C. F., Shindorf, Z. R., Holter, O. (2017). School-based considerations for supporting Arab American youths' mental health. *Contemporary School Psychology*, 21(3), 191–2000. doi:10.1007/s40688-016-0117-7.

Haboush, K. L. (2007). Working with Arab American families: Culturally competent practice for school psychologists. *Psychology in the Schools*, 44(2), 183–198.

Ikizler, A. S. & Szymanski, D. M. (2017). Discrimination, religious and cultural factors, and Middle Eastern/Arab Americans' psychological distress. *Journal of Clinical Psychology*, 74, 1219–1233. doi:10.1002/jclp.22584.

Khouri, L. Z. (2016). On belonging: The American adolescent of Arab descent. *Journal of Clinical Psychology*, 72(8), 818–826. doi:10.1002/jclp.22363.

Kim, S. Y., Chen, Q., Wang, Y., Shen, Y., & Orozco-Lapray, D. (2013). Longitudinal linkages among parent-child acculturation discrepancy, parenting, parent-child sense of alienation, and adolescent adjustment in Chinese immigrant families. *Developmental Psychology*, 49(5), 900–912. doi:10.1037/a0029169.

Kissil, K., Davey, M., & Davey, A. (2013). Therapists in a foreign land: Acculturation, language proficiency and counseling self-efficacy among foreign-born therapists practicing in the United States. *International Journal of Advanced Counseling*, 35, 216–233.

Kumar, R., Seay, N, & Karabenick, S. A. (2015). Immigrant Arab adolescents in ethnic enclaves: Physical and phenomenological contexts of identity negotiation. *Cultural Diversity and Ethnic Minority Psychology*, 21(2), 201–212. doi:10.1037/a0037748.

Landreth, G. L. (2012). *Play therapy: The art of the relationship*. Routledge.

Lichtblau, E. (2016, September 17). Hate crimes against American Muslims most since post-9/11 era. *The New York Times*. www.nytimes.com/2016/09/18/us/politics/hate-crimes-american-muslims-rise.html.

Lipson, J. G., Reizian, A. E., & Meleis, A. I. (1987). Arab-American patients: A medical record review. *Social Science and Medicine*, 24(2).

Manning, M. L. & Baruth, L. G. (2004). *Multicultural education of children and adolescents* (4th ed.). Pearson.

Marvasti, A. & McKinney, K. D. (2004). *Middle Eastern lives in America*. Rowman & Littlefield.

Measher, L. (2020, May 21). The 2020 census continues the whitewashing of Middle Eastern Americans. *NBC News THINK*. www.nbcnews.com/think/opinion/2020-census-continues-whitewashing-middle-eastern-americans-ncna1212051.

Mechammil, M., Boghosian, S., & Cruz, R. A. (2019). Mental health attitudes among Middle Easter/North African individuals in the United States. *Mental Health, Religion, and Culture*, 22(7), 724–737. doi:10.1080/13674676.2019.1644302.

Moosa, S., Karabenick, S. A., & Adams, L. (2001). Teacher perceptions of Arab parent involvement in elementary schools. *The School Community Journal*, 11, 7–26. www.adi.org/journal/fw01/Moosa%20et%20al.pdf.

Nassar-McMillan, S. C. & Hakim-Larson, J. (2003). Counseling considerations among Arab Americans. *Journal of Counseling and Development*, 81(2), 150–159. doi:10.1002/j.1556-6678.2003.tb00236.x.

Paige, S., Hatfield, E., & Liang, L. (2015). Iranian-American perceptions of prejudice and discrimination: Differences between Muslim, Jewish, and non-religious Iranian-Americans. *An International Journal of Personal Relationships*, 9(2), 236–252. doi:10.5964/ijpr.v9i2.194.

Patterson, C. H. (1996). Multicultural counseling: From diversity to universality. *Journal of Counseling and Development*, 74, 227–231.

Ray, D. C. (2011). *Advanced play therapy: Essential conditions, knowledge, and skills for child practice*. Routledge.

Said, E. W. (1997). *Covering Islam*. Pantheon Books.

Sue, D. & Sue, D. (2003). *Counseling the culturally diverse: Theory and practice* (4th ed.). Wiley.

Tabbah, R., Miranda, A. H., & Wheaton, J. E. (2012). Self-concept in Arab-American adolescents: Implications of social support and experiences in the schools. *Psychology in the Schools*, 49(9), 817–827. doi:10.1002/pits.21640.

Tabbah, R., Miranda, A. H., & Wheaton, J. E. (2016). Intricacies of school relationships and the well-being of Arab American youth: Implications for school psychologists. *Contemporary School Psychology*, 20, 315–326. doi:10.1007/s40688.

Tehranian, J. (2009). *Whitewashed: America's invisible Middle Eastern minority*. New York University Press.

Vang, C. T. (2010). *An educational psychology of methods in multicultural counseling*. Peter Lang.

Wingfield, M. & Karaman, B. (1995). Arab stereotypes and American educators. *Social Studies and Young Learners*, 7(4), 7–10.

12 Becoming a Culturally Inclusive White Play Therapist

Kristie Opiola and Alyssa Swan

Carl Rogers (1980) regarded the self-actualizing tendency as a naturally occurring, ongoing process of human growth, not a designation to achieve nor a destination at which one eventually arrives. Similarly, we believe that becoming a culturally inclusive White play therapist is a continual journey. Because everyone is unique in their experiences and intersecting identities, each White play therapist acknowledges and witnesses the impact of their whiteness in different ways. In this chapter, we explore the journey of becoming culturally inclusive White play therapists and how to practice with cultural humility. We narrowed our focus to play therapy-specific scenarios in this chapter.

This chapter is not a how-to manual but a reflection on our processes of becoming more culturally inclusive as humans and play therapists. We found this chapter exciting to talk about but challenging to write. We struggled to ensure our words reflected our intentions. Nevertheless, we worry about being misunderstood, our intentions missed, or unintentionally writing a microaggressive statement without engaging the reader. We attempt to counteract our fear by regularly processing our experiences and sharing our thoughts, experiences, and ideas. This gave us opportunities to challenge each other to think deeper or differently about culturally inclusive practices. This discomfort was consistent throughout the writing process as we tried to express our thoughts and ideas fully.

Our journeys have required us to reflect, take risks, be vulnerable, embrace discomfort, and challenge ourselves to hold courageous conversations. We have certainly not arrived at a full culturally inclusive/anti-racist destination but continue to travel as we serve and support others on their life journeys. We encourage the reader to slow down, reflect, and respond to their experiences with whiteness, positionalities, and racist mistakes they have made. We found that slowing down to experience has allowed us to become more intentional and sensitive in our interactions. Mistakes are part of this journey and we embrace them. We have hit many speed bumps and know we will make more mistakes as we strive to become more culturally and racially inclusive.

Second, we experienced various emotional reactions as we have read works on culturally inclusive practices and cultural humility. Our emotional

DOI: 10.4324/9781003190073-15

responses have included anger, guilt, shame, silence, withdrawal, and defensiveness. These emotional reactions are a disconnect between our thoughts, beliefs, attitudes, and behaviors. As we explored our reactions, we found them to be common reactions to challenge our ideologies, and at times we felt threatened. DiAngelo (2016) explained this reaction as "white fragility, the attempt to protect and shelter one's white privilege from honest exploration, racial discomfort, or racial stress" (p. 246). Our responses indicate discomfort and resistance to exploration or open communication. Our discomfort is healthy and will help us identify areas and thoughts that need attention. We believe that if we breathe into the discomfort, we can stay present, acknowledge our reaction, and examine our biases.

We want to share our experiences and clinical stories with you. As we discussed the creation of this chapter, we worried that our examples might escalate our whiteness. We have thoughtfully and carefully tried to honor the children and families we serve. However, we are aware that we are invoking power by sharing stories and clinical cases by deciding how much, when, and what we address. We attempt to share our stories' raw, authentic sides while also staying accountable for our roles.

Characteristics of White Play Therapists

The Association of Play Therapy's (APT) most recent growth report stated roughly 7,518 members, with an average length of membership of 16.2 years (APT, n.d.). APT collects demographic information from members on a voluntary basis. Current APT demographic data includes membership status, gender, credentials, discipline, generation, and race/origin. Roughly 75% of current members identified their race/ethnicity field, 95% identified their discipline field, 44% identified their gender field, and 66% of members identified their work settings. According to APT (2021), 73.9% identified as White, 6.8% identified as First Nations, 6.7% identified as Latinx, 6.3% identified as Black or African American, 3% identified as Asian, 3% identified as biracial, and less than 0.01% identified as multiracial. Play therapists are primarily women, with 92.4% identifying as female, 6.7% identifying as male, and 0.9% identifying as other or preferring not to answer. The demographic information is slightly more diverse than previous studies (Ryan et al., 2002; Kranz et al., 1998; Phillips & Landreth, 1998; Phillips & Landreth, 1995), but the landscape of play therapy lacks diversity (Abrams et al., 2006). Ryan et al. (2002) explored education levels and found most of the population holding a master's degree (76.9%) and some members obtaining doctorate degrees (18.8%). Diversity does exist with professional licensure identity, with 53.3% reporting as counselors, 25.8% as social workers, 6% as psychologists, and 12.3% as marriage and family therapists (APT, 2021).

From our experiences, most Association for Play Therapy (APT) national conference attendees and presenters are White and female. We know many play therapists of color, but overall the landscape of the profession is White. The same is true if we explore authorship. Although we have found more articles from authors of color recently, White professionals have written most articles on play therapy since its development. Parallel to other related fields (e.g. psychology, counseling, medicine, development), major play therapy theories were developed and written by White play therapists and are still used today. For example, Child-Centered (Axline; Landreth), Adlerian (Kottman), Gestalt (Oaklander), Jungian (Allen), Prescriptive (Schaefer), and Filial (Guerneys). All play therapists can (1) appreciate the extent to which generational and culture shape theoretical frameworks and (2) ensure conceptualization from these theories include voices of color. Although White authors permeate the play therapy field, there are researchers targeting outcomes with populations of color. According to Lin and Bratton (2015), 29% of child-centered play therapy (CCPT) research studies targeted non-Caucasian populations and found CCPT "is particularly responsive to the needs of diverse populations of children" (p. 50) and suggests CCPT is a culturally responsive counseling intervention for diverse populations. These studies show the positive impacts of play therapy with children from diverse cultural backgrounds and help play therapists explore cultural considerations and limitations within clinical practices.

The above points are important to note because knowledge is socially constructed and therefore reflects the values and interests of the authors (Banks, 1993). If knowledge is socially constructed, much of our learning may be rooted in White values, White practices, White customs, White language, etc. This was surprising as I (KO) was always taught that learning and education were neutral, universal, and objective. Unfortunately, this narrative upholds Western "mainstream" views of knowledge (Banks, 1993). If our professional writings and learned play therapy experiences primarily come from White presenters and White authors, then many of the concepts learned to carry the values, frame of reference, and normative positions of whiteness. This is an area of concern and further reflection when working with individuals from diverse backgrounds and experiences.

As noted above, whiteness and being White have advantages that are scarcely acknowledged and often unconscious. The death of George Floyd has brought the disadvantages and injustices of persons of color (POC) to the forefront of mainstream discussions and thoughts. However, there have been racial injustice incidents throughout history. In the George Floyd killing, the American public saw firsthand the brutality, police violence, and disregard towards POC. For me (KO), this was an incident where no other plausible factors could explain the officers' actions. This incident, coupled with the death of Breonna Taylor, opened my eyes to systemic practices that targeted POC and the level of injustices they experience. People of all colors flooded the streets and demanded justice and equality for individuals, specifically for POC. Individuals and institutions began to learn more about anti-racist beliefs and how White society was complicit in maintaining racism in U.S. society. Many play therapists in my community saw a rise of book clubs and suggestions on anti-racist readings to help White professionals take intentional steps to acknowledge, dismantle, and confront White supremacy and White privilege.

So, what does it mean to be White? This may seem like a strange question and one that White therapists might find challenging to answer. White people are often blind to color, and this is reflected in the literature. Kendall (2012) highlights White culture's blindness to seeing color and the relevance of being White in America. When asked about being White, I (KO) struggled to describe it because whiteness is the norm and unnamed in my culture. Instead, terms like "individual" were used when describing race-related topics for White individuals. I see myself utilizing the term "individual" often when describing clients and families. Not seeing color or using non-racial language to describe White clients prevents White therapists and individuals from recognizing and acknowledging their own racial biases, unearned privileges, and the impact of institutional racism (Sue & Sue, 2016). Additionally, hesitation to see color and a lack of awareness of colorblindness put White therapists at greater risk for discriminating based on color and harming clients (Baima & Sude, 2019).

I (KO) have found DiAngelo's work on White fragility informative and personally insightful. I have experienced defensiveness when talking about race but lacked the awareness of where my defensiveness was stemming from. DiAngelo's (2018) six reasons White individuals experience racial defensiveness helped me explore my reactions and lean into the discomfort. For example, I worried about others' thoughts about me because I had a dualist belief that being racist was bad and relatable to being a member of the White supremacy group, the Ku Klux Klan (KKK). Additionally, I was taught that talking about race was politically incorrect and seen as taboo. Lastly, I was socialized to see myself as an individual instead of part of a group. My group membership shaped me in profound ways (Sensoy & DiAngelo, 2017). I would get defensive out of fear of being called racist, shut down, and disengage from the interaction. DiAngelo's work indicates that my White defensive reactions may protect me from exploring racism, create an environment of social comfort, and perpetuate my systematic benefits. My White comfort makes me less tolerant of racial stress in the future instead of an entry point to acknowledge my blind spots and prejudices (Sensoy & DiAngelo, 2017).

According to McIntosh (1989), the color of our (KO and AS) White skin offers us a privilege that our friends of color do not experience. Therefore, our White skin is an unearned asset. Whiteness benefits us by allowing us to speak and act freely without fear of criticism based on race; protecting us from hostility, harm, or distress based on race; allowing us to identify and choose people to socialize and work alongside; receiving opportunities and advantages that are not available to all. These are not conditions that we have earned, but instead those passed down to us due to being White and a system that empowered our White cultural group. Suchet (2007) described being White as an ideological lived experience that created beliefs, policies, and practices. These lived experiences have enabled White people to maintain power and control (Colombo, 2015). Whiteness and White superiority are embedded in American culture and have afforded White individuals unearned advantages over people and communities of color. Whiteness is the silent norm and "silence is central to [its] power" (Suchet, 2007, p. 868).

Color is not the only characteristic that affords power and privilege. Intersectionality (also referred to as positionality) acknowledges the unique lived experiences of people and the complex, multidimensional aspects of our lives (Mullan, 2021). Mullan shared that a single identity cannot define a person and people are a complex mix of different identities. Each identity has a different level of power. Intersectionality was first coined by Kimberlé Williams Crenshaw (1989) and allows individuals to explore their lives and how different social dynamics give them advantages. Table 12.1 illustrates the spectrum of different identities and characteristics by which someone has unearned privilege or experienced oppression. Individuals can best understand one's positionality/intersectionality through self-reflection. Self-reflection allows individuals to explore themselves as well as one's relationships with others. Through self-reflection, I (KO) better understand my

Table 12.1 Chart of power/privilege

	Privilege		Marginalized
Gender	Cisgendered male	Cisgendered female	Trans, intersex, non-binary
Skin color	White	Different shades	Dark
Ability	Able bodied	Health issues	Living with a disability
Sexuality	Heterosexual	Gay man	Lesbian, gay, queer, pan, bi, asexual
Age	Middle-aged	Youth	Elderly
Neurodiversity	Neurotypical	Some neurodiversity	Significant neurodivergence
Body size	Slim	Average	Large
Socio-economic status	Rich	Middle-class	Poor
Language	English	Some English	Non-English monolingual
Citizenship	Citizen	Documented	Undocumented
Indigenous	Non-indigenous		Indigenous

Adapted from ccrweb.ca and Canadian Council of Refugees

positionality and become more inclusive of different dynamics that impact the children and families with whom I work. This has allowed me to confront and challenge the conscious and unconscious attitudes and beliefs I hold of clients (Sensoy & DiAngelo, 2017).

I (KO) have found that being White requires me to own the injustices and oppression that my ancestors and contemporaries have caused, intentionally or unintentionally. Because I am likely to see myself more as an individual, this makes that level of accountability challenging, yet I believe it is imperative to my work as a play therapist because I need to increase my openness to others' experiences and counteract my natural tendencies to normalize my White values, beliefs, ideals, and standards and interject my worldview on all clients (Kendall, 2012). According to Andersen (2019), the current culture of whiteness reproduces itself by normalizing White behaviors and mutating the rules when they want to maintain superiority, power, and control. Unfortunately, this creates unequal standards, overtly and covertly, and reproduced superiority in our society's institutions, including health care and mental health practices. For example, play therapy was founded and developed by White therapists and had centralized White middle-class cultural norms as healthy standards for all children.

Lastly, White play therapists must evaluate if their intentions or actions are part of the White Savior Complex. White saviorism is a practice where individuals intentionally or unintentionally believe they can (1) help POC in ways that can negatively affect POC due to a lack of understanding of client needs; (2) rescue or heal POC; or (3) support POC because they lack the resources, willpower, and intelligence to help themselves. White saviorism reinforces colonist beliefs of White people as authority figures and that POC need strong, capable White helpers to rescue POC from their current situations. This does not mean all acts of support or help are White saviorism. I (KO) have found that asking myself the following questions helps me identify if I am providing a meaningful form of allyship or acting out of White saviorism: (1) Is my help serving a need or does it make me feel better? (2) Do I have the skills needed for this job? and (3) Am I providing the help the client wants or operating from my assumptions about their need? We will now discuss ways to confront our assumptions, biases, and stereotypes by raising our awareness, shifting our focus from cultural competence to cultural humility, and identifying cultural opportunities in our practices and the community.

Awareness

Perhaps, like us, you grew up with an implicit understanding, veiled by terminology of political correctness, that it is taboo or political for White people to discuss race. DiAngelo (2011) described this experience as part of White fragility, which sustains White supremacy. If race is only talked about as othered or non-White experiences, then White individuals are shielded or excused societally from discussions related to race; this is one example of privilege. Guided by this racially engrained principle and implicit bias, a White play therapist may feel uncertain how, when, or if to communicate about race when racial experiences may be impacting play therapy, inside or outside of the playroom. As a culturally inclusive play therapist, it is essential not to perpetuate oppressive structures in play therapy relationships and practices. White play therapists can intentionally and routinely set aside time to familiarize themselves with sources of biases. Sincere reflective practice of identifying biases towards clients, considering alternative perspectives, and practicing empathic perspective-taking can lead to fewer oppressive clinical attributions and biased dispositions with clients (Chen et al., 1997).

Awareness on the part of a White play therapist goes beyond direct clinical interactions, including continual self-evaluation of potential for racial and/or cultural bias in conceptualization, treatment planning, and assessment. Accurate self-evaluation of the therapist's view of the client and assessment of a client's experiences and identity leads to play therapists' more accurate use of reflections and limit-setting, engagement in advocacy efforts in children's lives (i.e. teachers, administration), and measurement of outcomes and progress. For example, a White play therapist may view a Black child's assertive behavior as pathological or a personal defect without investigating the situation in which the behavior is embedded. As the play therapist, this requires me to reflect on my relationship with the child, my interpretation of the behavior, and how the child's assertiveness impacts me. If I view assertiveness as pathological behavior, I will likely respond to eliminate the behavior or judge the child. Assessing a child's assertive nature as an asset rather than a pathological behavior, for example, directly influences the nature of the therapist's tolerance of a child's world without therapist countertransference supporting the avoidance of the child from actual lived experiences and feelings. Perhaps a shift from limit-setting to an acceptance of the child's feelings, such as "you are mad about that" or "you are deciding which one you want to wear," may suffice and subdue the need for the limit in the first place. Similarly, accurate assessment of a child's world can support a White play therapist to identify play themes most accurately for each child (perhaps, a shift from power/control theme to relationship-seeking) during play therapy.

According to the Experience-Expression Congruence Model (EECM; Ray et al., 2014), play therapists' perceptions of emerging experiences in play therapy guide their intentional expression of congruence. The EECM can be expanded to address culture and has helped us become more culturally inclusive play therapists and grow in our cultural awareness and skills development. For us, the EECM model helps us as White play therapists to (a) be aware of racially or culturally situated experiences during play therapy with children and (b) allow congruent awareness of content into consciousness, without implicitly avoiding due to race-related stress that may thwart authenticity, then White play therapists can most congruently assess the situation and its impact on the therapeutic relationship to respond accordingly.

To manage race-related stress, White play therapists may use defense mechanisms, such as avoidance and rationalization (Utsey & Gernat, 2002), which impair the accuracy of self and other awareness. For example, Cartwright et al. (2008) found that White clinicians reported inflated rates of self-reported multicultural counseling competence compared to independent observer ratings of videotaped multicultural counseling scenarios. With or without intention, making assumptions can confirm the cultural mistrust that clients experience with White mental health providers (Carlisle & Murray, 2020). For example, a White play therapist assumes a client's experience based on a racial stereotype or they miss an essential element of a child's story based on a color-blind fallacy. In both cases, the child may validly detect contradiction between the therapist's stated professional identity or theoretical orientation and client-observed therapist behavior. For example, a play therapist laughs when a child tells a racist joke in the playroom because the play therapist does not understand the context of the joke, and the child is laughing. The play therapist laughs and believes this to convey acceptance of the child's humor; yet the child could feel confused or hurt that the play therapist (whom they view as accepting and non-judgmental) would laugh at such a joke. When White play therapists aim to manage race-related stress rather than authentically embracing an opportunity for growth in understanding social positioning, they risk unknowingly amplifying the power differential from clients and exercising privilege to maintain the status quo.

Cultural Humility

A significant shift from cultural competence to cultural humility (Tervalon & Murray-García, 1998) requires a lifelong commitment to evaluating and critiquing self to amend power imbalances in therapeutic relationships. Making biases explicit and promoting respect for all clients, core aspects of operating from a cultural humility framework, can result in mutual empowerment and authentic partnerships (Foronda, 2019). Cultural humility is not equivalent to avoidance. The play therapist may not be comfortable but can develop a tolerance for ambiguity, paired with an authentic acceptance that they do not know all the answers and the courage to initiate and sustain culturally pertinent conversations and experiences.

For context application, White play therapists need to understand and identify racial microaggressions, ideally preemptively and certainly if they commit a microaggression. Self-evaluation is the first step; the next step requires a commitment to cultural humility from the White play therapist. Subsequent actions will likely, and are not limited to, include a combination of the following: (1) discontinuing use of oppressive statement or behavior, (2) seeking supervision/consultation to discuss a racial-relevant clinical event and seek advice, (3) initiating conversation to address the offense with the client or parent, (4) understanding microaggressions from the perspectives of racial minority clients as well as White clients, while considering individual client context and intersecting identities to avoid stereotypes, and (5) safeguarding clients from future unintentional racial microaggressions through ongoing reflective practice and intentional commitment to continue learning about how consequences of the White-based internal frame of reference. The intersection of cultural and racial factors also, undoubtedly, influences the work and perspective of a play therapist.

Although education about racial groups and cultures similar and different from the play therapist is essential, play therapists must avoid unnecessary stereotypes of a particular client based on working knowledge of cultural norms. A part of cultural humility is an appreciation for learning about the person in front of you (i.e. child, parent, family) from their unique worldview. Asking a parent about their values, preferences, impact of racial/ethnic identity, and experiences with injustices is a solid place to begin understanding a particular family's experiences and inviting dialogue related to race into the therapeutic relationship. Lekas et al. (2020) regarded the shift from cultural competence to cultural humility as a focus of training buffers providers, like play therapists, from disregarding intersectionality. Clients hold multiple social statuses and identities that shape their lived experiences, perceptions of the play therapist, values, and behaviors. At the core of their model of cultural humility, Zhu and colleagues (2021) designated the foundational principle of cultural humility as a way of being. Zhu et al. (2021) proposed a grounded theory of cultural humility enactment and development, illustrated by a figure representing the ongoing, cyclical nature of related factors: precipitating events, contextual factors, intervening factors, action/interaction strategies, and consequences (p. 78). White play therapists who espouse a cultural humility framework embrace cultural opportunities with children of similar or different races.

Embracing Cultural Opportunities

White play therapists will serve clients who identify as part of a majority group and racially or culturally oppressed groups. It is not unlikely that White play therapists might miss cultural opportunities inside and outside of the playroom due to the above factors. Thus, we describe how White play therapists can embrace more racially and/or culturally situated opportunities with clients, in supervision, and within systemic contexts.

With Clients

In play therapy, children are not reliant on verbal communication nor conscious awareness to express inner experiences to the therapist. A child may play out direct expressions of racial awareness. For example, a five-year-old Latinx child was in the playroom looking through the medical bag; they found several band-aids. Upon opening a brown color band-aid, they exclaimed, "Hey, this band-aid is my color!" They handed the White play therapist a tan color band-aid, "This one's for you." A child may process observed racial differences between child and therapist with less overt play expression. For example, during the fifth weekly play therapy session, a four-year-old Black child drew a picture of her and the White play therapist. The play therapist watched as she carefully selected a yellow marker and began drawing. When she finished, she looked up at the therapist and proudly declared, "There we are. It is you, and that is me" (the child pointed to each figure in the drawing). The drawing was two yellow stick figures with matching yellow hair.

Nevertheless, a child may still enact play behavior like the examples provided and not communicate or process about race. Because play therapy allows children to communicate and relate through play, often nonverbal exchanges via play behavior and play themes are witnessed by the play therapist. Play therapists decide how to respond to children in the playroom based on theoretical orientation, core conditions, and in-the-moment relational contact.

The above examples occur in the playroom; and have occurred in the playroom when I (AS) was the play therapist. In either case, I did not question the child to confirm if they were demonstrating race-related play; instead, I reflected and engaged in the moment. From a person-centered perspective, I understand that the process of children's play can be more important than the product of their play. No rule book exists for relationships. As such, I rely on the relationship to respond to children in the playroom with genuineness, congruence, and empathic understanding; all of which are derived from my professional and personal experiences as a human being and, therefore, susceptible to bias. As a White therapist, I went to supervision and processed these experiences. In supervision, I processed if, from my White lens, I was making assumptions of race-related play that were not accurately reflective of the child's experience. For example, perhaps the child's parent had verbalized the last time they bought band-aids at the store that the color matched this child's skin color; the child in the playroom could have been repeating her mother's observation and less so making note of her skin color for the therapist.

As a therapist, I sometimes feel worried that I might miss an important opportunity to convey more complete acceptance to this child while balancing concern of not wanting to pathologize characteristics of play that are common for all children. In processing my feelings openly with my supervisor, I can work through my own anxieties as a play therapist who is unsure at times in the play therapy session. I have wondered aloud in supervision, "What if I missed a cultural exploration opportunity to most accurately understand what the child was processing through play... how could I broach cultural opportunities that I missed... should I be more directive in this moment?" It is unsettling at times to "trust the process" without controlling the child's self-directed process and simultaneously to wonder if I am "hearing" a child's play accurately from their lens.

Similarly, in the following example, the child may have chosen to create both stick figures in yellow because they prefer the color yellow, rather than communicating the skin color differences between child and therapist. Using supervision as a place for processing, the White play therapist can form a complete conceptualization of the therapeutic relationship and child. Understanding contextual factors that impact the child, in combination with in-session interactions, helps any play therapist to most accurately reflect children's feelings and intentions in play therapy. If, based on my White lens and potential for White saviorism, I make assumptions that the child is processing race-related content, when in fact they are playing just as any child their age may in the playroom, I might inaccurately reflect the child's experience at the moment. Conceptually, these assumptions can interfere with the core condition of empathic understanding.

Conversely, if I did not process the potential for race-related play to enter the playroom and therapeutic relationship (e.g. using the example above, I assume that yellow is their favorite color with no indication of racial identity processing), then I might not bring these interactions into supervision or into my awareness to process. If conceptualization is that the child appears to like yellow, I might reflect, "You like us both being yellow." If conceptualization is that the child has internalized that darker color skin is bad and light color/blonde is good, I might reflect, "You wanted us both to look just like this," while pointing to the figures. The latter reflection can open up the child's exploration of wanting to "look like" the therapist or valuing the therapist's skin color. Avoiding cultural opportunities for the sake of convenience or assuming the absence of culturally related play, the White play therapist can unintentionally enact conditional regard for the child; which impacts the authenticity felt by the child in the play therapy room (e.g. is all of the child's experience being heard and accepted by the therapist?).

Imagine the following parent consultation meeting. I listen to a parent tearfully share frustration and exhaustion related to the school-reported struggles at school. She shared with me that the evening before, her young son cried to his mother, "My teacher does not like me." She disclosed fear of being a burden to the predominantly White school. She shared concerns that the administrators and teacher had not taken time to get to know her son before issuing consequences and pending dismissal for behavior issues. This parent and her son identified as Black American; I am a White play therapist.

In response, I could avoid the discussion and focus on the child's behavior; I have the privilege to evade racial discourse as a White individual (Singleton & Hays, 2006). Alternatively, I could ask this parent to sign a release of information to consult with the school administration, counselor, or teacher; my privileges and connections at the school might move beyond the mother's position. Or I could ask her about other students' racial/ethnic composition and the teachers in her son's classroom. All of these responses may be professionally appropriate and helpful in different ways. I believe there is no one "right" way to respond in sessions. Guided by a person-centered orientation, I hope to be most authentic in my relationship with this parent.

In this particular meeting, I was attuned to the mother's tearful disposition and her mention of not wanting to seem like a burden to school administration. Her experience as a Black woman with a Black son in a White school felt prevalent. I decided to reflect on her hesitation and ask this mother about the racial composition of her child's classroom. I learned that they are the only Black family in the school. This mother shared that she had not considered the impact of race in this situation until I asked. Parents in other cases might have shared that they did not believe race plays a significant role in this situation. Parents in other cases might bring up the topic of race during the next parent-teacher conference. Other parents may ask for assistance in planning the next steps in advocating for and supporting her son at this school. This mother seemed to appreciate that racism was being openly discussed as a possible factor. Consistent with classroom management and behavioral approaches, the school and teacher were focused on improving this child's behavior. Therefore, the mother approached parent consultation from a behavior lens: help me help my son improve his behavior. This parent shared in our first meeting that the school, teacher, and mother had tried nearly every available behavior modification strategy. The child felt "bad" about themselves, and their behavior, and the mother and school system felt helpless. I understood that broaching race in session with this mother was not equivalent to an easy fix behavior "save all" strategy. However, it was an honest reflection of my observation of the system.

Singleton and Hays (2006) encouraged professionals to facilitate courageous conversations about race, encouraging professionals to increase comfort in broaching race and cultural discourse. White play therapists also may ask parents to describe their experiences with questions such as, what is a normal (week, day, visit) for *your* family; what will it be like to work with a White therapist; and what pieces of your family and culture do you want this therapist to know?

In Supervision

Beliefs about race are often misconceptions (Singleton & Hays, 2006). Professionals can inspect their racial identities and personal race history to provide context for their most natural worldview, which may counter the lens of clients. Through honest efforts to understand clients' racial identities and personal history from their perspectives, the White play therapist can be willing to abandon old habits built through a lifetime of being White

(Singleton & Hays, 2006). Cultural humility can be enhanced and developed through supervision (e.g. Hook et al., 2016). A more in-depth look at supervision can be found in Chapter 14, but we wanted to address how to facilitate cultural development for White therapists in supervision specifically.

Supervision and/or consultation is an essential ingredient to ongoing professional growth as a White play therapist. Kleist and Hill (2003) cited the reflective model of triadic supervision (RMTS) as one context for fostering cultural humility. Hook et al. (2016) presented a two-component model for addressing cultural humility in clinical supervision, including (a) modeling and teaching cultural humility as part of the interpersonal nature of clinical supervision and (b) overt opportunities to teach cultural humility via learning experiences outside of clinical supervision sessions. Adopting an attitude of cultural humility during clinical supervision connects to providers' broaching of racial conversations and topics in counseling sessions (Jones & Branco, 2020). Supervision with video or audio recorded play sessions to review can allow supervisors to observe client or therapist behavior related to racial content in the session and/or point out missed cultural opportunities.

Working with the Systems

Social justice counseling requires a shift from awareness of individual clients' context in their environment and understanding the nuances of how clients are coping with systemic oppression or racism to facilitating concrete action to change or influence the environment around current and future clients (Ratts et al., 2015). I called a teen client to confirm our first appointment. We talked briefly about their experiences in their current out-of-home placement and new school and then hung up. When I met them at the clinic door the next day, I had hoped they could feel welcome at yet another new clinician's office. "Hi, it is nice to meet you in person!" Their response surprised me as they smirked and responded, "You did not have a White person's voice on the phone." I responded congruently, sharing a smile that matched their playfulness and my curiosity, yet honoring the seriousness in their observation, "I am different than you expected." They shared that they learned to judge White providers' authenticity early on by listening to them talk on the phone. Before meeting me, and unbeknownst to me, they were in a natural process of deciding if they could trust me. In this example, this teen overtly equated inauthenticity with whiteness. This teen verbalized what many individuals may not have words or safety to express in words; the impact of whiteness, separate from a White therapist's therapeutic intent and morality, in a system disguised as a helping, not oppressive, profession. Helping and oppressive contexts are not mutually exclusive. White play therapists can understand how their intention may be to help while their impact may be harmful, sometimes due to clients' experiences within White systems in the past.

Further, White allies use their own privilege to create more equitable systems (Spanierman & Smith, 2017) and not contribute to recapitulating paternalistic and White saviorism attitudes in play therapy practice or training. Clients of color are not objects of White humanitarianism and White play therapist allyship should not be cosmetic. White play therapists can outline a plan for participation in social justice-oriented action toward anti-racist practice. Malott et al. (2019) described backlashes of White allyship, namely relational conflict and burnout. As a White play therapist, I am likely to be in communities of White individuals outside of the play therapy office. White allyship crosses over into social justice actions in the personal lives of White individuals. For example, I may witness discrimination and microaggression in my daily life among family members and friends. My decision to intervene in systems of oppression is not restricted to the walls of the playroom; however, this reality of being an advocate may be difficult for White play therapists. Spanierman and Smith (2017) discussed the disruption of systems and environments that perpetuate oppression and color-blind ideology, extending impact to current and future clients' environments. Assuming an orientation of cultural humility can help White play therapists tolerate mistakes and take risks. We suggest for White play therapists to take a moment to consider their positioning in changing systems and list action-oriented commitments that they can make to support social justice as a reality in their lived experiences as play therapists. If White play therapists already engage in social justice-oriented work, consider ways to expand further or deepen areas of impact. Remember that operating with cultural humility means that play therapists commit to a lifelong learning process and grow as advocates.

Conclusion

As two White play therapists, we wrote this chapter to dialogue with play therapists of all backgrounds about the impact of whiteness in play therapy and supervision. Play therapists can conceptualize how racial and ethnic identity impacts the experiences of therapists, child clients, and caregivers during play therapy sessions, consultation, supervision, and advocacy. The effort to genuinely seize cultural opportunities is not often easy, to see the angst and hurt of others due to racial inequity or discrimination/bias; however, play therapists can support one another in leaning into courageous conversations and embracing cultural opportunities in the playroom.

Positionality Statements

Kristie

I grew up in a family structure with married parents and two siblings. My parents instilled traditional Catholic values of hard work, respect, obedience, commitment, honesty, and kindness. Early in my life, my father was a member of the U.S. Army and worked for an international firm that bounced us around the United States and internationally. In middle school, my family moved to a planned community in the Northeastern U.S., and this was the first time I remember living in a diverse community. This was when I learned to practice "political correctness," in other words, to say the right words that would not offend, exclude, or marginalize people that looked or lived differently from me. This experience had the most significant influence on my beliefs and the ways I interacted with others. Political correctness was challenging and caused me anxiety about how I interacted with others and how others perceived me. I was told not to ask or point out differences which caused me to lose opportunities to learn from diverse individuals and grow in accepting others' way of living, believing, or thinking.

My anti-racist journey focuses on counteracting my beliefs, values, and color-blindness. I find it hard to define my White privilege, values, and beliefs. I get tongue-tied when I attempt to define my beliefs and values because I have not had to verbalize them before, and I worry that I might sound racist. I am still surprised by my lack of awareness of differences and quick judgment to compare or relate their experiences to my relationship with others. As a White play therapist, I see my judgment arise most around parenting and discipline practices. I consistently remind myself that all beliefs and experiences are valued and accurate. In sessions with children and families, I resist my urge to withdrawal from initiating or partaking in cultural conversations. Instead, I attempt to reflect and open dialogue. When I am aware of racist, insensitive statements or behaviors I make, I wrestle not to become defensive or argue my viewpoint. Instead, I attempt to repair and invite feedback. I am still blind to different aspects of my privilege and continue to be open and engaged in relationships. I am working on having greater awareness of my way of being and challenging my biases around whiteness and privilege and my actions that unintentionally discriminate against others.

Alyssa

I am a White American-born woman who identifies as a cisgender, heterosexual, college-educated, employed, middle-class individual. Until I moved to attend college, I spent my formative years living in the same small, rural Midwestern town that mainly consisted of White working-class families. My parents encouraged hard work and community; I still have dear friends that I met in grade school. I understand many times when my whiteness has impacted my work as a play therapist. Although I can articulate examples of both embraced and missed cultural opportunities, there are and will be times when my implicit bias or socialized White identity shields me from awareness or clear cultural inclusiveness. I am committed to being in relationships with individuals, communities, and myself in ways that continue to deepen with sincere acknowledgment of the impact of cultural sameness or differences inherent to being in relationships. While this commitment is honest, I will continue to fumble over my socialized values, biases, and ignorance as I strive to continue embracing cultural opportunities.

References

Abrams, L. P., Post, P., Algozzine, B., Miller, T., Scott, R., Gomory, T., & Cooper, J. B. (2006). Clinical experiences of play therapists: Does race/ethnicity matter? *International Journal of Play Therapy*, 15(2), 11–34. doi:10.1037/h0088913.

Andersen, K. (2019). White fragility: Why it's so hard for White people to talk about racism. *Journal of College and Character*, 20(2), 187–189. doi:10.1080/2194587X.2019.1591288.

Association for Play Therapy (n.d.). APT Annual Growth Report by CEO. https://cdn.ymaws.com/www.a4pt.org/resource/resmgr/about_apt/growth_report.pdf.

Baima, T., & Sude, M. E. (2019). What White mental health professionals need to understand about Whiteness: A Delphi study. *Journal of Marital and Family Therapy*, 46(1), 62–80. doi:10.1111/jmft.12385.

Banks, J. A. (1993). The canon debate, knowledge construction, and multicultural education. *Educational Researcher*, 22(5), 4–14. doi:10.3102/0013189X022005004.

Bartoli, E., Bentley-Edwards, K. L., Garcia, A. M., Michael, A., & Ervin, A. (2015). What do White counselors and psychotherapists need to know about race? White racial socialization in counseling and psychotherapy training programs. *Women & Therapy*, 38(3–4), 246–262. doi:10.1080/02703149.2015.1059206.

Carlisle, B., & Murray, C. (2020). The role of cultural mistrust in health disparities. In S. Bird Gulliver & L. Cohen (Eds.)., *The Wiley Encyclopedia of Health Psychology*. Wiley.

Cartwright, B., Daniels, J., Zhung, S. (2008). Assessing multicultural competence: perceived versus demonstrated performance. *Journal of Counseling and Development*, 86(3), 318–322.

Chen, M.-W., Froehle, T., & Morran, K. (1997). Deconstructing dispositional bias in clinical inference: Two interventions. *Journal of Counseling & Development*, 76(1), 74–81. doi:10.1002/j.1556-6676.1997.tb02378.x.

Chouinard, J. A., & Cram, F. (2020). *Culturally responsive approaches to evaluation*. Sage.

Colombo E. (2015). Multiculturalism: An overview of multicultural debates in western societies. *Current Sociological Review*, 63(6), 800–824. doi:10.1177/0011392115586802.

Crenshaw, K. (1989). Demarginalizing the Intersection of race and sex: A black feminist critique of antidiscrimination doctrine, feminist theory and antiracist politics. *University of Chicago Legal Forum*, 1(8). Available at: https://chicagounbound.uchicago.edu/uclf/vol1989/iss1/8.

DiAngelo, R. (2011). White fragility. *International Journal of Critical Pedagogy*, 3(3), 54–70.

DiAngelo, R. (2016). White fragility. In P. Lang (Ed.), *What Does It Mean to Be White? Developing White Racial Literacy* (Revised Edition, 245–253). Retrieved from www.jstor.org/stable/45157307.

DiAngelo, R. (2018). *White fragility: Why it's so hard for White people to talk about racism*. Beacon Press.

Foronda C. (2019). A theory of cultural humility. *Journal of Transcultural Nursing*, 31(1), 7–12.

Hook J., Farrell J., Davis, D., DeBlaere, C., Van Tongeren, D., & Utsey, S. (2016). Cultural humility and racial microaggressions in counseling. *Journal of Counseling Psychology*, 63(3), 269–277.

Jones, C. T., & Branco, S. F. (2020). Trauma-informed supervision: Clinical supervision of addictions counselors. *Journal of Addictions and Offender Counseling*, 41, 2–17. doi:10.1002/jaoc.12072.

Kendall, F. (2012). *Understanding White privilege: Creating pathways to authentic relationships across race*. Routledge.

Kleist, D., & Hill, N. (2003). *The reflective model of triadic supervision*. Unpublished manuscript.

Kranz, P., Kottman, T., & Lund, N. (1998). Play therapists' opinions concerning education, training, and practices of play therapists. *International Journal of Play Therapy*, 7(1), 73–87.

Lekas, H.-M., Pahl, K., & Fuller Lewis, C. (2020). *Rethinking Cultural Competence: Shifting to Cultural Humility*. Health Services Insights. https://doi.org/10.1177/1178632920970580.

Lin, Y-W., & Bratton, S. C. (2015). A meta-analytic review of child-centered play therapy approaches. *Journal of Counseling and Development*, 93(1), 45–58. doi:10.1002/j.1556-6676.2015.00180.x.

Malott, K. M., Schaefle, S., Paone, T. R., Cates, J., & Haizlip, B. (2019). Challenges and coping mechanisms of Whites committed to anti-racism. *Journal of Counseling & Development*, 97(1), 86–97. doi:10.1002/jcad.12238.

McIntosh, P. (1989). White privilege: Unpacking the invisible knapsack. *Peace and Freedom Magazine*, July/August, 10–12.

Mullan, J. (2021, April 25). *Race-based traumatic stress [3 hour Intensive Session]*. 2021 Annual Children's Mental Health Symposium, Alberta, Canada (virtual).

Olcon, K. (2020). Confronting Whiteness: White U.S. social work students' experiences studying abroad in West Africa. *Journal of Teaching in Social Work*, 40 (4), 318–335. doi:10.1080/08841233.2020.1790472.

Phillips, R. D., & Landreth, G. L. (1995). Play therapists on play therapy I: A report of methods, demographics and professional practices. *International Journal of Play Therapy*, 4(1), 1–26.

Phillips, R. D., & Landreth, G. L. (1998). Play therapists on play therapy II: Clinical issues in play therapy. *International Journal of Play Therapy*, 6(2), 1–24.

Ratts*et al.* (2015). Multicultural and social justice competencies. American Counseling Association. Retrieved from www.counseling.org/docs/default-source/comp etencies/multicultural-and-social-justice-counseling-competencies.pdf?sfvrsn=20.

Ray, D. C., Jayne, K. M., & Stulmaker, H. L. (2014). A way of being in the playroom: Experience-expression congruence model (EECM). *International Journal of Play Therapy*, 23(1), 18–30. doi:10.1037/a0035512.

Rogers, C. (1980). *A way of being*. Houghton-Mifflin Co.

Ryan, S. D., Gomory, T., & Lacasse, J. R. (2002). Who are we? Examining the results of the Association for Play Therapy membership survey. *International Journal of Play Therapy*, 11(2), 11–41. doi:10.1037/h0088863.

Sensoy, O., & DiAngelo, R. (2017). *Is everyone really equal? An introduction to key concepts in social justice education* (2nd ed.). Teacher College Press.

Singleton, G., & Hays, C. (2006). Beginning courageous conversations about race. In G. Singleton & C. Linton (Eds.), *Courageous Conversations about Race: A Field Guide for Achieving Equity in Schools*. Corwin Press.

Spanierman, L. B., & Smith, L. (2017). Roles and responsibilities of White allies: Implications for research, teaching, and practice. *The Counseling Psychologist*, 45(5), 606–617. doi:10.1177/0011000017717712.

Suchet, M. (2007). Unraveling Whiteness. *Psychoanalytic Dialogues*, 17(6) 867–886. doi:10.1080/10481880703730.

Sue, D. W., & Sue, D. (2016). *Counseling the culturally diverse*. Wiley.

Tervalon, M., & Murray-García, J. (1998). Cultural humility versus cultural competence: A critical distinction in defining physician training outcomes in multicultural education. *Journal of Health Care for Poor Underserved*, 9 (2), 117–125.

Utsey, S. O., & Gernat, C. A. (2002). White racial identity attitudes and the ego defense mechanisms used by White counselor trainees in racially provocative counseling situations. *Journal of Counseling & Development*, 80(4), 475–483. doi:10.1002/j.1556-6678.2002.tb00214.x.

Zhu, P., Luke, M., & Bellini, J. (2021). A grounded theory analysis of cultural humility in counseling and counselor education. *Counselor Education and Supervision*, 60, 73–89.

13 Play Therapy with Children in Poverty

Sarah Tucker

At the onset of this chapter, I wish to clarify any misconceptions that could arise from the inclusion of poverty considerations in this book with the following assertion: poverty does not represent a culture in and of itself. Although references to poverty culture have been made across disciplines, data does not support the notion that those in poverty demonstrate shared characteristics or beliefs, as do distinct cultures (Seale, 2020). Conceptualizing poverty as a culture may perpetuate a damaging perception that those in poverty create their condition through commonalities in values, traits, and behaviors (Gorski, 2008; Ladson-Billings, 2017). Instead, poverty can be understood as a circumstance that intersects with an individual's cultural identity to create complexity within their phenomenal field. Hence, I have chosen to title this chapter slightly differently than other population chapters.

Across theories of play therapy, the play therapist's communication of empathic understanding towards the child is considered an essential component of the change process (Garza & Bruhn, 2011). I have had several opportunities to witness play therapy colleagues, supervisees, and students intentionally engage in empathy-building efforts. I have heard presentations of case conceptualizations informed by a child's presenting concern, family structure, racial and ethnic identity, and development as part of play therapists' sincere attempts to gain a clearer understanding of a child's inner world. Yet, even when working in high poverty contexts such as Title I funded schools (i.e. schools with 40% or more of their student population living in low-income families) and community agencies, I found it to be a rare occurrence that a play therapist would explore the influence socioeconomic factors may have on a child's experience.

Poverty impacts social, emotional, physical, behavioral, and cognitive facets of a child's life. When considering a child's identity in isolation from their socioeconomic context, the play therapist risks missing critical opportunities to accurately empathize with key aspects of the child's inner world. The primary aim of this chapter is to support the reader in enhancing both their awareness and empathic understanding of poverty in childhood while offering recommendations for translating awareness into action within clinical practice.

DOI: 10.4324/9781003190073-16

Childhood Poverty: Definitions and Demographics

What is poverty, exactly? While general definitions reference a "lack" or "scarcity" in resources, the construct of poverty is described in varying ways across the literature. In navigating the intricacies of different measures and definitions, it is beneficial to distinguish between two primary categories of poverty measurement: absolute and relative. Absolute poverty refers to financial means falling below a threshold of what is necessary to access life-sustaining resources, including food and shelter (Notten & de Neubourg, 2011). Much of the available data related to poverty statistics, including those represented in this chapter, are gathered through absolute measurements. By contrast, relative poverty is more fluid in nature, accounting instead for access to financial resources that allow for a societally average way of living (Townsend, 1979). Using a relative definition, one begins to recognize how the impact of poverty is far more prevalent than most official measures could ever capture. Considering various definitions globally and nationally can provide a holistic perspective into the prevalence of childhood poverty and allow play therapists to conceptualize the impact of poverty on children who are not captured by traditional measurement methods.

To measure extreme poverty worldwide, the World Bank developed an absolute measure of global poverty. By this measure, set at the United States equivalent of $1.90 per day, 689 million individuals were in extreme global poverty in 2018 (World Bank, 2020). Nearly half of those in poverty were 15 years old and younger, demonstrating an overrepresentation of children in poverty across the world (World Bank, 2020). Within the United States, national poverty is measured utilizing absolute income thresholds that vary by family size and composition. For reference, the weighted average poverty threshold in 2019 for a family of four was $26,172, and for a family of two was $16,521 (Semega et al., 2020). By this definition, approximately 34 million people lived below the poverty line in 2019, including 10.5 million children under 18 years old (Semega et al., 2020). Young children are disproportionately impacted by poverty in the U.S., with approximately one in five children under nine years old living in poverty (Koball et al., 2021).

Just as young children are overrepresented in poverty, so too are children of color. Researchers estimate that of all children in poverty, 71% are children of color (Children's Defense Fund, 2021). The racial disparities in poverty are glaringly evident in the demographic breakdown, with 26.5% of Black children, 20.8% of Hispanic children, 20.6% of American Indian/Alaska Native children, 8.3% of White, non-Hispanic children, and 7.7% of Asian, Native Hawaiian, and other Pacific Islander children living in poverty (Children's Defense Fund, 2021). Systemic oppression and racial discrimination have long created disparities in access to economic resources for people of color, which perpetuates the experience of poverty and inhibits economic mobility (Lin & Harris, 2008). Play therapists must remain attentive to how a child's marginalized identities related to social class and race may intersect to compound their experiences of discrimination and oppression.

Poverty and COVID-19

The aforementioned numbers alone would be enough to illustrate the concerning prevalence of childhood poverty; however, as of July 2021, most official poverty measures have not yet captured the impact of the presently unfolding COVID-19 pandemic. For the first time in over two decades, this pandemic has triggered a rise in extreme global poverty (World Bank, 2020). Researchers project that up to 163 million people worldwide will become newly impoverished due to the impact of the COVID-19 crisis (World Bank, 2021). Within the United States, researchers estimate that over 8 million additional individuals, including 2.5 million children, fell into poverty following the start of the pandemic (Parolin et al., 2020). As the COVID-19 pandemic continues to unfold, these numbers are expected to trend upwards (Parolin et al., 2020).

Considerations for Children in Poverty

Childhood Poverty Outcomes

In addition to the stressors of economic uncertainty, children living within the context of poverty experience higher rates of various childhood adversities (Steele et al., 2016). Community violence, food insecurity, and residential instability are among the many concerns highly correlated with living in poverty (Carlson, 2006; Ihrke & Faber, 2012; U.S. Department of Agriculture, n.d.). Considering the intensity of these compounding stressors, it stands to reason that childhood poverty would also be associated with poor mental health outcomes. Research confirms this presumption.

In a systematic review of 55 research studies, Reiss (2013) found that low-income children were twice as likely to experience mental health concerns as their economically privileged peers. These impacts were most substantial for children younger than 12 years of age (Reiss, 2013). Further research illustrates that the adverse effects of childhood poverty persist across the lifespan, with economic disadvantage in childhood serving as a significant predictor of the onset of mental health concerns in adulthood (McLaughlin et al., 2011).

Poverty also contributes to disruptions in academic achievement, compounding poor psychological outcomes. The topic of educational outcomes holds particular relevance for children in poverty, as education attainment plays a role in disrupting the cycle of poverty. Children who experience diminished academic achievement may face challenges obtaining employment in adulthood. Those who do may earn less than those with more favorable educational outcomes, thus perpetuating their experience of poverty (Reardon, 2011; Reiss, 2013). Scholars propose that poor mental health contributes to poor academic achievement and suggest that interventions supporting mental health may aid in achievement gains for children in poverty (Le Floch et al., 2018; Reiss, 2013). These outcomes underscore the importance of providing developmentally responsive mental health interventions for children in poverty.

Developmental Considerations

A child's development informs the social-emotional and cognitive structures through which they perceive the world. As such, children may process their understanding of their poverty context in various ways across different stages of development. As adults have lost contact with these developmental lenses, it can be challenging for adults to accurately perceive the developmentally unique ways children understand themselves and the world. While there are implications for a child's perception at each developmental stage, I highlight two key ages to illustrate the considerations present. The developmental overviews provided are brief, and play therapists are encouraged to seek further information regarding child development to strengthen their understanding.

Five-year-old

The brain of a five-year-old child is in a stage of rapid development (Sprenger, 2008). Cognitively, five-year-olds are increasingly able to apply causality to events around them; however, their perceptions of causal relationships overlap with developmentally appropriate egocentrism and magical thinking (Dillman Taylor, 2016). The simultaneous presence of these cognitive processes may result in the five-year-old child misattributing adverse outcomes to their own actions (Dillman Taylor, 2016). As children in poverty experience this period of development contextualized by chronic stressors, children in this stage may mistakenly perceive a sense of responsibility for the challenges they are facing.

I have witnessed children actively explore themes related to this causality in the playroom. In one instance of a child experiencing residential instability, the child played out a scene of packing up the dollhouse to move. This play repeated throughout several sessions, with few verbalizations, before the child transitioned to play at the craft table to self-soothe. Finally, in one iteration of the dollhouse play, the child gave voice to the dolls as they left the home. "You should have listened! Now we have to go!" the older doll shouted to the younger one. It seemed that the child was expressing their internal association of their behaviors as contributing to the cause for the upcoming move.

Seven-year-old

At seven years of age, children are increasingly concerned with heavier topics, including money and finances (Stulmaker, 2016). This stage also marks a heightened period of comparison between self and others (Stul-maker, 2016). As these two considerations overlap with a child's experience of poverty, children may begin processing the ways in which money impacts their experience while also noticing the disparity in the resources between themselves and their economically advantaged peers.

In my own experiences, the expression of this preoccupation has mani-fested clearly in the playroom. In one instance, an ordinarily upbeat and playful child entered the playroom, looking particularly distressed. After several minutes of silence and disengagement from play, the child asked if we could stop our special playtimes. When I reflected what I understood as a newfound disinterest in being there, the child shook their head and said, "It costs my mom a lot for me to come here." In another occurrence, a child engaging in puppet play shared a narrative of a baby puppet bringing different items to a father puppet. Each time, the father puppet would shout a new rejection of the request: "Put that back, we can't afford it!" "I'm not made out of money!" "Don't be so selfish!"

Play therapists should maintain an awareness of the ways in which development structures a child's cognitive and emotional processes. By overlapping developmental considerations with poverty awareness, the play therapist is increasingly equipped to communicate an enhanced under-standing of the child's experience.

Opportunities in Play Therapy to Attend to Children in Poverty

The necessity for adequate mental health supports for children in poverty is apparent. Given this, play therapists working with children in poverty should endeavor to ensure that the services they provide are optimized to address the needs of this population. This section outlines several opportu-nities for play therapists to enhance their facilitation of the therapeutic pro-cess for children in poverty.

Increasing Empathic Accuracy

A primary opportunity for the play therapist working with children in poverty is leveraging socioeconomic considerations to increase the accuracy of their empathic understanding. This requires the play therapist to integrate their foun-dational knowledge of poverty implications with their understanding of each individual child. In my work with children across the socioeconomic spectrum, I have witnessed many children engage in the exploration of themes related to poverty within their play. Most often, it is not the child's play behavior itself that signals an expression of poverty-related concerns. On the surface, the play may present as a child putting on a puppet show or trying on dress-up clothes. Yet, to an empathically connected play therapist, the play may communicate experi-ences of powerlessness or scarcity connected to low-income circumstances.

Play therapists who neglect socioeconomic considerations risk missing critical components of a child's experience, which may disrupt the development of accurate empathic understanding. On the other hand, play therapists who generalize themes of poverty are also at risk for making errors in empathy. For example, a play therapist fixated on a child's low-income status may misperceive a child using play money each session as related to themes of financial scarcity, when it may more accurately display a child's desire for mastery. Play therapists should evaluate socioeconomic considerations on a case-by-case basis to avoid generalizing poverty awareness across work with economically disadvantaged children. Seeking clinical supervision or consultation for routine discussions of case conceptualizations may support in minimizing errors on either side of the spectrum.

Selecting Facilitative Therapeutic Responses

Play therapists across the theoretical spectrum utilize foundational verbal skills as part of the therapeutic process (Kottman, 2011). Primary categories of these facilitative responses include tracking, reflecting content and feeling, limit setting, returning responsibility, and esteem-building responses (Ray, 2011). Throughout the therapeutic process, the play therapist aims to implement those responses that they believe will support a movement towards therapeutic objectives. Informed by an enhanced empathic understanding, play therapists working with children in poverty have the opportunity to increase the intentionality in the selection of their verbal responses.

In reviewing the many factors that inform the play therapist's selection of facilitative skills, Kottman (2011) emphasizes the need to consider each child and their unique life context. As is true with any child, each category of verbal skills holds potential for therapeutic benefit for children in poverty; however, play therapists can increase the intentionality in their selection of verbal responses by more closely attuning to the ways in which children may be expressing and exploring their experiences related to poverty. I offer the following fictional example to illustrate what the process of response selection may look like in session.

Case Scenario: Ally

I was facilitating play therapy with a six-year-old, Ally, whose mother reported concerns of anxiety and social isolation. The issues were present for approximately one year, beginning when Ally's mother was first laid off from work. Since that time, Ally had appeared disconnected from peers at school and increasingly preoccupied with what was happening at home. For several consecutive sessions, Ally frequently returned to the kitchen set in the playroom, taking out one piece of toy food after another and pretending to cook. She rotated between feeding the baby dolls, puppets, herself, and me, each time smiling in satisfaction. How might I respond with intention?

Discussion

It could be sufficient to reflect in ways that facilitate decision-making, "You decided to make something new," or provide encouragement, "You're working hard at that." After all, these statements align with the primary objectives of a humanistic approach to play therapy by acknowledging the child's autonomy and effort. Yet, after considering the unique socioeconomic experience of the child, these reflections may not fully speak to the motive behind the play behaviors. Knowing how poverty influences a child's context, I might instead provide reflections of meaning: "You wanted to make sure everyone had enough to eat," or "You're working hard to give us as much food as we need." These responses may communicate a deeper understanding of the significance within the child's play.

Emphasizing Esteem-Building

While conveying accurate empathy is one goal of intentional response selection, the play therapist may also find utility in conceptualizing how certain categories of responses are uniquely positioned to address the therapeutic needs of children in poverty. Children in poverty often experience a decreased sense of self-esteem due to the psychosocial factors associated with poverty (Fujiwara et al., 2019). The nature of poverty can be self-defeating and is often accompanied by negative feedback related to a child's capabilities by teachers and peers (Jensen, 2009). With this in mind, one category of response that holds particular relevance for children in poverty is that of esteem-building. Once again, the following fictitious example may provide insight into the process of emphasizing esteem-building.

Case Scenario: Josh

An eight-year-old boy, Josh, was referred to play therapy for displaying disruptive behaviors in the classroom. Josh's teachers described him as lagging behind academically and described him as caring less about his learning than other children his age. Josh's parents shared that he had experienced teasing from his peers for his low grades and noted difficulties in accessing the same outside tutoring resources as other children in his class due to financial concerns. In his sixth session, Josh engaged in his usual routine of constructive play with toy blocks, working to stack them as high as possible, when suddenly they came crashing down. In previous sessions, Josh had demonstrated low frustration tolerance when the blocks fall and moves on to another task. In this session, while Josh disconnected from the task momentarily, he returned to the blocks again before the session ended. This time, he stacked them successfully. He turned to look at me to ensure I witnessed his success. How might I respond?

Discussion

As before, various facilitative responses could be appropriate in this scenario. A tracking response: "You stacked them as high as you wanted," or reflection of feeling: "You felt mad when they fell, but now you're excited!" could also serve to progress the therapeutic process. Yet, a play therapist striving to emphasize esteem-building could instead reflect: "You kept working until you figured it out!" or "You didn't give up, even when it was hard." As esteem-building responses aim to facilitate an enhanced sense of capability within the child separate from external praise, these responses may best align with the child's unique therapeutic needs.

Providing Resources

While play therapy supports a child's process of healing from and navigating through stressors associated with living in poverty, it should not be the final step of a play therapist. After all, if a child had been burned by a fire, one would not simply bandage the child and send them back into the flames. Instead, the play therapist must recognize that a child's need for resources will inevitably extend past what the therapist can provide in the context of the therapeutic relationship.

To be responsive to the variety of needs a child in poverty may present with, the play therapist should be well acquainted with social support resources within their community. Food pantries, childcare services, and subsidized housing programs are just a few of the many resources that families in poverty may need to access. In addition to community resources, the play therapist can also cultivate a familiarity with government programs. For example, in the United States, programs such as the Supplemental Nutrition Assistance Program (SNAP), Temporary Assistance for Needy Families (TANF), and Child's Health Insurance Program (CHIP) are designed to support the varied needs of families in poverty. By facilitating connections to resources the family may not otherwise access, play therapists are able to advocate for addressing the holistic needs of the child and family system.

In the United States and Canada, a simple way for play therapists and clients alike to identify support services is by calling the number 211. Through the 211 social service line, callers will be connected to local agencies designed to help identify available resources within their community (United Way Worldwide, 2021). Readers can learn more about this service by visiting www.211.org.

Working with Families

While no family structure is immune from experiencing poverty, some are more vulnerable than others. For example, children in poverty are twice as likely to live in single-parent households than their economically privileged peers (National Center for Poverty, 2018). Single parents are often the sole wage-earners for their family and can carry the heightened economic burden of childcare costs due to competing caregiving and employment demands (Maldonado & Nieuwenhuis, 2015). Further, children in poverty are more likely to have grandparents serving as their primary caregivers (Pew Research Center, 2013).

Regardless of the family structure, the play therapist must consider how the same chronic stressors impacting children in poverty also disrupt the wellness of the child's parents and caregivers. Researchers found that parents in poverty were nearly five times more likely to fall in the clinical score range on formal measures of parental stress than middle-income parents (Steele et al., 2016). Not only is this concerning for the parent's mental health outcomes, but also for those of the child. High levels of parental stress are associated with increased parental use of harsh discipline approaches, increased externalizing and internalizing behaviors in children, and disruptions in the parent-child attachment (O'Brien Caughy, Huang, & Lima, 2009; Lohaus et al., 2017; Sturge-Apple, Suor, & Skibo, 2014). Scholars have emphasized the importance of addressing the emotional needs of parents to promote positive emotional outcomes for children (Hajal & Paley, 2020).

The importance of maintaining a strong therapeutic relationship with parents has been reiterated throughout play therapy literature (Ray, 2011; Kottman, 2003). Intake sessions and parent consultations present an opportune time for the play therapist to provide parental support. Play therapists working with families impacted by poverty can stay mindful of emphasizing empathic understanding towards parents/caregivers while delivering targeted strategies and resources to support a stress reduction in the caregiving relationship. The following case study demonstrates how these goals can unfold simultaneously.

Case Scenario: Jaxson

Tanya, the mother of my new seven-year-old client, Jaxson, presented to the first parent consultation session in a state of distress. She received persistent calls from the school regarding Jaxon's disruptive behavior. She experienced similar behaviors at home and struggled to identify effective strategies to respond. Tanya became visibly frustrated, exclaiming that she has tried everything that has been suggested. She shared that, between the stress of constant phone calls from school, the two jobs she is working, and concerns about providing for her family, she needs a strategy that will work immediately.

Discussion

The needs of this parent are multifaceted. While there was an apparent urgency to identify an effective support strategy, there was also a need to address parental stress to support the family system fully. Moving straight into providing support strategies and resources without acknowledging the parents' stressors may communicate a lack of understanding of their efforts to support their child.

To address this parent's need, I first spent time communicating empathic understanding. For example, I reflected: "You're trying your very best to care for your family, but at this point, you're feeling overwhelmed and discouraged." Leading with empathy allows the play therapist to support the parent's own emotional needs while simultaneously modeling the responses that they endeavor for the parent to utilize with the child. As appropriate, the play therapist can transition empathic responses into therapeutic strategies that the parent may integrate at home with their child. "I noticed how relieved you seemed when I shared some responses that showed I understood where you were coming from. Jaxson can benefit from this too. Often, the disruptive behaviors you described can start with feeling emotionally distressed, and having those emotions acknowledged can be one way to address those behaviors. Let's practice how you might use similar kinds of responses with Jaxson."

Finally, the play therapist can facilitate connection to resources that can support a reduction in parental stress. In identifying appropriate supports, a poverty-informed play therapist should conceptualize all aspects of what contributes to the distress in a family system. As noted previously in the chapter, the needs of those in poverty extend beyond mental health support. While providing parents and caregivers with referrals for individual counseling services is strongly recommended, doing this in isolation risks dismissing the complexity of the needs they are facing. In the previous example, the parent communicated challenges in meeting concrete needs at home. In addition to therapeutic supports, the play therapist may coordinate the parents' connection to local food pantries, housing resources, or employment services.

Working Within Systems

Screening for Poverty

Children in poverty present for therapeutic services across mental health settings. To adequately address the needs of a child in poverty, the play therapist must first identify that poverty is a part of the child's experience. Though some parents may openly discuss their socioeconomic experiences, many will not. Parents may not perceive this as being relevant to the child's presenting concern or may be hesitant to disclose due to previous experiences of social stigma.

To adequately identify and address the needs of children in poverty, scholars have emphasized the importance of screening for poverty-related concerns using multifaceted measurement techniques (Berman et al., 2018). Berman et al. (2018) outlines numerous screening tools which explore various facets of poverty, including the Health Leads (2016) Social Needs

Screening Toolkit, IHELLP (Kenyon et al., 2007), and WE CARE (Garg et al., 2007). Integrating poverty screeners as a standard part of a counseling intake can broaden a therapist's awareness of the psychosocial factors that may be informing the child's outcomes. Play therapists can advocate for the inclusion of poverty-related screeners in their place of practice to ensure that these concerns are not overlooked.

Address Logistical Challenges

Accessibility is a primary issue in providing play therapy services to children in poverty. Children in poverty are critically underserved in mental health services, and scholars cite several barriers to accessing services (Hodgkinson et al., 2017). First and foremost, high costs associated with mental health services may prevent those in poverty from seeking care. Compounding these financial barriers, individuals in poverty may face logistical challenges, such as transportation, changing vocational demands, and scheduling difficulties (Hodgkinson et al., 2017). These barriers can quickly impede a caregiver's ability to access therapeutic services for their child.

Therapists have the opportunity to advocate for accessibility in many ways. Providing pro-bono or sliding scale therapeutic services is one direct way to remove a primary barrier for families in poverty. Play therapists working in community agencies can advocate for financial accessibility by exploring opportunities for grant-based funding and becoming knowledgeable in state and federal legislation related to funding for mental health.

Play therapists should also familiarize themselves with available services within the client's community that may address logistical barriers. For example, providing families with information regarding available public transportation services may benefit those who may lack access to consistent means of travel. Further, coordinating session times and locations in alignment with local public transportation schedules and routes can ease related logistical challenges.

Finally, play therapists have the opportunity to advocate for embedding services within a child's context. Scholars have emphasized a need to provide services that can be integrated into existing settings such as public schools (Cappella et al., 2008). Play therapists seeking to serve this population effectively may propose the implementation of play therapy services in schools, childcare centers, and pediatric health care practices.

Play Therapist Wellness

When reflecting on the weight of life in poverty, and the systemic barriers that prevent shifting circumstances for children and their families, a sense of powerlessness can set in. During one poverty awareness presentation I facilitated, I was asked, "Doesn't counseling children in these circumstances feel like putting a bandage on a bullet wound?" To what seemed like the attendee's surprise, I began my response with a simple, "Yes." Though I went on to reiterate the critical role of counseling within a multilevel approach to caring for those impacted by poverty, I am keenly aware of the limitations of my reach as a play therapist.

As with many concerns that play therapists encounter in their work with clients, the realities of a childhood poverty are heavy. The difference, perhaps, is that many stressors children present with may be considered acute, while poverty and the concerns associated with it are often pervasive and chronic. Working to support children through these persistent stressors can be consuming and necessitate painful reflections on one's own class privilege and resources. For this reason, it is important for play therapists to identify methods of maintaining their own wellness to support the children they serve effectively.

Wellness is a multifaceted concept, involving mental, emotional, physical, social, and spiritual considerations (Myers & Sweeney, 2004). No one self-care strategy can address the individual wellness needs for all play therapists; however, research regarding play therapists' self-care strategies reveals categories of wellness activities that play therapists often implement (Meany-Walen et al., 2018). These themes included engaging in a myriad of activities that promote wellness at individual, interpersonal, and professional levels (Meany-Walen et al., 2018). Examples provided by participants included engaging in physical activity, spiritual practices, social engagement, professional consultations, and playful/creative activities (Meany-Walen et al., 2018). Participants emphasized the importance of engaging in such practices with intentionality, deliberately integrating wellness practices within their routine (Meany-Walen et al., 2018). Though there is no "one-size-fit-all" approach to maintaining wellness when providing services children in poverty, it may benefit play therapists to consider how they can concretely integrate individualized strategies that incorporate each of the aforementioned themes into their own wellness repertoire.

Conclusion

As with all aspects of identity, poverty is only one of many components contributing to a child's inner world. Considering the impact of poverty in isolation from other aspects of a child's identity may be just as damaging as disregarding the experience completely. While I am hopeful that this chapter can begin to illuminate a less frequently explored component of a child's experience, I encourage the play therapist to avoid generalization and contextualize this information within their experience of each unique child.

Positionality Statement

Sarah

The person of the play therapist is a critical component of the play therapy process. Play therapists previously or currently impacted by the context of poverty may find it challenging to bracket their own lived experiences of socioeconomic disadvantage in the playroom. As a play therapist who grew up in a low-income household myself, I admit that it can be challenging to avoid over-identification with the experiences of my child clients in poverty. Transitioning from a child in low-income circumstances to an adult professional in the middle class, feelings of guilt and shame have intruded on my work with children in poverty, rooted in a fear that my current financial stability equates to the abandonment of those still living in poverty. I also feel a strong sense of urgency to address any systemic barriers present for the families I serve. Though advocacy is essential and encouraged, I often find myself reflecting on this in session, which can prevent me from being as therapeutically present in the playroom as I believe necessary.

For fellow play therapists personally impacted by poverty, I share the same recommendations that I have utilized myself. First, it is essential to connect with play therapy colleagues and supervisors committed to socioeconomic awareness. Having others in the field with whom to process socioeconomic considerations can aid in maintaining awareness of how your own experiences may be disrupting the therapeutic process, promoting therapeutic efficacy and professional wellness. Additionally, exploring individual poverty-related concerns in the context of personal counseling may allow for enhanced awareness of the psychological impacts of poverty.

References

Berman, R. S., Patel, M. R., Belamarich, P. F., & Gross, R. S. (2018). Screening for poverty and poverty-related social determinants of health. *Pediatrics in Review*, 39 (5), 235–246. doi:10.1542/pir.2017-0123.

Cappella, E., Frazier, S. L., Atkins, M. S., Schoenwald, S. K., & Glisson, C. (2008). Enhancing schools' capacity to support children in poverty: An ecological model of school-based mental health services. *Administration and Policy in Mental Health and Mental Health Services Research*, 35(5), 395. doi:10.1007/s10488-008-0182-y.

Carlson, K. T. (2006). Poverty and youth violence exposure: Experiences in rural communities. *Children & Schools*, 28(2), 87–96. doi:10.1093/cs/28.2.87.

Children's Defense Fund (2021). The state of America's children: 2021. Children's Defense. www.childrensdefense.org/wp-content/uploads/2021/04/The-State-of-Americas-Children-2021.pdf.

Cochran, J. L., & Cochran, N. H. (2017). Effects of child-centered play therapy for students with highly-disruptive behavior in high-poverty schools. *International Journal of Play Therapy*, 26(2), 59–72. doi:10.1037/pla0000052.

Dillman Taylor, D. (2016). The extraordinary 5-year-old. In D. C. Ray (Ed.), *A therapist's guide to child development: The extraordinarily normal years*. Routledge.

Feeding America (2021). The impact of the coronavirus on food insecurity in 2020 & 2021. Feeding America. www.feedingamerica.org/sites/default/files/2021-03/National%20Projections%20Brief_3.9.2021_0.pdf.

Fujiwara, T., Isumi, A., & Ochi, M. (2019). Pathway of the association between child poverty and low self-esteem: Results from a population-based study of adolescents in Japan. *Frontiers in Psychology*, 10, 937. doi:10.3389/fpsyg.2019.00937.

Garg, A., Butz, A. M., Dworkin, P. H., Lewis, R. A., Thompson, R. E., & Serwint, J. R. (2007). Improving the management of family psychosocial problems at low-income children's well-child care visits: the WE CARE Project. *Pediatrics*, 120(3), 547–558. doi:10.1542/peds.2007-0398.

Garza, Y., & Bruhn, R. (2011). Empathy in play therapy: A case analysis through two theoretical perspectives. In D. J. Scapaletti (Ed.), *Psychology of empathy* (pp. 167–184). Nova Publishers.

Gorski, P. (2008). The myth of the "culture of poverty". *Educational Leadership*, 65 (7), 32.

Hajal, N. J., & Paley, B. (2020). Parental emotion and emotion regulation: A critical target of study for research and intervention to promote child emotion socialization. *Developmental Psychology*, 56(3), 403–417. doi:10.1037/dev0000864.

Health Leads (2018). The health leads screening toolkit. Health Leads USA: Resource Library. https://healthleadsusa.org/resources/the-health-leads-screening-toolkit.

Ho, C. S., Lempers, J. D., & Clark-Lempers, D. (1995). Effects of economic hardship on adolescent self-esteem: A family mediation model. *Adolescence*, 30(117), 117–131.

Hodgkinson, S., Godoy, L., Beers, L. S., & Lewin, A. (2017). Improving mental health access for low-income children and families in the primary care setting. *Pediatrics*, 139(1). doi:10.1542/peds.2015-1175.

Ihrke, D. K., & Faber, C. S. (2012). *Geographical mobility: 2005 to 2010*. U.S. Department of Commerce, Economics and Statistics Administration, U.S. Census Bureau.

Jensen, E. (2009). *Teaching with poverty in mind: What being poor does to kids' brains and what schools can do about it*. ASCD.

Kenyon, C., Sandel, M., Silverstein, M., Shakir, A., & Zuckerman, B. (2007). Revisiting the social history for child health. *Pediatrics*, 120(3), 734–738. doi:10.1542/peds.2006-2495.

Koball, H., Moore, A, & Hernandez, J. (2021). *Basic facts about low-income children: Children under 9 years, 2019*. National Center for Children in Poverty, Bank Street College of Education.

Kottman, T. (2003). *Partners in play: An Adlerian approach to play therapy*. American Counseling Association.

Kottman, T. (2011). *Play therapy: Basics and beyond*. John Wiley & Sons.

Ladson-Billings, G. (2017). Makes me wanna holler: Refuting the "Culture of poverty" discourse in urban schooling. *The Annals of the American Academy of Political and Social Science*, 673(1), 80–90. doi:10.1177/0002716217718793.

Le Floch, K. C., Levin, J., Atchison, D., Tanenbaum, C., Hurlburt, S., Manship, K., & Stullich, S. (2018). *Study of Title I Schoolwide and Targeted Assistance Programs*. Office of Planning, Evaluation and Policy Development, US Department of Education.

Lin, A. C., & Harris, D. R. (Eds.) (2008). *The colors of poverty: Why racial and ethnic disparities persist*. Russell Sage Foundation.

Lohaus, A., Chodura, S., Möller, C., Symanzik, T., Ehrenberg, D., Job, A.-K., Reindl, V., Konrad, K., & Heinrichs, N. (2017). Children's mental health problems and their relation to parental stress in foster mothers and fathers. *Child and Adolescent Psychiatry and Mental Health*, 11(1). doi:10.1186/s13034-017-0180-5.

Maldonado, L. C., & Nieuwenhuis, R. (2015). Family policies and single parent poverty in 18 OECD countries, 1978–2008. *Community, Work & Family*, 18(4), 395–415. doi:10.1080/13668803.2015.1080661.

McLaughlin, K. A., Breslau, J., Green, J. G., Lakoma, M. D., Sampson, N. A., Zaslavsky, A. M., & Kessler, R. C. (2011). Childhood socio-economic status and the onset, persistence, and severity of DSM-IV mental disorders in a US national sample. *Social Science & Medicine*, 73(7), 1088–1096. doi:10.1016/j.socscimed.2011.06.011.

Meany-Walen, K. K., Cobie-Nuss, A., Eittreim, E., Teeling, S., Wilson, S., & Xander, C. (2018). Play therapists' perceptions of wellness and self-care practices. *International Journal of Play Therapy*, 27(3), 176–186. doi:10.1037/pla0000067.

Myers, J. E., & Sweeney, T. J. (2004). The indivisible self: an evidence-based model of wellness. *Journal of Individual Psychology*, 60(3), 234–245.

National Center for Children in Poverty (2018). *Basic facts about low-income children: Children under 9 years* [Fact sheet].

Notten, G., & De Neubourg, C. (2011). Monitoring absolute and relative poverty: "Not enough" is not the same as "much less". *Review of Income and Wealth*, 57 (2), 247–269. doi:10.1111/j.1475-4991.2011.00443.x.

O'Brien Caughy, M., Huang, K. Y., & Lima, J. (2009). Patterns of conflict interaction in mother-toddler dyads: Differences between depressed and non-depressed mothers. *Journal of Child and Family Studies*, 18(1), 10–20. doi:10.1007/s10826-008-9201-6.

Parolin. Z, Curran, M., Matsudaira, J., Waldfogel, J. & Wimer, C. (2020) *Monthly Poverty Rates in the United States during the COVID-19 Pandemic (Poverty and Social Policy Working Paper)*. Center on Poverty & Social Policy, School of Social Work, Columbia University.

Pew Research Center (2013). At grandmother's house we stay: Children living with or being cared for by a grandparent. *Pew Research Center: Social and Demographic Trends*. www.pewresearch.org/social-trends/2013/09/04/children-living-with-or-being-cared-for-by-a-grandparent/#fn-19039-5.

Ray, D. C. (2011). *Advanced play therapy: Essential conditions, knowledge, and skills for child practice*. Routledge.

Reardon, S. F. (2011). The widening academic achievement gap between the rich and the poor: New evidence and possible explanations. In G. Duncan & R. J. Murnane (Eds.), *Whither opportunity: Rising inequality, schools, and children's life chances* (pp. 91–116). Russell Sage Foundation.

Reiss, F. (2013). Socioeconomic inequalities and mental health problems in children and adolescents: a systematic review. *Social science & medicine*, 90, 24–31. doi:10.1016/j.socscimed.2013.04.026.

Seale, E. (2020). Strategies for conducting post-culture-of-poverty research on poverty, meaning, and behavior. *The American Sociologist*, 51(4), 402. doi:10.1007/s12108-020-09460-2.

Semega, J., Kollar, M., Shrider, E., and Creamer, J. (2020). Income and poverty in the United States: 2019. United States Census Bureau. www.census.gov/content/dam/Census/library/publications/2020/demo/p60-270.pdf.

Sprenger, M. (2008). *The developing brain: Birth to age eight*. Corwin Press.

Steele, H., Bate, J., Steele, M., Dube, S. R., Danskin, K., Knafo, H., … Murphy, A. (2016). Adverse childhood experiences, poverty, and parenting stress. *Canadian Journal of Behavioural Science*, 48 (1), 32–38. doi:10.1037/cbs0000034.

Stulmaker, H. (2016). The extraordinary 7-year-old. In D. C. Ray (Ed.), *A therapist's guide to child development: The extraordinarily normal years*. Routledge.

Sturge-Apple, M. L., Suor, J. H., & Skibo, M. A. (2014). Maternal child-centered attributions and harsh discipline: The moderating role of maternal working memory across socioeconomic contexts. *Journal of Family Psychology*, 28(5), 645–654. doi:10.1037/fam0000023.

Townsend, P. (1979). *Poverty in the United Kingdom: A survey of household resources and standards of living.* University of California Press.

United Way Worldwide (2021). About 211. www.211.org/about-us.

U.S. Department of Agriculture Economic Research Service (n.d.). Definitions of Food Security. www.ers.usda.gov/topics/food-nutrition-assistance/food-security-in-the-us/definitions-of-food-security.aspx.

World Bank (2020). *Poverty and Shared Prosperity 2020: Reversals of Fortune.* World Bank. doi:10.1596/978-1-4648-1602-4.

World Bank (2021). Updated estimates of the impact of COVID-19 on global poverty:Looking back at 2020 and the outlook for 2021. *World Bank Blogs.* https://blogs.worldbank.org/opendata/updated-estimates-impact-covid-19-global-poverty-looking-back-2020-and-outlook-2021?cid=pov_tt_poverty_en_ext.

Part 3

Special Topics in Multicultural Play Therapy

DOI: 10.4324/9781003190073-17

14 Inclusive Play Therapy Supervision

Natalya A. Lindo

Growing up in Jamaica, I did not have to *think* about my race. At least, not in the ways I do now. I knew I was Black, a descendant of slaves, born in a country forged from colonialism. The majority of people around me looked like me, so I was not forced to examine my race unless I interacted with a White tourist, for example. However, in those situations, I was the norm and they were the other. It was not until I immigrated to the United States to pursue a master's in counseling that I was confronted daily with *my otherness*. While there were various cultural differences that set me apart (like not knowing what kind of detergent one uses in a dishwasher), the most noticeable source of difference was the color of my skin. Twenty years later, I vividly remember the rapid sequence of emotions – confusion, shock, and anger that I felt when I first heard a racial slur, directed at *me*. That afternoon, I came to the realization that as long as I lived in the U.S., my race and my otherness would define me. However, I was not prepared for the visible and invisible ways it would impact my personal relationships, as well as my professional life.

During one of my first play therapy sessions, I made what I thought was a spot-on reflection, but a confused look was apparent on my client's face as he turned to me and brusquely asked, "What did you say?" Although shocked, I quickly recovered and found myself repeating the statement, but ensuring that I added a hint of an *American* (read: Southern) accent. As I willingly engaged in code-switching, a wave of sadness passed over me. I realized that this was the first of many adjustments I would need to make in order to accommodate others and help them feel more at ease with my difference.

In my master's internship, during a parent consultation, an African American parent described her struggles as a Black parent in a White-centric society and stated, "You know how *they* are." It took me a moment to realize that "they" really meant White people. In that moment, despite my non-American accent, she saw our point of connection – the color of our skin and our cultural disconnection from White people. While I do not recall my exact response, I do remember feeling a great deal of discomfort. How does one respond to such a comment?

DOI: 10.4324/9781003190073-18

While I had been well prepared to facilitate play therapy sessions and conduct parent consultations, I was not as prepared to engage in open dialogue with clients about race and culture. I carried memories of clinical cultural faux pas for years and never discussed them with any of my White supervisors in my practicum and internship experiences. In fact, in all my years of supervision, discussions about culture were glaringly absent, although my culture and my race permeated all of my encounters. In my play therapy sessions, the children noticed, and as children do, commented on the color of my skin. Sometimes it was a point of connection, like the time my White eight-year-old client told me that she had a boyfriend who looked like me, as she shyly pointed to the skin on my forearm. In my supervision sessions, I would often stare at faces that did not look like me, and would discuss worldviews and training protocols that did not align with my cultural framework. In those spaces, I never felt the room to question, and I was not asked about the impact of my culture on my learning process and my work with clients. I was often forced to leave my cultural identity on the outside of the room, only to dust it off when my client was racially or ethnically diverse, their differences coming to the fore, thus forcing us to pay attention.

During my play therapy experiences, I saw myself as a cultural being, and because most of my clients were culturally different from me, I consciously and unconsciously examined clients' cultural perspectives in a bid to serve them more appropriately. However, in supervision, I must admit that I never spent much time wondering about my supervisors' culture. Perhaps because the norm is often unexamined. More likely, I was too focused on my own cultural makeup and what it meant for me to be a Black international play therapist in the Southern U.S. Regardless, over time, I have come to understand the dynamic relationships within the play therapy supervision triad, and the importance of understanding what each member brings to the experience. This includes an examination of each member's cultural framework, its impact on the supervision triad, and the therapeutic process (Mitchell & Butler, 2021; Phillips et al., 2017).

The Play Therapy Supervision Triad

The play therapy supervision triad is a dynamic system comprised of the supervisor, supervisee, and client system; the latter includes parent(s), primary caregiver(s), and/or the family unit (Perryman et al., 2016). The main purpose of supervision is to foster the development of junior therapists (Bernard & Goodyear, 2019; Morrison & Lent, 2018; Tracey et al., 2012), with the implication being that the play therapy supervisor should be more experienced than the supervisee. The supervisor's role is multifaceted and includes both instructional and evaluative components (Bernard & Goodyear, 2019) not limited to: play therapy knowledge, skills, attitudes, legal and ethical issues, theory development, cultural competence (Perryman et al., 2016), and cultural humility (Hook et al., 2013). This latter role highlights the importance of facilitating a healthy supervisory relationship (Wilson et al., 2016).

The supervisory relationship is an integral part of the therapeutic process as it sets the tone for the supervisee's clinical development (Bernard & Goodyear, 2019; Morrison & Lent, 2018). Like any healthy relationship, there needs to be a sense of safety grounded in authenticity and open communication (Wilson et al., 2016). In addition to an exploration of compatible goals and supervision style, the supervisor should attend to the personal comfort of the supervisee (Starr et al., 2013). Within the context of safety, the supervisor can facilitate discussions related to cultural experiences, cultural identity, and their impact on the therapeutic process.

Best Practices in Play Therapy Supervision

Several professional associations indicate best practices for engaging in multicultural clinical supervision. The National Association of Social Workers (NASW) standards delineate the importance of cultural awareness, noting that supervisors "have specialized knowledge and understanding about the culture of the client population served by the supervisee" (NASW, 2013, p. 11). Similarly, the American Psychological Association (APA) states that

> competent supervision attends to a broad range of diversity dimensions (e.g., age, gender, gender identity, race, ethnicity, culture, national origin, religion, sexual orientation, disability, language, and socio-economic status), and includes sensitivity to diversity of supervisees, clients/ patients, and the supervisor.
>
> (APA, 2014, p. 11)

According to the Association for Counselor Education and Supervision (2011), best practices in supervision include guidelines for working with supervisees within the context of diversity, equity and inclusion:

- 6.b.iii. The supervisor encourages the supervisee to be aware of and address issues of culture, power, and privilege that may serve as barriers to clients from diverse populations seeking or receiving services.
- 6.a.v. The supervisor is aware of issues of privilege and oppression and how they affect the supervision process with each supervisee, with particular attention to supervisees and clients with minority statutes.

Throughout the play therapy supervision experience, it is incumbent upon supervisors to facilitate the development of supervisees' cultural competence through discussion of cultural issues that are potential barriers to serving diverse clients effectively. Further, supervisors should be aware of the potential impact of systemic discrimination and oppressive forces on the supervisee, the supervisory relationship, and the supervisee's ability to provide effective service to minoritized clients and families. By understanding the impact of social oppression on individuals, supervisors can enhance their empathy for their culturally diverse supervisees and facilitate supervisees' empathy for their marginalized clients (Fickling et al., 2019; Laher & Cockcroft, 2017). This perspective attends to the cultural framework of each member of the play therapy supervision triad.

Culturally Attuned Play Therapy Supervision

Inman and DeBoer Kreider (2013) define *multicultural supervision and counseling competence* as "the development of an understanding of the influence of contextual and systemic issues on each member of the client-counselor-supervisor triad as well as the process and outcome of counseling and supervision" (p. 346). Each member of the play therapy supervision triad holds visible and invisible cultural identities such as race, ethnicity, socioeconomic status, age, gender identity, sexual identity, religion/spirituality, and ability. In essence, all play therapy supervision is cross-cultural, and supervision can be considered a culturally centered triadic relationship (Tohidian & Quek, 2017).

Since cultural identities of each member of the supervision triad consciously and unconsciously impact both the content and process of supervision and clinical experiences (Peters, 2017), it is imperative that play therapy supervisors directly attend to cultural variables. This includes taking a broader view of culture while acknowledging any way in which an individual identifies themselves through their own lived experiences (Mitchell & Butler, 2021). Not only does this center the voices of marginalized supervisees in particular, but it also allows for an examination of the socioemotional impact of systemic issues on the play therapy supervisor, play therapist, and by extension, the client system (Ceballos et al., 2012; Parikh et al., 2013).

Broaching in Play Therapy Supervision

Within the counseling setting, *broaching* refers to "the counselor's deliberate and intentional efforts to discuss those racial, ethnic, and cultural concerns that may impact the client's presenting concerns" (Day-Vines et al., 2020, p. 107). Broaching can and should also take place in supervision (Jones et al., 2019). Within this context, broaching is the supervisor's intentional effort to discuss racial, ethnic, and cultural concerns that may impact the supervisee, the supervisory relationship, and therapeutic progress (King & Jones, 2019).

There is always a degree of discomfort when discussing cultural issues. When engaging in difficult dialogue, we, as supervisors, often conflate discomfort with a lack of safety, and unintentionally absolve ourselves of the need to dig deeper or to address cultural conflicts. However, there is a difference between comfort and safety. While a play therapy supervisor who initiates cultural conversations cannot ensure comfort, they can cultivate safety by engaging in culturally attuned interventions that are appropriate and facilitative for all members of the supervision triad. This requires reflexivity on the part of supervisors; the belief that they can therapeutically engage in use of self to facilitate relational depth (Calvert et al., 2016).

Providing a supervisor has effectively set the stage for safety and feels competent to manage the responses that may arise from broaching, here are some questions that one can use to initiate a discussion with supervisees about cultural dimensions:

- How comfortable are you discussing cultural issues during our supervision session?
- How do you describe your racial and or ethnic identity?
- What are the various cultural groups to which you belong?
- How do you think your culture affects the way you see your roles as a play therapist?
- How do you think your culture impacts your relationship with children and their parents or families?
- Can you think of ways in which cultural differences or similarities may impact your relationship with clients?
- Can you identify ways in which our cultural differences or similarities may impact our supervisory relationship?
- What was it like to engage in discussions about culture during our supervision session?

In my experience, when utilizing some of these questions in play therapy supervision, I have found it helpful to broach the topic by first disclosing my conception of my racial/ethnic identity and how it has influenced my work with clients, both in terms of cultural differences as well as perceived shared cultural experiences. This models an openness to cultural discussions, and makes me more accessible to supervisees. As a Black woman with a very visible cultural dimension, this approach works for me, but may not work for others.

Whatever approach is taken, supervisors need to pay keen attention to a supervisee's body language, attending to discomfort while facilitating safety. This was highlighted for me during a play therapy supervision session with a White supervisee. When I initially spoke about my race and related play therapy experiences, she seemed relatively comfortable. However, once I asked about *her* culture, her body language shifted and she seemed very uncomfortable with the discussion. I gently commented on her apparent discomfort, at which point she shyly smiled and noted that as a White woman, before entering the counseling field, she was not asked about her culture, and had difficulty identifying her cultural dimensions beyond race. Voicing this concern seemed to strengthen her resolve; she stated that she struggled to talk about her race as it often led to even more uncomfortable conversations about privilege. While initially hesitant to open up, this supervisee's willingness to disclose that she had difficulty naming her cultural dimensions, set the tone for more in-depth conversation about our respective cultural identities, and their potential impact on the supervisory relationship and play therapy clients.

While it is important for play therapy supervisors to become adept at broaching with their supervisees, and utilize some of the suggested cultural discussion questions, it is essential that they engage in their own reflective process beforehand (Singh & Chun, 2010; Upshaw et al., 2020). In fact, supervisors should be intentional about answering these questions before posing them in supervision. Moreover, supervisors could model appropriate self-disclosure by describing their own cultural dimensions or allowing the space for supervisees to ask them questions about their cultural identity as well.

Self-Exploration and Engaged Humility

Our worldview has a direct impact on the supervisory relationship and potentially impacts the therapeutic choices that our supervisees make (Borders, 2014; Cook et al., 2020). Therefore, a thorough examination of one's worldview, cultural framework, implicit biases, and assumptions are an essential prerequisite to engaging in culturally inclusive supervision (Hook et al., 2016; Watkins et al., 2019). It is also imperative for play therapy supervisors to move from insight to action, from the intellectual to the personal, and from cultural awareness to cultural humility.

Cultural awareness is "a cognitive phenomenon in which culturally relevant content is brought into awareness and processed intellectually" (Christiansen et al., 2011, p. 110). In building cultural awareness, play therapy supervisors participate in essential cognitive work and acquisition of knowledge through independent research and multicultural training. Cultural awareness should be distinguished from *cultural humility*, which Hook et al. (2013) conceptualize as the "ability to maintain an interpersonal stance that is other-oriented in relation to aspects of cultural identity that are most important to the [person]" (p. 2). Supervisors who wish to develop cultural humility actively seek out opportunities to engage in culture-specific dialogue, illuminate implicit bias, and challenge ways in which they consciously and unconsciously participate in perpetuating systems of oppression (Fickling et al., 2019).

Cultural awareness is a prerequisite to facilitating cultural humility (Cook et al., 2020); the latter requiring in-depth self-exploration, a keen awareness of one's impact on others, a commitment to change, and "the courage to be imperfect" (Lazarfeld, 1966, p. 163–165). As play therapy supervisors engender cultural awareness and cultural humility, they can engage in the following self-exploration questions (A. Cyr, personal communication, June 19, 2017):

- Through what lens do I view the world?
- What is my definition of culture?
- With which cultural groups do I primarily identify?
- What cultural values, beliefs, and attitudes do I hold, and how do these fit with the dominant culture?
- How did I learn my cultural values?
- What has been my experience with other cultures, and what has been my perception of these cultures?
- How might my beliefs affect my ability to supervise effectively?

Play therapy supervisors can also utilize Sensoy and DiAngelo's (2014) challenge to social justice education, and apply these principles to play therapy supervision. These guidelines for engaged humility can assist play therapy supervisors in the development of cultural awareness and cultural humility:

- Strive for intellectual humility with a willingness to grapple with challenging ideas.
- Differentiate between opinion – which everyone has – and informed knowledge, which comes from sustained experience, study, and practice. Hold your opinions lightly and with humility.
- Let go of personal anecdotal evidence and look at broader group-level patterns.
- Notice your own defensive reactions and attempt to use them as an opportunity to gain deeper self-knowledge, rather than as a reason for closing off.
- Recognize how your own positionality (e.g. race, class, gender, sexuality, ability) informs your perspectives and reactions.
- Differentiate between safety and comfort. Accept discomfort as necessary for social justice growth.
- Identify your learning edge and push it. For example, whenever you think, "I already know this," ask yourself, "How can I take this deeper?" You can also ask, "How am I applying in practice what I already know?"

As mentioned, the path from cultural awareness to cultural/engaged humility takes courage and a commitment to change. Depending on one's background and life experiences, this can be a particularly challenging, and even painful process as one comes to terms with unconscious bias, generational trauma, and maladaptive internalized cultural messages.

Race Evasiveness

Over the years, I have made it a point in my teaching and supervision to openly discuss issues surrounding race and racism. As a Black woman, and often the only Person of Color in a group, it is my way of naming the unnamed, using (my) race as a bridge to discuss power, privilege, systems of oppression, and their impact on the therapeutic process. However, I have noticed a trend, particularly among White people in the room. It happens so subtly that the shift is almost imperceptible. Although the conversation initially centers on race, inevitably, someone brings up another cultural dimension, such as socioeconomic status. While race and class often intersect, race is a visible, salient identity that warrants special attention.

Race is a social construct (Kendi, 2019), but it is also a lived reality for those who routinely experience discrimination solely based on their skin color. Due to the complexity of race relations in the U.S., discussions about race have the power to elicit deep-rooted emotions such as guilt, fear, and anger (Kendi, 2016). In fact, Spanierman and Cabrera (2014) delineate the spectrum of emotions of White racism – apathy, fear, melancholia, rage, guilt, and shame – noting how integral such emotions are to understanding how race is experienced and understood within the U.S. context. Even within a therapeutic setting, therapists' and supervisors' lived experiences, cultural worldviews, and conscious and unconscious biases have a direct impact on the supervisory and clinical process (Cook et al., 2020). This may dictate the degree to which they are willing to engage in race-related discussions.

One of the biggest barriers to talking about race is fear (Nnawulezi et al., 2020). Even experienced play therapy supervisors may fear saying the wrong thing. I often tell my students and supervisees that even with my experience and training, I make mistakes all the time, and have unintentionally committed microaggressions. I have been lucky to have colleagues and friends who are willing to call me out, and over time I have learned to accept my imperfections, make amends when the situation calls for it, and find opportunities to grow and learn.

Fear of being hurtful or offensive can prevent play therapy supervisors from engaging in race-related discussions with their supervisees. A White supervisor who wants to understand the cultural framework of their supervisee of color may be hesitant to ask direct questions for fear of unintentionally causing offense or being misunderstood. This fear may also extend to direct questions related to client care. For example, a White supervisor overseeing a case of a Chinese client who was recently adopted by White parents may want to know the perspective of their Chinese supervisee, and yet may be hesitant to broach the conversation. This highlights the importance of engaging in discussions about race and other cultural dimensions of the supervisor and supervisee at the onset of the supervision process (Jendrusina & Martinez, 2019), setting the tone for future interactions, and allowing room for deeper exploration regarding culturally diverse clients.

I have found the greatest barrier to engaging in race-related discussions is simply not knowing what to say. Unfortunately, silence can be detrimental, especially within the context of a cross-racial supervisory relationship. When the COVID-19 pandemic intersected with racial conflict and protests in the U.S. in May 2020, in addition to concerns about appropriate client care and clinical skill development, a Black supervisee entering a supervision session with a White supervisor likely also grappled with personal experiences and emotions related to disproportionate illness and death among People of Color, health-care disparities, police brutality, and racial conflict. A supervisor experiencing White empathy (Spanierman & Cabrera, 2014) may have felt anger and sadness about the events of 2020 and wanted to express their concern for their Black supervisee. However, not knowing what to say, they may have opted to remain silent on the issue altogether. In this case, the supervisee may have interpreted the supervisor's silence for apathy, perceiving a lack of safety to discuss issues of race in supervision (Jendrusina & Martinez, 2019).

Despite past mistakes or fears regarding conversations about race, play therapy supervisors need to talk about race because we cannot challenge racism if we are unable to talk about it. Race is a huge, salient part of who we are, yet it is the elephant in the room, especially in a cross-racial supervisory relationship (Burkard et al., 2014; Estrada et al., 2004). Even when supervisors and supervisees are from the same race, such discussions are crucial (Phillips et al., 2017) so that supervisees are well-equipped to serve play therapy clients and families from minoritized racial groups.

While it is important to address race evasiveness (Nnawulezi et al., 2020), ensuring that issues of race are discussed during supervision, it is also vital to examine the intersection of multiple cultural dimensions (Mitchell & Butler, 2021; Peters, 2017). It is likely supervisors will encounter supervisees with multiple intersecting marginalized identities and/or who work with clients who hold multiple intersecting marginalized identities. Therefore, simply discussing race (or any other marginalized identity) in isolation creates missed opportunities for dialogue, engagement, and understanding. This highlights the importance of openly addressing intersecting identities as well (Collins & Bilge, 2020).

Intersectionality and Identity Salience

Intersectionality is the multidimensionality and interdependence of intersecting identities such as race, sexual identity, gender identity, and ability status, which creates modes of power and discrimination (Collins, 2019; Collins & Bilge, 2020). Because intersectionality identity development begins in childhood (Ecklund, 2012), it is essential that play therapists and play therapy supervisors develop the knowledge and skills related to intersectionality and its impact on the play therapy and supervision process. Intersectionality of identity allows us to understand fluidity of identity – how one cultural identity becomes more salient within an individual when in certain contexts, whereas other cultural identities may be more salient in the same person when in different situations (Yakushko et al., 2009). Emphasis should be placed on the awareness of this dynamic in cross-cultural

supervisory relationships and/or when discussing cross-cultural client-coun-
selor relationships (Burkard et al., 2014).

Othering takes place when we focus on salient characteristics of those we
perceive as being different, and view or treat them according to these perceived differences. In the context of culture, othering perpetuates societal
disparities and is a common pitfall when discussing cultural dimensions and
intersectional identities (Edgell & Tranby, 2010). In play therapy supervision, the focus should be on climate – the systems within which the
supervisee functions – rather than unintentionally othering minoritized
groups. One possible approach to avoiding othering is to examine our own
cultural dimensions, identity salience, and intersectional identities (Yakushko
et al., 2009). This includes noting our biases, assumptions, interpersonal interactions, and possible ways we unintentionally perpetuate systems of oppression.

Supervision regarding intersectional identities may vary depending on the
experience of the supervisor and supervisee (Peters, 2017). A good starting
point might be to engage in the following identity salience exercise, which
can be done independently or during a play therapy supervision session.
When engaging in the exercise:

1   Take a piece of paper and fold it in two or draw a line down the
middle.
2   On one side make a list of the various identities you hold:

  a   Race/Ethnicity
  b   Sex
  c   Gender Identity
  d   Ability Status
  e   Class/Socioeconomic Status
  f   Religion/Spirituality
  g   Sexual Identity
  h   Other (e.g. Parent/Partner)

3   On the other side of the paper, draw a circle into segments or slices.

  i   Each slice represents a different cultural dimension or identity.
  ii   The largest slices represent the identities you think about the most
       and that are most meaningful to you.
  iii The smallest slices represent the identities you think about the least
       or that are least meaningful to you.
  iv   How might these "parts of you" show up in, and impact the play
       therapy supervision relationship?

When processing this activity with a supervisee, the supervisor should bear in
mind the key difference between those identities that are salient because of
external social factors (e.g. race), versus those identities that the supervisee
desires to be salient (e.g. play therapist). It should be considered that identity

Personal Identity/Cultural Dimension

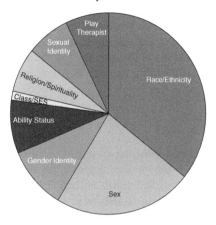

Figure 14.1 An example of an identity salience map. Whether conducting this activity alone or in a play therapy supervision session, it is important to remember that there is no value judgment. The goal of this activity is to determine one's personal identity and role salience.

salience shifts depending on setting (Yakushko et al, 2009). For example, one's identity salience as a play therapist might be greater within the context of an academic program or convention than within a church community setting.

When conducting this activity, the play therapy supervisor should also be aware of the potential impact of their cultural dimensions on the identity salience map of their supervisee. For example, I have yet to engage in this activity with a supervisee who does not list race as a salient identity. I sometimes wonder to what degree my visible identity as a Black woman influences this choice. This may be especially significant for White supervisees who may not typically view their race as a salient identity.

Because intersectionality refers to the interconnected nature of social categories that create overlapping systems of advantage and disadvantage (Collins & Bilge, 2020), it also entails an examination of power and privilege. In exploring our cultural dimensions, we may be faced with subordinated identities (e.g. being a member of a minoritized racial group) or privileged identities (e.g. class privilege). The reality is that everyone has some privilege, and some people have more privilege than others (Collins, 2019). Rather than viewing an exploration of privilege as a negative experience, play therapy supervisors can facilitate this conversation as an opportunity for a supervisee to identify unexamined blind spots in their counseling practice.

I once initiated a discussion about privilege with a Black supervisee. After noting her initial surprise that two Black women were having a conversation about privilege, she realized that her class and related educational opportunities were clear points of privilege for her. She also recognized that her client base was predominantly racial/ethnic minority and from traditionally marginalized communities, further highlighting her privilege in relation to her clients. As such, a supervisee can ask themselves, "When working with children and families, what do I think about? What don't I think about?" Answers to these questions are a good litmus test for privileged identities, and can help a supervisee be more aware of their own cultural dimensions as well as their perceptions of and attitudes toward the cultural identities of their clients.

Equality vs Equity

In addition to an examination of the spectrum of emotions of White racism, Spanierman and Cabrera (2014) also describe the emotions of White anti-racism, which include empathy, moral outrage, compassion, joy, and hope, noting how these emotions lead to anti-racist action. Play therapy supervisors who strive for increased cultural awareness and the development of cultural humility should determine ways to engage in anti-racist actions in their personal lives as well as their professional practice. At the foundation of anti-racism is the acknowledgment of systemic oppression as well as the key differences between equality and equity within the context of a biased system (Kendi, 2019).

In an examination of the systems of advantage and disadvantage inherent in a biased society, we often commingle equality with equity. While equality refers to providing the same treatment to all (Hero & Levy, 2016), we should in fact aim for equity, which refers to treating people differently based on what they need (Myers, 2015). Sometimes to be truly equitable it means providing extra support and resources to those who start out at a disadvantage, those with limited resources, less access, and lack of privilege. Play therapy supervisors should consider what this might mean for them in their daily lives as well as with their supervisory work. Appropriately assessing the unique needs of each supervisee (and client system) can ensure that play therapy supervisors provide resources and support that best meet those needs. For instance, this might include allowing a supervisee without a designated playroom or who has limited play materials to utilize the supervisor's facilities at a reduced or free cost. Supervisors could also offer sliding scale services to supervisees who might otherwise be unable to afford the supervision fees. Similarly, supervisors could offer pro bono supervision services to select supervisees. Equity in practice often requires creative problem-solving and an adjustment of rigid boundaries.

Anti-racist action in one's daily life and play therapy supervision practice also includes the following tips adapted from Pendakur (2020):

- Maintain focus on yourself – *what does this mean for me and my life? What does this mean for my play therapy or supervision practice?*
- Ask questions – find safe people you can process with and learn from.
- Reflect on yourself to identify blind spots – remember, everyone has them. *What are my cultural blind spots with my play therapy supervisees?*

- Examine where those blind spots are unintentionally embedded in the everyday fabric of your play therapy supervision practice and tear that fabric apart thread by thread.
- Be in authentic community with those affected by historic and current forms of marginalization.
- Develop relationships, in your personal life as well as play therapy and supervision practice, with people who will challenge your cultural assumptions.
- Move from the intellectual to the interpersonal. Move from cultural awareness to cultural humility.
- Reflect again… and again.
- Keep doing the work.

Conclusion

Play therapy supervision is a culturally centered triad; intersecting how the identities of the supervisor, the supervisee(s), and client system interact and impact the clinical process (Tohidian & Quek, 2017). This is particularly salient when the supervisee or client hold one or more marginalized identities. While the instructional and evaluative components of supervision are essential to the supervisee's clinical development (Bernard & Goodyear, 2019), so are the relational elements, particularly the supervisee's perceived sense of safety and trust in the supervisory relationship (Wilson et al., 2016). In addition to facilitating skill development, culturally inclusive play therapy supervision incorporates culturally attuned interventions, acknowledging cultural dimensions of each member of the supervision triad, and their potential influence on the supervisory relationship and therapeutic outcomes (Jendrusina & Martinez, 2019).

Positionality Statement

Natalya

I identify as an Afro-Caribbean immigrant, middle-class, straight woman. My cultural dimensions are salient pieces of my identity as a counselor, play therapist, supervisor, researcher, and educator. These multiple intersecting identities inform my activities as an academician, practitioner, and citizen. Woven throughout my community and school-based interventions, collaborative scholarship, play therapy, and supervisory experiences is a commitment to serving systematically minoritized communities, and centralizing marginalized voices.

References

American Psychological Association (2014). Guidelines for Clinical Supervision in Health Service Psychology. Retrieved from http://apa.org/about/policy/guidelines-supervision.pdf.

Association for Counselor Education and Supervision Taskforce on Best Practices in Clinical Supervision (2011, April). Best practices in clinical supervision. Retrieved June 9, 2021, from https://acesonline.net/wp-content/uploads/2018/11/ACES-Best-Practices-in-Clinical-Supervision-2011.pdf.

Bernard, J.M., & Goodyear, R. K. (2019). *Fundamentals of clinical supervision* (6th ed.). Pearson.

Borders, L. D. (2014). Best practices in clinical supervision: Another step in delineating effective supervision practice. *American Journal of Psychotherapy*, 68(2), 151–162. doi:10.1176/appi.psychotherapy.2014.68.2.151.

Burkard, A. W., Knox, S., Clarke, R. D., Phelps, D. L., & Inman, A. G. (2014). Supervisors' experiences of providing difficult feedback in cross-ethnic/racial supervision. *The Counseling Psychologist*, 42(3), 14–344. doi:10.1177/0011000012461157.

Calvert, F. L., Crowe, T. P., & Grenyer, B. F. S. (2016). Dialogical reflexivity in supervision: An experiential learning process for enhancing reflective and relational competencies. *The Clinical Supervisor*, 35(1), 1–21. doi:10.1080/07325223.2015.1135840.

Ceballos, P. L., Parikh, S., & Post, P. B. (2012). Examining social justice attitudes among play therapists: Implications for multicultural supervision and training. *International Journal of Play Therapy*, 21(4), 232–243. doi:10.1037/a0028540.

Christiansen, A. T., Thomas, V., Kafescioglu, N., Karakurt, G., Lowe, W., Smith, W., & Wittenborn, A. (2011). Multicultural supervision: Lessons learned about an ongoing struggle. *Journal of Marital and Family Therapy*, 37, 109–119.

Collins, P. H. (2019). *Intersectionality as critical social theory*. Duke University Press.

Collins, P. H., & Bilge, S. (2020). *Intersectionality* (2nd ed.). Polity Press.

Cook, R. M., Jones, C. T., & Welfare, L. E. (2020). Supervisor cultural humility predicts intentional nondisclosure by Post-Master's counselors. *Counselor Education and Supervision*, 59(2), 160–167. doi:10.1002/ceas.12173.

Day-Vines, N. L., Cluxton-Keller, F., Agorsor, C., Gubara, S., & Otabil, N. A. A. (2020). The multidimensional model of broaching behavior. *Journal of Counseling and Development*, 98(1), 107–118. doi:10.1002/jcad.12304.

Ecklund, K. (2012). Intersectionality of identity in children: A case study. *Professional Psychology, Research and Practice*, 43(3), 256–264. doi:10.1037/a0028654.

Edgell, P., & Tranby, E. (2010). Shared visions? Diversity and cultural membership in American life. *Social Problems*, 57(2), 175–204. doi:10.1525/sp.2010.57.2.175.

Estrada, D., Frame, M. W., & Williams, C. B. (2004). Cross-cultural supervision: guiding the conversation toward race and ethnicity. *Journal of Multicultural Counseling and Development*, 32, 307–319.

Fickling, M. J., Tangen, J. L., Graden, M. W., & Grays, D. (2019). Multicultural and social justice competence in clinical supervision. *Counselor Education and Supervision*, 58(4), 309–316. doi:10.1002/ceas.12159.

Hero, R. E., & Levy, M. E. (2016). The racial structure of economic inequality in the United States: Understanding change and continuity in an era of "Great divergence". *Social Science Quarterly*, 97(3), 491–505. doi:10.1111/ssqu.12327.

Hook, J. N., Davis, D. E., Owen, J., Worthington, E. L., & Utsey, S. O. (2013). Cultural humility: Measuring openness to culturally diverse clients. *Journal of Counseling Psychology*, 60(3), 353–366. doi:10.1037/a0032595.

Hook, J. N., Watkins, J., C Edward, Davis, D. E., Owen, J., Van Tongeren, D. R., & Ramos, M. J. (2016). Cultural humility in psychotherapy supervision. *American*

Journal of Psychotherapy, 70(2), 149–166. doi:10.1176/appi.psychotherapy.2016.70.2.149.

Inman, A. G., & DeBoer Kreider, E. (2013). Multicultural competence: Psychotherapy practice and supervision. *Psychotherapy*, 50(3), 346–350. doi:10.1037/a0032029.

Jendrusina, A. A., & Martinez, J. H. (2019). Hello from the other side: Student of color perspectives in supervision. *Training and Education in Professional Psychology*, 13(3), 160–166. doi:10.1037/tep0000255.

Jones, C. T., Welfare, L. E., Melchior, S., & Cash, R. M. (2019). Broaching as a strategy for intercultural understanding in clinical supervision. *The Clinical Supervisor*, 38(1), 1–16. doi:10.1080/07325223.2018.1560384.

Kendi, I. X. (2019). *How to be an Antiracist*. Random House.

Kendi, I. X. (2016). *Stamped from the beginning*. Avalon.

King, K. M., & Jones, K. (2019). An autoethnography of broaching in supervision: Joining supervisee and supervisor perspectives on addressing identity, power, and difference. *The Clinical Supervisor*, 38(1), 17–37. doi:10.1080/07325223.2018.1525597.

Laher, S., & Cockcroft, K. (2017). Moving from culturally biased to culturally responsive assessment practices in low-resource, multicultural settings. *Professional Psychology, Research and Practice*, 48(2), 115–121. doi:10.1037/pro0000102.

Lazarfeld, S. (1966). The courage for imperfection. *American Journal of Individual Psychology*, 22(2), 163–165.

Mitchell, M. D., & Butler, S. K. (2021). Acknowledging intersectional identity in supervision: The multicultural integrated supervision model. *Journal of Multicultural Counseling and Development*, 49(2), 101–115. doi:10.1002/jmcd.12209.

Morrison, M. A., & Lent, R. W. (2018). The working alliance, beliefs about the supervisor, and counseling self-efficacy: Applying the relational efficacy model to counselor supervision. *Journal of Counseling Psychology*, 65(4), 512–522. doi:10.1037/cou0000267.

Myers, D. (2015). Mutual benefits and equity amid racial diversity: A generational strategy for growing a broader base of support for social equity. *Journal of Planning Education and Research*, 35(3), 369–375. doi:10.1177/0739456X15596579.

National Association of Social Workers (2013). Best practice standards in social work supervision. Retrieved from www.socialworkers.org/LinkClick.aspx?fileticket=GBrLbl4BuwI%3D&portalid=0.

Nnawulezi, N., Case, K. A., & Settles, I. H. (2020). Ambivalent white racial consciousness: Examining intersectional reflection and complexity in practitioner graduate training. *Women & Therapy*, 43(3–4), 365–388. doi:10.1080/02703149.2020.1729476.

Parikh, S. B., Ceballos, P., & Post, P. (2013). Factors related to play therapists' social justice advocacy attitudes. *Journal of Multicultural Counseling and Development*, 41(4), 240–253. doi:10.1002/j.2161-1912.2013.00039.x.

Pendakur, S. L. (2020, October 6). *Unpacking internal and institutional racism* [Conference session]. USC Race and Equity Center's Equity NOW! Conference, Los Angeles, CA, United States.

Perryman, K. L., Moss, R. C., & Anderson, L. (2016). Sandtray supervision: An integrated model for play therapy supervision. *International Journal of Play Therapy*, 25(4), 186–196. doi:10.1037/pla0040288.

Peters, H. C. (2017). Multicultural complexity: An intersectional lens for clinical supervision. *International Journal for the Advancement of Counselling*, 39(2), 176–187. doi:10.1007/s10447-017-9290-2.

Phillips, J. C., Parent, M. C., Dozier, V. C., & Jackson, P. L. (2017). Depth of discussion of multicultural identities in supervision and supervisory outcomes. *Counselling Psychology Quarterly*, 30(2), 188–210. doi:10.1080/09515070.2016.1169995.

Sensoy, O., & DiAngelo, R. (2014). Respect differences? Challenging the common guidelines in social justice education. *Democracy & Education*, 22(2), 1–10.

Singh, A., & Chun, K. Y. S. (2010). "From the margins to the center": Moving towards a resilience-based model of supervision for queer people of color supervisors. *Training and Education in Professional Psychology*, 4(1), 36–46. doi:10.1037/a0017373.

Spanierman, L.B., & Cabrera, N.L. (2014). The emotions of white racism and anti-racism. In V. Watson, D. Howard-Wagner & L. Spanierman (Eds.), *Unveiling whiteness in the twenty-first century*, pp. 9–28. Lexington Books.

Starr, F., Ciclitira, K., Marzano, L., Brunswick, N., & Costa, A. (2013). Comfort and challenge: A thematic analysis of female clinicians' experiences of supervision. *Psychology and Psychotherapy*, 86(3), 334–351. doi:10.1111/j.2044-8341.2012.02063.x.

Tohidian, N. B., & Quek, K. M. (2017). Processes that inform multicultural supervision: A qualitative meta-analysis. *Journal of Marital and Family Therapy*, 43(4), 573–590. doi:10.1111/jmft.12219.

Tracey, T. J. G., Bludworth, J., & Glidden-Tracey, C. E. (2012). Are there parallel processes in psychotherapy supervision? An empirical examination. *Psychotherapy*, 49(3), 330–343. doi:10.1037/a0026246.

Upshaw, N. C., Lewis, D. E., & Nelson, A. L. (2020). Cultural humility in action: Reflective and process-oriented supervision with black trainees. *Training and Education in Professional Psychology*, 14(4), 277–284. doi:10.1037/tep0000284.

Watkins, C. E., Hook, J. N., Mosher, D. K., & Callahan, J. L. (2019). Humility in clinical supervision: Fundamental, foundational, and transformational. *The Clinical Supervisor*, 38(1), 58–78. doi:10.1080/07325223.2018.1487355.

Wilson, H. M. N., Davies, J. S., & Weatherhead, S. (2016). Trainee therapists' experiences of supervision during training: A meta-synthesis. *Clinical Psychology and Psychotherapy*, 23(4), 340–351. doi:10.1002/cpp.1957.

Yakushko, O., Davidson, M. M., & Williams, E. N. (2009). Identity salience model: A paradigm for integrating multiple identities in clinical practice. *Psychotherapy*, 46(2), 180–192. doi:10.1037/a0016080.

15 The Multicultural Playroom

A Delphi Study

Dee C. Ray, Regine K. Chung, Krystal K. Turner and Elizabeth V. Aguilar

Concerning the needs for mental health intervention within an increasingly diverse younger population, there is a need for play therapists to ensure cultural inclusivity in their clinical practice. Apart from application of treatment modalities and skills with specific populations, play therapy that fosters multicultural inclusivity also involves the process of constructing the therapeutic environment – the playroom. We are particularly concerned with structuring a playroom that is inviting to children of varying identities and backgrounds. For this chapter, we sought to explore the potential of enhancing the multicultural inclusivity of the playroom for play therapy through research and discussion of outcomes related to a research project designed specifically for the purpose of building knowledge regarding play therapy rooms. In this chapter, we will present the methods and results of a recent research study conducted with play therapy experts on increasing the inclusivity of the playroom through attention to the attitudes, structure, and materials that comprise a playroom.

In the release of the 2020 census results, the U.S. Bureau of the Census introduced a new concept labeled as the Diversity Index (DI), which indicates the probability that two people chosen at random will be from different race or ethnicity groups. It was shown that in 25 out of 51 states, the DI is above 50%; and among these states, eight have a high DI ranging from 65.8% to 76% (U.S. Census Bureau, 2021), indicating the nation is diversifying rapidly. Taking a closer look at the population trend in the United States over the last two decades, the percentage of the population under age 16 who identified as a racial or ethnic minority grew from 39.2% to 50%. This group is comprised of U.S. residents identifying as Latino or Hispanic, Black, Asian American, American Indian Alaska Native, and "2+ and other races" (Frey, 2020). Race/ethnicity is only one aspect of cultural diversity. In play therapy, we are attuned to cultural aspects of gender, sexual identity, socioeconomic status, religion, and ability status, among many other diverse identities. Growing diversity in the U.S. child population also means that cultural sensitivity and inclusivity in play therapy is needed now more than ever.

Child-centered play therapy (CCPT; Landreth, 2012) is a developmentally responsive and evidence-based child therapy intervention for

DOI: 10.4324/9781003190073-19

children who experience social, emotional, behavioral, and relational disorders supported by multiple meta-analytic studies (Bratton et al., 2005; Lin & Bratton, 2015; Ray et al., 2015). Growing empirical research supports the efficacy of CCPT with children across ethnicities, gender, and ability levels (e.g. Garza & Bratton, 2005; Ogawa, 2007; Lin & Bratton, 2015; Schottelkorb et al., 2020; Taylor & Ray, 2021). Because toys are seen as children's medium of expression in the therapeutic process, the selection of toys and materials requires careful attention (Axline, 1974; Landreth, 2012). Axline (1974) suggested multiple toys and play items that facilitate children's imagination, free expression, and allow symbolic representation of significant relationships and experiences. Landreth (2012) offered a more systematic discussion on the playroom setting, such as the size of the playroom and choice of materials. Landreth recommended that toys and materials should be selected in order to facilitate seven essentials in play therapy including: establishment of a positive relationship with the child, expression of a wide range of feelings, exploration of real-life experiences, reality testing of limits, development of a positive self-image, development of self-understanding, and opportunity to develop self-control. Landreth further emphasized the importance of intentional selection of toys/materials.

Based on these principles, Landreth (2012) suggested three categories of toys and materials: real-life toys, acting-out aggressive-release toys, and toys for creative expression and emotional release. Real-life toys such as dolls, cars, and chalkboards provide the opportunity for children to play out events and experiences that occur for them in everyday life. Acting-out aggressive-release toys such as bop bags, rubber knives, and aggressive animals allow children to express intense anger or aggressive-related feelings. Creative expression and emotional release toys such as sand, water, and paints offer the least structure in order for children to project or create limitless possibilities. VanFleet et al. (2010) recommended the following categories for the CCPT playroom: Family/Nurturance, Communication, Aggression, Mastery, and Creative Expression. Finally, Cochran et al. (2010) identified the need for materials allowing for sociodramatic play, creative expression, aggressive release, and nurturing to support the CCPT stage process. Cochran et al. further cautioned against an imbalance of toys that are more appealing to specific genders or cultures and suggested a variety of toys for multicultural populations.

Landreth (2012) underscored the importance for play therapists to be sensitive to culture and diversity issues in the toy selection process. However, limited literature exists on in-depth exploration of culturally appropriate/ adaptive play therapy settings. Notably, limited research has been conducted to explore the structure of the therapeutic space, i.e. the playroom environment and the choice of toys and play materials to enhance multicultural sensitivity throughout the CCPT process. In the only study to date on multicultural items in the playroom, Chang et al. (2005) surveyed Association for Play Therapy members on items they included in their playrooms to represent diverse cultures. Chang et al.'s participants identified culturally based play and differences in play within ethnic minority children and suggested the need for selecting multicultural play items to enhance the therapeutic process in play therapy. Participants most frequently reported the use of ethnic dolls, sandtray items, and puppets as representative of diverse cultures. A few participants noted the use of religious items, dress-up clothes specific to race/ethnicity, and foods specific to cultures. Although Chang et al. provided an initial exploration of multicultural items, there was limited discussion of items that are typically included and recommended for playrooms.

In individual studies on the effectiveness of play therapy with specific populations, researchers have noted the need to modify playroom materials to meet the needs of the population served. In their study on the effectiveness of CCPT with Hispanic children, Garza and Bratton (2005) observed that the inclusion of culturally relevant craft materials and toys strengthened the communication between the therapist and the child and fostered a sense of familiarity, particularly at the beginning of the therapeutic relationship. Garza and Bratton also documented children's preference for the "culturally responsive" toys/materials such as Mexican instruments, foods, darker skin-toned dolls, and religious items. Taylor and Ray (2021) highlighted the need for culturally responsive toys in their study on the effectiveness of CCPT with African American children. Specifically, the researchers noted the use of dolls that were truly representative of African American individuals rather than dolls that had a darker skin tone but Eurocentric features, as well as representative play figures and religious items.

Recently, researchers examined the use of toys in CCPT (Ray et al., 2013) and gendered language associated with toys in play therapy (Stutey et al., 2020). Based on the utilization of toys in session by children of both genders and different ages, Ray and colleagues (2013) suggested that traditional toy categories identified by Kottman (2003) including Family/Nurture, Aggressive/Scary, Expressive, and Pretend/Fantasy toys are necessary for CCPT because children of all ages and genders play with them frequently in sessions. However, the frequency of toys being played with may vary among children of different genders, suggesting gender differences exist in the expressions through play (Ray et al., 2013). For example, Ray et al. found that females tended to gravitate towards family/nurturing toys more, while males tended to play with aggressive/scary toys more often, and children of both genders play with expressive and pretend/fantasy toys equally.

Stutey et al. (2020) further explored children's gendered language and toy preference among 22 children in play therapy. Stutey's team found that males were more likely to play with masculine toys while females played with a wider variety of toys. Findings from Ray et al. (2013) and Stutey et al. (2020) support the conclusion that culture affects play behaviors and highlight the importance for play therapists to consider how toys and materials can better represent the culture and development of the children they serve. Yet, consensus among play therapists related to the selection of play materials to enhance multicultural sensitivity has not yet been empirically explored or validated. Although researchers who have conducted play therapy studies with specific populations often note the modification or need for modification of playroom materials, there has not been a study explicitly focused on playroom materials and settings to meet diversity needs in over 15 years. Additionally, researchers have typically limited their focus to racial/ethnic diversity in their studies. The limitation in existing literature suggests that research is needed to inform play therapists' decision-making in designing a multicultural playroom that fits the needs of a rapidly diversifying society.

The purpose of this study was to define and identify what comprises a playroom that is multiculturally inclusive, as well as identify how play therapists can enhance the inclusivity of their playrooms. We used the Delphi technique to gain a consensus of opinion from experts in the field of play therapy regarding definition of a multicultural playroom, ways in which a play therapist can ensure that a playroom is multiculturally inclusive, and identification of toys and materials that comprise a multicultural playroom. This study was guided by three research questions:

1   What is the definition of a multicultural playroom?
2   How can play therapists make the playroom more multiculturally inclusive?
3   What materials should be included to increase the multicultural inclusiveness of the playroom?

Method

The primary purpose of the Delphi method is to form a consensus in areas of study that are beyond existing knowledge (Jünger et al., 2017). We chose to use the Delphi method as a philosophical fit for our focus on multicultural inclusion. The goal of the Delphi method is to form group consensus in which all voices are heard and considered in iterative rounds of data collection. Highlighting a consensus focus is also consistent with the CCPT humanistic approach to ensuring that each person's perspective is valued and worthy of inclusion. The Delphi method structures data collection to allow participants to provide information, opinions, and feedback anonymously in a systematic procedure of multiple rounds of inquiry. Delphi is characterized by four features including: (1) participants are a group of experts; (2) process is anonymous to avoid undue pressure on participants; (3) procedure is iterative in nature; and (4) the design of subsequent rounds is informed by previous rounds (Jünger et al., 2017).

Participants

The Delphi method allows for purposive sampling which allowed us to identify expert panelists who held both play therapy expertise and a multicultural expertise, as well as varying intersectional identities. Criteria for panelists included: (1) has identified as a CCPT therapist for at least five years; (2) has published or presented on CCPT; and (3) has previously set up at least one CCPT playroom. We intentionally sought expert panelists who met these criteria and who represented multiple intersectional identities. There is no agreement in the Delphi literature regarding an optimal number of panelists resulting in varied numbers; however, eight to ten and ten to 50 have been typically cited numbers for smaller studies (Keeney et al., 2011). Using purposive sampling, we identified 25 potential panelists. Individual emails were sent to the potential experts asking them to participate in the study, along with an explanation of study procedures. Of the 25 potential panelists, 22 participated in the study.

Table 15.1 presents demographic data on all participants. Due to the multicultural focus of the study, we chose to use open-ended responses to all demographic descriptors. Based on open-ended responses, there were diverse descriptors regarding race, gender, sexual orientation, and other salient identities. We chose to report all the descriptors in order to remain consistent with our goal of inclusivity. Although the Association for Play Therapy reports 76% members identify as female and 76% as White (APT, 2021), we sought to diversify our panel, resulting in 32% (n=7) reporting as White women and 45% (n=10) reporting as White.

Research Team

The research team consisted of four team members who hold various intersectional identities. Additionally, all four team members are author contributors to this book, play therapists, identify as theoretically aligned with CCPT, and are committed to a multicultural focus in play therapy. Positionality statements for each research team member can be found in previous chapters of the book (see Introduction and Chapters 8, 9, and 10).

Procedures

Following human subjects approval, we sent out emails to 25 potential participants inviting them to participate in the study and informing them of study procedures. Of the 22 who agreed to participate, 21 completed Round 1 (95% response rate). Rounds 2 and 3 were completed by all 22 panelists (100% response rate). Round 1 consisted of a demographic questionnaire, two open-ended questions, and a third question with a listing of playroom items. The first open-ended question consisted of: "The purpose of the proposed study is to use the Delphi technique to gain a consensus of

Table 15.1 Self-identified characteristics of participants (N=22)

Demographic characteristics	n	%
Age		
26–35	6	27.3
36–45	8	36.4
46–60	5	22.7
>60	3	13.6
Race		
African American	1	4.5
Asian	2	9
Black	2	9
Hispanic	1	4.5
Latinx	1	4.5
Middle Eastern/Caucasian	1	4.5
Mestizo/Latino	1	4.5
Native American rural tribal member	1	4.5
White	10	45.5
White (brown)	1	4.5
White/Native American of the Salish-Flathead Nation	1	4.5
Gender		
Cisgender	1	4.5
Cisgender woman	1	4.5
Cis-male	1	4.5
Female	15	68.2
Male/man	4	18.2
Sexual orientation		
Cisgender	1	4.5
Gay	1	4.5
Heterosexual/straight	19	86.4
Unidentified	1	4.5
Other personally salient identity		
Christian, Black	1	4.5
ENFJ (Myers-Briggs Type)	1	4.5
Family of origin; low social class/poverty	1	4.5
First gen. U.S.-born; bicultural; Spanish speaking	1	4.5
Immigrant	2	9.1
Immigrant, English as second language	1	4.5
International/non-American; Taiwanese; middle class; mother/parent	1	4.5

Demographic characteristics	*n*	%
Jewish	1	4.5
My ethnicity; Latina	1	4.5
Unidentified	12	54.5
Number of years as a play therapist		
5–9	6	27.3
10–14	3	13.6
15–19	4	18.2
20–24	2	9.1
25–29	3	13.6
≥30	4	18.2
Number of years teaching play therapy		
<5	8	36.4
5–9	3	13.6
10–14	3	13.6
15–19	3	13.6
20–24	2	9.1
25–29	2	9.1
≥30	1	4.5
Number of play therapy rooms worked in as a play therapist or play therapist supervisor		
5–9	9	40.9
10–14	8	36.4
15–19	2	9.1
20–24	2	9.1
25–29	0	0
≥30	1	4.5
Highest degree		
Masters	4	18.2
PhD	18	81.8

opinion from experts in the field of play therapy to define and identify what constitutes a multicultural playroom, specifically meaning a playroom that is designed for all children. Given your experience and knowledge of the field, please provide your definition of a multicultural playroom." The second open-ended question was: "Given your experience and knowledge of the field, please address how play therapists make the playroom more multiculturally inclusive?" For the final group of items, panelists were provided with a list from Landreth's (2012) list of 69 playroom materials and asked to rate each item on a five-point Likert scale from Not Essential to

Essential to a Multicultural Playroom (i.e. 1=Not Essential, 5= Essential). They were also provided with an open-ended response category to add comments about any of the items. The informed consent and questionnaire were distributed through Qualtrics.

Following Round 1, the research team conducted a content analysis of the responses from the two open-ended questions. Content analysis steps consisted of open coding conducted independently by the four research team members. Following the completion of open coding, all data was recorded and examined in an axial coding process. During the axial coding phase, the research team met to examine relationships among the open codes through a consensus process. Finally, we conducted selective coding to ensure that all data was included in final codes (i.e. statements). In order to remain consistent with our focus on multicultural process, we as the research team believed it was most inclusive to complete the axial and final selective coding processes as a team. For the final item of the Round 1 questionnaire, we compiled the results regarding level of essentialism for each of the playroom materials.

For Round 2, we presented participants with statements regarding the definition of the multicultural playroom based on content analysis results. We asked participants to rate each statement on a five-point Likert scale regarding how important the statement was to being a part of a multicultural playroom definition (i.e. 1=Not Important at All, 5=Very Important). We also presented statements regarding how play therapists can better create multiculturally inclusive playrooms based on content analysis results with the same Likert scale instructions. Additionally, in Round 2, we asked participants to rate playroom materials for which consensus had not been reached in Round 1. Comments were solicited throughout the Round 2 questionnaire to allow for open-ended responses.

For Round 3, any statements or playroom materials that had not reached consensus in the first two rounds were listed and participants were asked to rate each of the items on the same Likert scale categories. For Rounds 2 and 3, participants were provided with their individual ratings for each statement/item, along with the group mean. We asked participants to consider their rating in the context of the group and invited them to make changes to their original ratings if desired. Finally, in Round 3, we asked participants to provide a rationale for a rating of 3 on playroom materials/toys in order to have a better understanding of their perceptions of not having a strong opinion of that material's inclusion.

In accordance with standard practices in Delphi methods (Jünger et al., 2017), the desired agreement level for a response to reach consensus in this study was set at 80% of responses for each individual item achieving a median response score of greater than or equal to 4, or less than or equal to 2. Playroom materials that failed to reach the 80% consensus rating following Round 1 were included in Round 2. Statements and playroom materials that failed to reach the 80% consensus in Round 2 were included in Round 3. All items following Round 3 that reached the 80% threshold were considered to be consensus items.

Results

Multicultural Definition

Content analysis from Round 1 yielded six statements that encompassed the definition of a multicultural playroom. In Round 2, participants rated the six statements based on their importance regarding being part of the definition. Table 15.2 presents the statements, consensus results, and the round in which consensus was reached. Results from Round 2 resulted in consensus on four of the statements. Two of the statements did not reach consensus. Based on feedback from participants in Round 2, statements were edited to include concepts shared by participants. The original statement for 1c. was: "Cultural expression includes those within the context of gender, race, ethnicity, sexual orientation, ability, social class, language, nationality, citizenship status, religion, childhood, generation, family structure, and community type (i.e. urban/rural/suburban)." Participants reported discomfort with a finite list of identities, as well as preference for the term sexual identity rather than sexual orientation. The statement was modified for Round 3 by adding the phrase, "but not limited to," and replacing the word orientation with the word identity. The original statement for 1e, "Materials in the multicultural playroom are developmentally appropriate and representative of the micro and macro culture, allow for cultural challenges and pride, open-ended to allow for child's own interpretation, and represent contemporary childhood," resulted in feedback regarding wording confusion. Due to limited comments on rationale for lack of importance of this statement, we made a slight word change by replacing the word contemporary with the phrase "present-day." Both modified statements reached consensus in Round 3. The final definition of a multicultural playroom based on consensus was the following:

> A multicultural playroom is intentionally designed to facilitate a child's free expression and exploration of self, including all cultural aspects of self. A multicultural playroom allows for expression and exploration of a child's cultural experiences on both the local and broader community level. Cultural expression includes those within the context of, but not limited to, gender, race, ethnicity, sexual identity, ability, social class, language, nationality, citizenship status, religion, childhood, generation, family structure, and community type (i.e. urban/rural/suburban). Materials and structural design in the multicultural playroom are intentionally selected to provide a sense of familiarity to children in

Table 15.2 Multicultural playroom definition statements that gained consensus

Statement	Mean (SD)	Consensus Level (%)	Round Consensus Reached
1a. A multicultural playroom is intentionally designed to facilitate a child's free expression and exploration of self, including all cultural aspects of self.	4.86 (.35)	100	2
1b. A multicultural playroom allows for expression and exploration of a child's cultural experiences on both the local and broader community level.	4.36 (.79)	81.8	2
1c. Cultural expression includes those within the context of, but not limited to, gender, race, ethnicity, sexual identity, ability, social class, language, nationality, citizenship status, religion, childhood, generation, family structure, and community type (i.e. urban/rural/suburban).	4.60 (.50)	100	3
1d. Materials and structural design in the multicultural playroom are intentionally selected to provide a sense of familiarity to children in reflecting their everyday interactions, leading to a sense of belonging and safety in the room.	4.55 (.67)	90.9	2
1e. Materials in the multicultural playroom are developmentally appropriate and representative of the micro and macro culture, allow for cultural challenges and pride, open-ended to allow for child's own interpretation, and represent present-day childhood.	4.41 (.59)	95.5	3
1f. Although materials and structural elements of a playroom are essential to cultural inclusivity, the play therapist is primary to the process of a child's sense of safety in cultural expression. The play therapist actively facilitates cultural expression and acceptance through attitudinal conditions of congruence, unconditional positive regard, and empathic understanding; cultural humility; responsibility for responding to cultural opportunities; and commitment to ongoing learning and development of diverse cultures, systemic oppression, and self-awareness of bias.	4.82 (.39)	100	2

reflecting their everyday interactions, leading to a sense of belonging and safety in the room. Materials in the multicultural playroom are developmentally appropriate and representative of the micro and macro culture, allow for cultural challenges and pride, open-ended to allow for child's own interpretation, and represent present-day childhood. Although materials and structural elements of a playroom are essential to cultural inclusivity, the play therapist is primary to the process of a child's sense of safety in cultural expression. The play therapist actively facilitates cultural expression and acceptance through attitudinal conditions of congruence, unconditional positive regard, and empathic under-standing; cultural humility; responsibility for responding to cultural opportunities; and commitment to ongoing learning and development of diverse cultures, systemic oppression, and self-awareness of bias.

Ways Play Therapists Create More Culturally Inclusive Playrooms

Content analysis from Round 1 yielded seven statements that represented the data on ways in which play therapists can create more culturally inclusive playrooms. In Round 2, participants rated the seven statements based on their importance. Table 15.3 presents the statements, consensus results, and the round in which consensus was reached. Results from Round 2 resulted in consensus on all seven statements.

Playroom Materials/Toys

In Round 1, we listed the 69 playroom materials suggested by Landreth (2012) and asked participants to rate their essentialism in a multicultural playroom. Of the 69 materials, participants reached positive consensus on 40 of the 69 materials, indicating support for these materials in the playroom. For Round 2, we included the 29 non-consensus items and asked partici-pants to rate the items in the context of their previous individual rating and the group mean rating. Round 2 resulted in a positive consensus on 6 items and a negative consensus on one item (i.e. Gumby). Based on Round 2 feedback, the research team modified wording for a few items for Round 3 consideration. A modifier was added to Barbies (i.e. Barbies [varying physi-cal characteristics]), whiteboard was added to chalkboard item (i.e. chalk-board/whiteboard), Lone Ranger mask was changed to "black mask and other masks," and tinker toys was changed to interlocking construction toys. The remaining 22 items were included in Round 3 for which parti-cipants were asked to rate these items again based on previous individual ratings and group mean ratings. Round 3 resulted in consensus on two additional items. Final analysis resulted in the inclusion of 48 playroom material items, exclusion of one item (i.e. Gumby), and no consensus

Table 15.3 Consensus statements on ways Play Therapists create more culturally inclusive playrooms

Materials/Toys	Mean (SD)	Consensus Level	Round Consensus Reached
The play therapist intentionally structures the playroom and selects materials that are accessible, diverse, and representative of many cultures, including but not limited to materials for categories of household, kitchen, food, dolls and figures, expressive materials, costumes, and transportation, with particular attention to forms, textures and colors that are diverse and representative of many cultures.	4.31 (.89)	81.8	2
In order to serve children through culturally inclusive practices, the therapist seeks to understand and respond to local and broader communities through engaging with and learning from the local community, researching local neighborhoods, seeking cultural mentoring, printing materials in languages of the community, and staying engaged with local and broader social concerns.	4.73 (.63)	90.9	2
The play therapist engages in lifelong cultural development on a personal level through exploring personal biases, remaining curious, holding high sensitivity for cultural issues, seeking self-acceptance when feeling discomfort in cultural differences, and striving for cultural humility.	4.86 (.35)	100	2
In session, the play therapist maintains awareness of clients' intersectional identities, responds with openness to the child and child's use of materials, seizes cultural opportunities to respond empathically to clients, maintains awareness of cultural messages sent through body language and communication style, and engages in ongoing process of modifying playroom for clients.	4.36 (.85)	86.3	2

Materials/Toys	Mean (SD)	Consensus Level	Round Consensus Reached
The play therapist recognizes cultural implications of the play therapy environment and seeks to ensure that the waiting room is designed inclusively, the location of services is responsive to the client's community, and ensures that parents and members of the family structure are involved in the play therapy process.	4.36 (.95)	86.4	2
In order to provide effective services across the field of play therapy, the play therapist is involved in training on personal and professional cultural development, as well as actively advocates for the inclusion of play therapists from diverse identities and backgrounds and multicultural training for all play therapists.	4.43 (.75)	90.9	2
The child-centered play therapist recognizes the value of traditionally identified materials in the playroom (e.g. Landreth, 2012) as materials that allow for open interpretation and free expression of culture. In addition, the play therapist continues to adapt traditional lists to meet the cultural needs of clients through careful and intentional selection.	4.55 (.74)	86.4	2

reached on 20 items. Table 15.4 lists all resulting essential items, consensus results, and the round in which consensus was reached. Table 15.5 lists all items for which consensus was not reached.

Discussion

In this study, we attempted to explore the perceptions of 22 experts in CCPT and multiculturalism regarding the definition and materials/toys of a multicultural playroom, as well as ways play therapists can enhance the cultural inclusivity of playrooms. Participants represented a wide array of diverse identities across race/ethnicity, gender, sexual identity, religion, and immigration/international status, as well as other salient identities. Panelists were well-versed as play therapists ranging from five to over 30 years of

Table 15.4 Essential materials/toys for the multicultural playroom that gained consensus

Materials/Toys	Mean (SD)	Consensus Level (%)	Round Consensus Reached
Band-aids	4.12 (1.12)	84.2	1
Bendable doll family	2.65 (1.39)	95.2	1
Blunt scissors	4.65 (.59)	95	1
Bob (bop bag)	4.75 (.44)	95	1
Building blocks	4.62 (.67)	90.4	1
Construction paper	4.76 (.54)	95.3	1
Crayons, pencils, paper	4.81 (.40)	100	1
Dart gun	4.33 (1.11)	81	1
Dinosaurs, shark	4.67 (.58)	95.2	1
Dishes	4.76 (.44)	99.2	1
Doll bed, clothes, blanket	4.57 (.75)	85.7	1
Doll furniture	4.29 (.85)	85.7	1
Dollhouse (open-on-floor type)	4.71 (.46)	100	1
Dolls, baby clothes	4.81 (.51)	95.2	1
Dress-up clothes	4.62 (.67)	90.4	1
Drum	4.29 (1.06)	80.9	1
Empty fruit and vegetable cans	4.05 (1.07)	81	1
Erasable nontoxic markers	4.62 (.67)	90.4	1
Flashlight	4.38 (1.02)	85.7	1
Handcuffs	4.80 (.41)	100	1
Hats: firefighter, police, tiara, crown	4.50 (.83)	90	1
Medical kit	4.85 (.37)	100	1
Medical mask	4.57 (.98)	85.8	1
Nursing bottle (plastic)	4.75 (.44)	100	1
Pacifier	4.40 (.88)	85	1
Paints, easel, newsprint, brushes	4.75 (.55)	95	1
Play money and cash register	4.71 (.64)	90.5	1
Pot, pans, silverware	4.70 (.66)	90	1
Rope	4.43 (.81)	80.9	1
Rubber knife	4.70 (.66)	90	1
Rubber snake, alligator	4.50 (.76)	85	1
Sandbox, large spoon, funnel, sieve, pail	4.80 (.52)	95	1
School bus	4.25 (.72)	85	1
Spider and other insects	4.29 (.90)	81	1
Telephone (two)	4.55 (.83)	90	1

Table 15.4 (continued)

Materials/Toys	Mean (SD)	Consensus Level (%)	Round Consensus Reached
Tissues	4.57 (.81)	90.4	1
Toy soldiers and army equipment	4.55 (.69)	90	1
Transparent tape, nontoxic glue	4.80 (.41)	100	1
Truck, car, airplane, tractor, boat, ambulance	4.70 (.57)	95	1
Zoo animals and farm animal families	4.90 (.30)	100	1
Balls	4.14 (.56)	90.9	2
Hand puppets	4.23 (.92)	86.4	2
Purse and jewelry	4.09 (.68)	81.8	2
Stove	3.45 (.66)	91	2
Tongue depressors	3.91 (.68)	81.8	2
Watercolor paints	4.23 (.81)	86.4	2
Broom, dustpan	4.05 (.58)	86.4	3
Soap, brush, comb	3.91 (.68)	81.8	3

Table 15.5 List of non-consensus materials/toys

Barbies (varying physical characteristics)
Black mask and other masks (formerly Lone Ranger Mask)
Cereal boxes
Chalkboard/whiteboard
Colored chalk
Cymbals
Dishpans
Egg cartons
Interlocking construction toys (formerly known as tinker toys)
Pitcher
Play camera
Pounding bench and hammer
Puppet theater
Rags or old towels
Refrigerator
Sponge
Stuffed animals
Toy noise-making gun
Toy watch
Xylophone

experience and also experiences setting up playrooms ranging from setting up five to over 30 playrooms during their careers. Although panelists were diverse in their backgrounds, identities, and experiences, they all identified as theoretically aligned with CCPT, which may have led to early consensus on most statements and toys throughout the Delphi process. As the research team for this study, we observed notable patterns and outcomes throughout data collection and analysis, including panelists focus on intentionality, the responsibility and personhood of the play therapist as a key facilitator to a multiculturally inclusive playroom, the need to consider structure of the multicultural playroom as well as materials/toys, and the consensus that traditionally recommended materials/toys are essential to the multicultural playroom but need modifications.

Intentionality

In the content analysis process following Round 1, we identified a consistent theme and frequent use of the word "intentional" or variations thereof in participant responses regarding definition of a multicultural playroom and ways in which play therapists can enhance cultural inclusivity in the playroom. Panelists emphasized the need for play therapists to be intentionally aware and purposeful in their choices of playroom structure and materials. The first sentence in the multicultural playroom definition states that the "multicultural playroom is intentionally designed..." highlighting that the play therapist consciously attends to the design of the playroom to ensure that it is multiculturally inclusive. This sentence reached 100% consensus in the first round of ratings, indicating that panelists were enthusiastically in support of this concept. Given that traditional play therapy literature (e.g. Axline, 1974; Cochran et al., 2010; Landreth, 2012; Ray, 2011; VanFleet et al., 2010) provides little discussion of concrete steps to ensure cultural inclusivity for playroom structure and materials/toys, panelists may be particularly drawn to promoting the need for play therapists to be more intentional in their selections for the playroom. In addition to intentionality, panelists were also concerned with the play thera-pist's self and other-awareness. The integration of awareness with intentionality is likely to activate a therapist's behavior in playroom decision-making. It appeared that panelists were making the point that sticking with traditionally listed materials/toys without intentionally questioning their inclusion was not enough to ensure that the playroom is inclusive. The final consensus definition and ways in which therapists can create more culturally inclusive playrooms hold the therapist accountable to being intentional in designing, selecting, and structuring the playroom.

The Play Therapist

Although panelists appeared enthusiastic about identifying materials/toys for inclusivity, there was a consensus that the most important factor in making a playroom inclusive was the play therapist. Throughout rounds, panelists continued to provide feedback that materials/toys were essential to a multicultural playroom but not as essential as the attitude, knowledge, skills, and personhood of the play therapist. As the research team, we noted that panelists seemed to be concerned that this point regarding the essential nature of the play therapist would be lost to a focus on toys/materials. In the final section of the multicultural playroom definition, the statement, "Although materials and structural elements of playroom are essential to cultural inclusivity, the play therapist is primary to the process of a child's sense of safety in cultural expression," appeared to capture the sentiments of the panelists as evidenced by 100% consensus following the first round of statement ratings. Panelists continued to hold play therapists accountable in both the definition and ways to create culturally inclusive playrooms by highlighting therapist intentionality, awareness, cultural humility, responsibility for cultural opportunities, accountability for advocacy and training, and ongoing personal and professional exploration of cultural issues.

Playroom Toys, Materials, and Structure

The consensus statements revealed that panelists were mostly concerned with the responsibilities of the play therapist in selecting toys and materials for the playroom based on awareness of personal biases and attitudes as well as knowledge of cultural issues, systemic racism, oppression, and specific cultural information. However, panelists expressed interest and enthusiasm for the selection of toys and materials for the multicultural playroom as evidenced by the many comments providing feedback about materials. Because literature on CCPT toys/materials is fairly consistent in playroom item lists, we believed that Landreth's (2012) list of 69 toys/materials mostly represented the CCPT approach to the playroom. Given that panelists identified with CCPT, it is not surprising the consensus on the majority of items (n=40) was reached in the first round of ratings.

Of distinct interest was early consensus regarding aggressive toys. In fact, all listed aggressive toys reached consensus in the first round except for noisy guns. These aggressive toys included bop bag, dart gun, handcuffs, knife, aggressive animals, and soldiers. Consensus was never reached on noisy guns. CCPT literature is replete with rationale and research supporting the use of aggressive materials in play therapy (see Landreth, 2012; Ray, 2011). Panelists had few comments regarding the aggressive toys yet rated them as essential early in the consensus process, indicating that CCPT experts see the need for aggressive toys as essential across culture. Based on comments, lack of consensus on noisy guns seemed to be attributed to the perception that there is no need for multiple types of guns, and a preference for dart guns.

Ultimately, panelists reached consensus on 48 toys/materials that are traditionally listed as CCPT playroom materials as being essential in a multicultural playroom. The fact that panelists could only come to consensus on eight additional items after the first round indicates that panelists struggled with the necessity and/or inclusiveness of the remaining items. Non-consensus items that elicited the most feedback included Barbies, cereal boxes, camera, watches, bench and hammer, and chalkboard/whiteboard. Barbies were, by far, the item with the most comments. Panelists expressed concerns about the cultural messages sent by the inclusion of Barbies, including gender and race/ethnicity messages pertaining to cultural standards of beauty. Because some panelists expressed positive reports of using Barbies of various skin tones, we changed the wording of Barbies for Round 3 to include the modifier, "varying physical characteristics." The modification did not help the panelists reach consensus and Barbies remained a non-consensus item. Panelists were not in agreement regarding cereal boxes. Panelists with a focus on international diversity noted that cereal is not a common food outside of the United States while some panelists communicated that a variety of cereals could be used to address diversity. In the end, cereal boxes remained a non-consensus item. Items such as cameras and watches were identified by some panelists as outdated for the current U.S. culture in which phones have replaced the functions of cameras and watches. Items such as whiteboard/chalkboard and hammer and bench were noted by panelists as unnecessary yet not due to cultural inclusivity concerns.

Ratings on musical instruments resulted in the inclusion of drums but the two other musical instruments, xylophone and cymbals, did not reach consensus. Panelists expressed the need for musical instruments to be specific to the culture served or to multiple cultures. Xylophone and cymbals were identified as culturally specific and may not represent multiple cultures. Interestingly, the panelists found that drums were cross-cultural and reached consensus on their inclusion early in Round 1.

For the 48 items that reached consensus, panelists were intentional in adding modifications to many of the items in order to ensure cultural inclusivity. It was clear that panelists were uncomfortable with the item titles typically listed and wanted to provide clearer descriptors for cultural inclusivity. Items such as dolls, food, dress-up clothes, band-aids, crayons, puppets, and money were all identified by panelists as needing more description to ensure that play therapists are selecting materials in these categories that represent the cultures, communities, identities, and experiences of children being served. While some panelists suggested the need for a myriad of cultures for each toy category in order to serve diverse clients, other panelists recommended ensuring the inclusion of materials for the specific population served. As the research team, we found this result to be the most overwhelming when identifying implications of these outcomes. For play therapists who serve children from diverse backgrounds in one room, the inclusion of multiple types of the same toy/material may be limited by space and funding. In addition, the child may become overwhelmed with too many materials in the playroom. Alternately, if the play therapist serves mainly one specific population, does a playroom that only represents that culture allow for the full expression of that child's world, especially if that child is living in a diverse community? These are thoughts that we are continuing to reflect upon and refine for the purposes of providing clearer direction for play therapists.

Throughout the process of refining statements for the multicultural playroom definition and ways to create culturally inclusive playrooms, panelists emphasized the need to not only intentionally select items for the playroom, but to also intentionally design the structure of the playroom for needs of children with varying abilities. Panelists reported attention to space size, accessibility, and stimulation within the playroom, indicating the need for play therapists to recognize and structure the playroom for children with varying physical abilities. Shelf placement, wheelchair accessibility, and colors of the room were mentioned as considerations for the structure of the playroom.

Limitations

Because we explored a relatively uninvestigated area of research, there were limitations to this study. In designing the study, we intended to explicitly focus on the multicultural inclusiveness of toys/materials in the playroom. We framed the questionnaire for panelists to consider materials in the context of a multicultural playroom. However, because we used the traditional list of CCPT materials, the inclusion of materials based on a perception of necessity for a playroom versus their contribution to multicultural inclusivity may have become conflated for panelists. It appeared that panelists were deliberate in their attunement to multicultural considerations, yet some responses indicated that panelists did not see a toy/material as particularly inclusive but necessary. In our research team framework, we held that any material that was deemed necessary would also be multiculturally inclusive but this framework may not have been the same for panelists.

Additionally, in Round 1, we asked panelists to add any items to the list that they thought were multiculturally inclusive and necessary for a multicultural playroom. The panelists responded with many suggestions. Although most suggestions centered on adding descriptors to the traditional categories of toys/materials, we received many additional items for consideration. In order to include the items in the subsequent rounds for rating, we would have extended the questionnaire beyond the probable patience of the panelists. Hence, the final consensus does not include items suggested in addition to the traditional list. We plan to extend our exploration of these items as we continue our work toward a multicultural playroom.

Conclusion

The study presented in this chapter represents an intensive exploration of what constitutes a multicultural playroom. Because we were focused on and committed to consistency concerning the humanistic approach in play therapy and power of cultural inclusivity, we chose a method of inquiry that allowed for the individual voices of our diverse panelists to be heard and recorded. We also valued the process of consensus in which panelists were reflective and considerate of their fellow panelists in their decision-making and feedback. The results of this exploration provide the field of play therapy with a clear and detailed description of a multicultural playroom, active behaviors for play therapists to ensure cultural inclusivity in their playrooms, and a list of toys/materials that are essential to a multicultural playroom. Our sincere hope is that play therapists will use these outcomes to reflect upon their playrooms, including their own intentionality toward cultural inclusivity and the role of each selected toy/material.

References

Axline, V. M. (1974). *Play Therapy*. Ballantine Books.

Bratton, S. C., Ray, D., Rhine, T., & Jones, L. (2005). The efficacy of play therapy with children: A meta-analytic review of treatment outcomes. *Professional Psychology: Research and Practice*, 36(4), 367–390. doi:10.1037/0735-7028.36.4.376.

Chang, C. Y., Ritter, K. B., & Hays, D. G. (2005). Multicultural trends and toys in play therapy. *International Journal of Play Therapy*, 14(2), 69–85. doi:10.1037/h0088903.

Cochran, N. H., Nordling, W. J., & Cochran, J. L. (2010). *Child-centered play therapy: A practical guide to developing therapeutic relationships with children*. John Wiley & Sons.

Frey, W. H. (2020, July 1). The nation is diversifying even faster than predicted, according to new census data. *Brookings*. www.brookings.edu/research/new-census-data-shows-the-nation-is-diversifying-even-faster-than-predicted.

Garza, Y., & Bratton, S. C. (2005). School-based child-centered play therapy with Hispanic children: Outcomes and cultural considerations. *International Journal of Play Therapy*, 14(1), 51–80. doi:10.1037/h0088896.

Jünger, S., Payne, S. A., Brine, J., Radbruch, L., & Brearley, S.G. (2017). Guidance on conducting and Reporting Delphi studies (CREDES) in palliative care: Recommendations based on a methodological systematic review. *Palliative Medicine*, 31(8), 684–706. doi:10.1177/0269216317690685.

Keeney, S., Hasson, F., & McKenna, H. (2011). *The Delphi technique in nursing and health research*. Wiley-Blackwell.

Kottman, T. (2003). *Partners in play: An Adlerian approach to play therapy* (2nd ed.). American Counseling Association.

Landreth, G. L. (2012). *Play therapy: The art of the relationship* (3rd ed.). Routledge.

Lin, Y., & Bratton, S. C. (2015). A meta-analytic review of child-centered play therapy approaches. *Journal of Counseling and Development*, 93(1), 45–58. doi:10.1002/j.1556-6676.2015.00180.x.

Ogawa, Y. (2007). *Effectiveness of child-centered play therapy with Japanese children in the United States*. [Doctoral dissertation, University of North Texas]. ProQuest Dissertations and Theses Global.

Ray, D. C. (2011). *Advanced play therapy: Essential conditions, knowledge, and skills for child practice*. Routledge.

Ray, D. C., Armstrong, S. A., Balkin, R. S., & Jayne, K. M. (2015). Child-centered play therapy in the schools: Review and meta-analysis. *Psychology in the Schools*, 52 (2), 107–123. doi:10.1002/pits.21798.

Ray, D. C., Lee, K. R., Meany-Walen, K. K., Carlson, S. E., Carnes-Holt, K. L., & Ware, J. N. (2013). Use of toys in child-centered play therapy. *International Journal of Play Therapy*, 22(1), 43–57. doi:10.1037/a0031430.

Schottelkorb, A. A., Swan, K. L., & Ogawa, Y. (2020). Intensive child-centered play therapy for children on the autism spectrum: A pilot study. *Journal of Counseling & Development*, 98(1), 63–73. doi:10.1002/jcad.12300.

Stutey, D. M., Klein, D. E., Henninger, J., Crethar, H. C., & Hammer, T. R. (2020). Examining gender in play therapy. *International Journal of Play Therapy*, 29 (1), 20–32. doi:10.1037/pla0000108.

Taylor, L., & Ray, D. C. (2021). Child-centered play therapy and social–emotional competencies of African American children: A randomized controlled trial. *International Journal of Play Therapy*, 30(2), 74–85. doi:10.1037/pla0000152.

U.S. Census Bureau (2021). Racial and ethnic diversity in the United States: 2010 Census and 2020 Census. www.census.gov/library/visualizations/interactive/racial-and-ethnic-diversity-in-the-united-states-2010-and-2020-census.html.

VanFleet, R., Sywulak, A., & Sniscak, C. C. (2010). *Child-centered play therapy*. Guilford Press.

16 Research Across Diverse Races/ Ethnicities in Play Therapy

Yung-Wei Dennis Lin and Terence Yee

Teaching in mental health fields for more than ten years, we have noticed that most mental health students and clinicians tend to have low interest in research. Unfortunately, research does not belong to scientists or researchers only. Mental health professionals, including play therapists, have an ethical obligation to provide interventions and services based on established empirical or scientific evidence (American Counseling Association, 2014; American Psychological Association, 2017). Play therapists should thus develop a clear understanding about the research evidence of play therapy, particularly, the research findings on its therapeutic effectiveness based on rigorous study designs. In the long history of play therapy research, which can be dated back to 1940s (Lin & Bratton, 2015), play therapy researchers have employed a variety of both qualitative and quantitative research designs, such as single subject/group designs, quasi-experimental between group designs, randomized controlled trials, meta-analysis, qualitative case study designs, phenomenological designs, and mixed-method designs. Each of these different research designs has provided unique precious findings, and altogether have demonstrated clear evidence for the treatment effect of humanistic play therapy.

Diversity is an extremely broad term that can cover a wide variety of perspectives. Due to the limited amount of play therapy studies addressing all different perspectives of diversity, we would like to focus on racial/ethnic diversity in play therapy for this chapter. In this chapter, we would like to: (a) provide a brief summary to introduce the general treatment effectiveness of humanistic play therapy; (b) address the quantitative research findings that support the unique treatment effect of humanistic play therapy specifically on racially/ethnically diverse populations; and (c) discuss the qualitative research findings about humanistic play therapy to help play therapists learn from the voices of racially/ethnically diverse populations. Due to language limitations, we are able to only include research findings that were published in English within or outside of the United States. In addition, we include child-parent relationship therapy (CPRT)/filial therapy within humanistic play therapy approaches in this chapter because of its theoretical grounding in person-centered philosophy and its focus as a play-based intervention for young children.

DOI: 10.4324/9781003190073-20

Overall Play Therapy Effectiveness

Researchers generally believe the most stringent criteria for an evidence-supported intervention is the statistically significant superiority of the treatment condition as compared to a no-treatment, alternative treatment, or placebo condition in controlled outcome studies (Nezu & Nezu, 2008). Although many play therapy researchers have contributed research findings for play therapy effectiveness following such stringent criteria, these individual studies often utilized relatively small sample sizes (less than 60 participants in total) and accordingly suffered from the limited ability to generalize their findings in each individual study (Lin & Bratton, 2015). Actually, this limitation of small sample size is a common challenge in empirical studies in social science fields. To overcome this challenge, Glass (1976) developed meta-analysis, a quantitative and systematic research method that enables researchers to integrate research findings from a collection of quantitative studies. Due to the use of advanced statistical analysis techniques and the aggregated large sample size from individual studies, meta-analysis allows researchers to provide generalizable findings for the overall effectiveness for an intervention and further explore potential moderator variables to the overall intervention effect (Lipsey & Wilson, 2001; Whiston & Li, 2011).

Several play therapy researchers have conducted meta-analytical reviews on play therapy studies. These meta-analytic studies used Cohen's *d* or Hedge's *g* for the effect size estimation, and we followed Cohen's (1988) effect size interpretation guidelines, in which effect size ≤ 0.2, effect size = 0.5, and effect size ≥ 0.8 respectively represent small, medium, and large treatment effect. LeBlanc and Ritchie (2001) published the first play therapy meta-analysis based on 42 controlled outcome studies between 1947 and 1996. Although the total aggregated sample size was not reported, they estimated an overall effect size of 0.66 for play therapy. Bratton and colleagues (2005) conducted a meta-analytic review for 93 humanistic and non-humanistic (behavioral) play therapy studies between 1953 and 2000. These 93 studies together included 3,248 child participants in total, which makes their overall effect size finding (0.80) much more generalizable as the general play therapy effect. Lin and Bratton (2015) conducted a later meta-analysis to explore the effectiveness of child-centered play therapy (CCPT) based on 52 controlled outcome studies (totaling 1,848 child participants) between 1995 and 2010. By using more stringent effect size calculation formula, they suggested an overall effect size of 0.47 for the general CCPT effect. Similarly, Ray and colleagues (2015) conducted a meta-analytical review for 23 school-based CCPT controlled outcome studies between 1975 and 2011. Based on 1,106 child participants in these 23 studies, they suggested effect sizes ranging between 0.21 and 0.38 for the overall effectiveness of school-based play therapy. Although the values of overall effect sizes in these meta-analytic studies vary from 0.21 to 0.8, they are all statistically significantly larger than 0, indicating outcomes from play therapy interventions were found to be statistically significantly positive. More precisely, these effect sizes represent that children after play therapy treatment made statistically significantly greater improvement by 0.21 to 0.80 standard deviations than those in the control groups who did not receive play therapy treatment.

The overall effect size findings from these four meta-analytic studies have provided clear research evidence for the highly generalizable treatment effect of play therapy to all children based on the enormous total sample sizes. Thus, play therapy is undoubtedly an effective mental health intervention for children in general. However, is play therapy equally effective to children and families from each specific ethnicity/race? We will further discuss both the quantitative and qualitative findings in the effect of play therapy across different ethnicities/races in the following sections.

Quantitative Research Findings for Play Therapy Effect with Diverse Populations

Play therapy theoretically is a culturally inclusive mental health intervention for children given the use of play, noted as children's most natural expression method (Landreth, 2012). Lin and Bratton (2015) in their meta-analysis also suggested CCPT as a culturally inclusive counseling intervention for children with diverse ethnicity backgrounds. Specifically, Lin and Bratton found that the studies that included mostly children of underrepresented groups generated a mean effect size of 0.76, which is statistically significantly greater than the mean effect size of 0.33 generated from studies that included mostly White child participants. In addition to the meta-analysis support for CCPT as a culturally inclusive intervention, play therapy researchers have conducted many quantitative studies that specifically targeted racially/ethnically diverse populations.

Studies with African/African American Populations

Play therapists have recommended play therapy as a culturally inclusive intervention for African/African American children (Baggerly & Parker, 2005; Olson, 2016; Sheely-Moore & Ceballos, 2011); however, empirical quantitative studies that specifically target these populations are very limited in the play therapy literature. For example, Patterson and colleagues (2018) conducted a pilot study with 12 African American children aged between five and nine years old who had adverse childhood experiences. After six weeks of individual CCPT and six weeks of group CCPT, the 12 child participants' problematic behaviors, general worry, and negative intrusive thought patterns decreased significantly based on teachers' reports. Although their study did not include a control group and only relied on teachers' assessment reports, their findings still provided initial support for CCPT benefits to African American children. Taylor and Ray (2021) recently examined CCPT effect on African American children's social-emotional abilities by using a randomized controlled trial (RCT) study design. According to parents' reports, the 20 children in the experimental group demonstrated significant enhancement of their social-emotional abilities after the CCPT treatment compared with the 17 children in the control group. Their RCT study provided solid research evidence for CCPT effect on improving African American children's social and emotional competencies. In addition to CCPT, Sheely-Moore and Bratton (2010) were interested in the effect of child-parent relationship therapy (CPRT; Landreth & Bratton, 2020), the ten-week filial therapy model, on African American children's behavioral concerns as well as parenting stress. In their quasi-experimental study, they compared 13 parent-child dyads in the experiment group and ten parent-child dyads in the non-treatment control group. Their findings suggested large treatment effects of CPRT on decreasing African American children's behavioral problems and alleviating parenting stress of their parents. Outside of the United States, there has been one empirical study focusing on African children. Ojiambo and Bratton (2014) conducted a randomized controlled study to explore the effect of group activity play therapy on behavioral problems among 60 orphan pre-adolescents in Uganda. Their findings suggested moderate to large treatment effects of group activity play therapy for this specific population in Uganda.

Studies with Latino/Hispanic Populations

The number of empirical quantitative play therapy studies specially focusing on Latino/Hispanic children and families compared to those focusing on African American children and families is relatively higher. As early as the 1980s, Trostle (1988) published a study investigating group CCPT effect on 48 Puerto Rican children aged three to five years. The findings in this RCT study suggested the effect of group CCPT on enhancing children's self-control and free play. Lopez (2000) also conducted a small-scale pilot study exploring CCPT effect on improving academic achievement, self-concept, and internal behavioral problems among Hispanic students in second grade. Although the 15 students in the experimental group did not demonstrate higher academic improvement compared with the 15 students in the control group, their self-concept and internal behavioral problems improved after 16 CCPT sessions. Despite the small sample size and non-significant results in statistical analysis, this pilot study brought researchers' attention to play therapy effects on Latino/Hispanic populations. Garza and Bratton (2005) were interested in the therapeutic effect of CCPT on Hispanic children compared to an evidence-based small group curriculum-based intervention. In their RCT, they randomly assigned 15 Hispanic elementary students to the CCPT group and the other 14 to the small group intervention. The students in CCPT group demonstrated significantly greater improvement in both externalizing and internalizing behavior problems over students in the small group intervention. Their findings suggested moderate and large treatment effects of CCPT for Hispanic children's internalizing and externalizing behavioral concerns.

Villarreal (2008) conducted a small-scale quasi-experimental study investigating the effect of CPRT on Hispanic children's externalizing and internalizing behavioral concerns. Based on parental reports, the seven Hispanic children whose parents received CPRT improved statistically significantly in their externalizing and internalizing behaviors compared with the six Hispanic children in the control group. Ceballos and Bratton (2010) conducted a RCT study with 48 Latino immigrant families to further confirm the effect of CPRT on both children's behavioral concerns and parents' parenting stress. Similar to Villarreal's (2008) findings, Ceballos and Bratton (2010) reported large treatment effects for CPRT in reducing Latino immigrant children's externalizing, internalizing, and overall behavior problems. In addition, the Latino immigrant parents in the experimental group also reported statistically significant decreases in their parenting stress, revealing a large treatment effect.

McGee (2010) conducted an interesting study exploring the effect of CCPT provided by English-speaking clinicians on Spanish-speaking Hispanic children. In this RCT study, 34 Spanish-speaking children were randomly assigned to experimental and wait-list control groups. According to teachers' reports, children in the experimental group after the eight-week CCPT intervention demonstrated statistically significant improvement in their overall and externalizing behavior problems compared to children in the wait-list control group. The findings in this study suggested that CCPT may allow counselors to surmount language barriers with non-English-speaking children. Barcenas Jaimez (2017) followed a similar research agenda and conducted another RCT study with three treatment conditions: CCPT with counselors who speak both Spanish and English, CCPT with counselors who speak only English, and active control condition. Among the 57 Latina/o children in this study, more than 70% of the children who received CCPT from either English-speaking or bilingual counselors improved their behaviors from clinical to normal functioning while only 15% of the children in the active control group demonstrated similar improvement. The findings in Barcenas Jaimez's study not only supported the promising treatment effect of CCPT to Latina/o children but again confirmed the unique benefit of CCPT, enabling counselors to overcome language barriers.

Studies with Asian/Asian American Populations

There are many more empirical quantitative studies investigating play therapy effect on Asian child populations compared with the previous two specific populations. Some of them targeted Asian immigrant families in the U.S., but the others were conducted in Asian countries. In this section, we are unable to address all empirical quantitative studies focusing on Asian/ Asian American child populations but will provide brief summaries for some example studies.

One of the earliest empirical quantitative studies exclusively focusing on Asian/Asian American families might be Chau and Landreth's (1997) quasi-experimental study. They investigated the effectiveness of CPRT with 36 Chinese families in the United States. Although they did not explore children's improvement, their findings suggested that CPRT enhanced parent-child relationships and decreased these Chinese parents' parenting stress. Similarly, Yuen and colleagues (2002) published their RCT study on the effect of CPRT with 35 Chinese immigrant families in Canada. Their findings suggested that those Chinese immigrant parents in the experimental group significantly enhanced their empathic interaction with and acceptance of their children and lowered their parenting stress compared with the parents in the control group. In addition, the children of those parents in the experimental group also demonstrated a significant decrease in their behavioral problems and a significant increase in their self-concept. Jang (2000) and Lee and Landreth (2003) were also interested in the effect of CPRT, focusing their studies on Korean immigrant families in the United States. The findings in their studies also supported the effect of CPRT on reducing Korean immigrant parents' parenting stress and enhancing their empathic interaction with and acceptance of their children.

Outside of the United States, there have also been many empirical play therapy studies conducted in many different Asian countries. For example, Shen (2002) investigated the effect of short-term CCPT for 65 Taiwanese children impacted by an earthquake. Shen found that the Taiwanese children in the experimental group showed a significant decrease in their anxiety and suicide risk after CCPT treatment while the children in control group did not. Kidron and Landreth (2010) explored the effects of CPRT in Israel, particularly parents and children who suffered from long-term stress and trauma. In their study, the 14 parents in the experimental group significantly enhanced their empathy and acceptance toward their children and lowered their parenting stress after participating in an intensive version of CPRT while the 13 parents in the control group did not. Children of those parents in the experimental group also demonstrated a significant improvement in their externalizing behavior problems compared to children of parents in the control group.

In play therapy literature, there have been many empirical studies conducted in India and Iran as compared to other Asian countries. For example, Shashi and colleagues (1999) published a RCT study evaluating the effect of nondirective play therapy in helping Indian children with emotional disturbance. Although their study was based on very small sample size (N=10), their encouraging findings suggested treatment effect of play therapy on reducing Indian children's emotional distress. In Iran, Ebrahimi and colleagues (2019) conducted the first RCT study that investigated the effect of

CPRT with mothers and their children diagnosed with cancer. Despite the relatively small sample size, the 16 mothers in the experimental group showed significant decrease in their depression, anxiety, and stress after the parenting intervention training while the other 16 mothers in the control group did not. Similarly, the depression level of the 16 children in the experimental group also decreased significantly while the other 16 children in the control group revealed no change.

Studies with Other Racially/Ethnically Diverse Populations

There are very limited empirical studies investigating play therapy effect on other diverse populations or cultures. We were able to identify only two studies in the play therapy literature, one targeting Native American families and the other one focusing on families in Germany and both focused on CPRT rather than CCPT. Glover and Landreth (2000) conducted a quasi-experimental study investigating the effect of CPRT on 21 Native American families. Despite the limited sample size, their findings suggested promising treatment effect of the parenting intervention on enhancing parental acceptance and empathy in Native American parents as well as increasing desirable play behaviors in their children. Grskovic and Goetze (2008) conducted a quasi-experimental study exploring the effect of an intense version of filial therapy on 33 pairs of German mothers and children. In their intense filial therapy, the parenting training program lasted for two weeks. In addition to the training, the mothers were required to provide five play sessions with their children within the two weeks. The findings in this quasi-experimental study suggested encouraging effect of this intense filial therapy on decreasing German children's internalizing and overall behavioral problems, enhancing German mothers' positive attention and nondirective response toward their children.

These quantitative research findings were brief summaries from either RCTs or quasi-experimental studies in the literature of humanistic play therapy. Although it is not a comprehensive review, the research findings in these individual studies clearly support the effectiveness of humanistic play therapy to racially/ethnically diverse children and parents. At the same time, we would like to also recognize the limitations of these quantitative research findings. First of all, the sample sizes in almost all of the aforementioned studies were small (less than 60 total participants). This small sample size issue may limit the generalization of the study results. Secondly, the majority of the studies we summarized utilized racially/ethnically diverse play therapists. We are thus unable to conclude whether or not there is a difference between the effect of humanistic play therapy provided by White therapists and therapists with other races or ethnicities. Thirdly, the majority of the empirical studies for humanistic play therapy were conducted within the United States. This also limits the generalizability of the findings in these studies to racially/ethnically diverse populations in other countries.

Qualitative Research Support for the Impact and Process of Play Therapy with Racially and Ethnically Diverse Populations

Although not as numerous as quantitative research, there exists a small amount of literature supporting the impact of humanistic play therapy with racially and ethnically diverse population using qualitative methodology, mainly from child-centered play therapy (CCPT) and child-parent relationship therapy (CPRT) approaches.

Child–Centered Play Therapy

Most qualitative studies in regard to child-centered play therapy were conducted utilizing group play therapy. For example, Su and Tsai (2016) examined the use of group play therapy with new immigrants in Taiwan using a mixed-method design. Eight children participated in the study, and they were divided into a treatment and control group. Children in the treatment group received (CCGPT) for 12-weeks. To collect qualitative data, the children and teachers were interviewed before and after the conclusion of group play therapy. Interview results revealed three themes: control, affection, and acceptance. Children who received group play therapy appeared to have more self-control and were better able to follow social norms at the end of treatment. Compared to the control group, children in the treatment group reported more positive feelings like happiness and having fun with friends after their treatment. Lastly, children who participated in group play therapy reported being better able to accept themselves, such as an increased acceptance in self-behavior, others, and increased confidence (Su & Tsai, 2016).

CCGPT has also been used with school-aged North Korean refugees living in South Korea (Kwon & Lee, 2018). Four North Korean refugee girls participated in group play therapy for 40 sessions. Data were collected by interviewing caregivers and teachers as well as changes in children's play. Overall, parents verbally reported that their children showed a reduction in their anxiety and depression symptoms, an improvement in their attention, and increased frequency of age-appropriate play after the intervention. Additionally, verbal reports indicated that children who showed externalizing behaviors exhibited a decrease in aggressive behaviors and increased empathy toward others. On the other hand, verbal reports also indicated that children who showed internalizing behaviors improved on their emotional expression as well as a decrease in withdrawal behaviors (Kwon & Lee, 2018).

Child–Parent Relationship Therapy (CPRT)/Filial Therapy

The process and impact of CPRT/filial therapy with racially/ethnically diverse populations appears to be positive when explored through qualitative methods.

For example, Solis and colleagues (2004) conducted a qualitative case study with an African American mother, Judy, and her six-year-old son, Dylan. Dylan's teacher raised some concerns regarding Dylan's restlessness, struggles with following rules, and difficulty focusing in class. Judy shared that she recently went through divorce and that Dylan is adjusting to the father's inconsistent presence in Dylan's life. Judy underwent filial therapy and was interviewed before and after the intervention. Judy also had to complete questionnaires and unstructured journals as additional data points. Solis et al. concluded that Dylan's self-esteem had improved at the end of filial therapy. Furthermore, Judy reported an increase in her awareness and understanding of Dylan's feelings and thoughts. However, Judy reported her struggle with maintaining a permissive and nondirective environment. She expressed wanting to be more directive when Dylan was playing aggressively and when she found herself bored in session (Solis et al., 2004). Discomfort with children's aggressive play is not unique to African American parents (e.g. Kale & Landreth, 1999). Thus, understanding parents' concern regarding creating and maintaining a permissive environment from their cultural context may strengthen the therapist-client relationship, which would then enhance the parent-child relationship.

In further exploration of the process of CPRT with African American parents, Socarras and colleagues (2015) recruited six African American parent-child dyads who completed a four-week CPRT program. Parents were interviewed before and after CPRT intervention. Apart from interviews, additional data points included videotaped segments of parents' play session and field notes taken by the research team. Themes that emerged from the interview included having a close bond to their children, applying CPRT skills to their parenting, and gaining a better understanding of their children's play (Socarras et al., 2015).

Edwards and colleagues (2007) also documented perceptions of filial therapy through a qualitative case study on an immigrant Jamaican mother, Patricia, and her four-year-old daughter, Jodi. Utilizing multiple data points (e.g. interviews, videotapes of play session, observation of parent-child interaction, parent's journal etc.), Edwards et al. investigated Patricia's perception of filial therapy. At the end of filial therapy, Patricia reported an increase in empathy and awareness to Jodi's needs, which strengthened the parent-child relationship. Despite Patricia's greater acceptance of skills learned in filial therapy, she also reported continuous use of spanking, which is considered an integral component to disciplining children among Jamaicans (Edwards et al., 2007). Therefore, it behooves play therapists to consider clients' cultural context and perhaps increase play therapists' acceptance and appreciation of different parenting practices, as opposed to imposing values onto parents.

Sangganjanavanich et al. (2010) conducted a phenomenological study on perceptions of effectiveness of filial therapy with monolingual Spanish-speaking mothers (Sangganjanavanich et al., 2010). Four mothers (three immigrated from Mexico and one from Peru) participated in a five-week filial therapy training. The mothers were interviewed after filial therapy to understand if there were changes in their child's behavior, any changes to mother's attitude, and changes in the child's relationship with others. Qualitative analysis revealed there was an improvement in parent-child relationships. However, mothers reported mixed findings in regards to their child's behavior after filial therapy with three of the mothers reporting either there was no change in child's behavior or behaviors worsened. Only one mother reported improvement in her child's behavior. Sangganjanavanich et al. concluded that the five-week training may have been too short a time to see changes in the child's behavior

Interestingly, Garza and colleagues (2009) found that Latinx parents who participated in CPRT reported changes in their children's behavior. In their study, three parents agreed to be interviewed after completing a ten-week CPRT program. All of the parents immigrated from Mexico and had been in the United States for at least nine years. Participants reported that their children were less resistant, calmer, and listened more after CPRT. Parents also reported increased warmth, decreased frustration, and increased sense of parenting self-efficacy which improved the overall parent-child relationship (Garza et al., 2009).

Hassey and colleagues (2016) provided support for CPRT with affluent Mexican immigrant parents. In their study, 14 parent-child dyads participated in a ten-session CPRT program. Incorporating a culturally inclusive component to intervention, a specialized time for *platica* (building trust via dialogues) was added to each session. Parents were interviewed in Spanish after the completion of CPRT program. All parents reported an increase in understanding their children's thoughts, emotions, and behaviors. Furthermore, all participants reported an improvement in the parent-child relationship. Interestingly, eight out of 14 parents expressed their appreciation for the program being conducted in their native language, Spanish (Hassey et al., 2016). Taken together, CPRT can be effective with this population when incorporating culturally inclusive elements (e.g. language, adding discussion time).

Extending the evidence of CPRT, Lim and Ogawa (2014) used a case study to investigate the perceived effect of CPRT with a Sudanese refugee family. John came to the United States as a refugee and had concerns about his son's behavior. According to John, his son, Chuol, exhibited aggressive behaviors, which was uncharacteristic of a Sudanese child. After attending eight weeks of CPRT, John noticed a positive change in Chuol's behavior at home. As Chuol felt more understood and accepted by John, there was a diminished need to exhibit problematic behaviors (Lim & Ogawa, 2014). This change was also captured via John's response on the behavioral assessment, which moved from the borderline/clinical ranges in a few areas (e.g. conduct problems, aggressive behaviors) to average ranges following CPRT.

Summary

To summarize our findings so far regarding qualitative research, we found two articles that documented the positive impact CCGPT (Kwon & Lee, 2018; Su and Tsai, 2016). Unfortunately, these studies were conducted outside the United States. Therefore, transferability of research findings (i.e. themes found in studies) to racially and ethnically diverse populations in the United States should be done with extreme caution. Surprisingly, there are more CPRT qualitative research studies that have been published as compared to CCPT studies, consistently documenting the positive effect of CPRT on improving the parent-child relationship (e.g. Hassey et al., 2016; Socarras et al., 2015). An important theme across the different CPRT research was the facilitators' intentions for cultural inclusivity, ranging from conducting sessions in participants' native language to considering participants' cultural context.

Conclusion

This chapter provided support for the effectiveness and impact of play therapy with racially and ethnically diverse populations. Based on both quantitative and qualitative research findings in the literature, humanistic play therapy appears to be an effective intervention with racially and ethnically diverse children. Our review in the quantitative research reveals that almost all the empirical play therapy studies that specifically targeted diverse populations were exploring the effects of CCPT and CPRT/filial therapy. We also noticed that although researchers have investigated play therapy effect on diverse populations within the United States, there have been a limited number of empirical play therapy studies conducted in other countries, with the majority of these studies conducted in India and Iran. In reviewing the qualitative research, we found that many practitioners incorporated some form of cultural inclusivity into their interventions including having culturally appropriate toys (e.g. Baggerly & Parker, 2005), conducting sessions in clients' native language (e.g. Hassey et al., 2016; Sangganjanavanich et al., 2010), and integrating clients' cultural background into delivery of intervention (e.g. Baggerly & Parker, 2005; Hassey et al., 2016). Although cultural inclusivity in itself (diverse toys, language) may not necessarily be the vehicle of change in the therapeutic process, we believe that a multicultural orientation conveys therapists' care in a meaningful and concrete manner, strengthens the therapeutic relationship, and results in greater likelihood of positive therapeutic outcomes.

To end this chapter, we offer a few directions for researchers in the field of play therapy to strengthen knowledge regarding serving children of diverse racial/ethnic backgrounds and broaden our knowledge to broader cultural considerations:

a   Conduct more quantitative research, particularly empirical studies, on the effectiveness of play therapy with diverse families. Studies identified and reviewed for this chapter were conducted mostly within the United States, indicating necessary attention to non-dominant racial/ethnic groups within the larger system. However, more empirical studies that explore the effectiveness of play therapy in other countries would provide deeper understanding of needs of children within and outside of the United States.

b   Conduct more quantitative research, particularly empirical studies, for the effect of other play therapy models on diverse populations. The majority of the empirical play therapy studies specifically on diverse populations were based on CCPT and CPRT/filial therapy. The play therapy literature needs empirical studies on cultural inclusivity of other humanistic play therapy interventions, such as Gestalt play therapy, Jungian play therapy, humanistic sandtray therapy, etc.

c   Conduct more qualitative and mixed-method research on the impact of play therapy with racially and ethnically diverse children. Our review found only two articles of CCGPT and those were conducted outside the United States. Increasing qualitative and mixed-method research on racially and ethnically diverse children in the United States will provide a richer and deeper understanding of themes that arise from humanistic play therapy. Qualitative data can be gathered from parents, teachers, caregivers, peers, and the client before and after play therapy. Interview techniques such as "Write, Draw, Show, and Tell" can be used to elicit information from children as part of data collection methods, which can greatly enhance our understanding of their healing process.

d   Increase research on the impact of culturally inclusive interventions. For example, a bilingual play therapist can provide CCPT to two different groups of children, with one group receiving therapy in their native language and the other in English. Comparing the effect size and clinical significance between the two groups could provide information regarding the importance of native language in the playroom. The same research design can be used to examine the inclusion of culturally diverse toys in the playroom.

e   Document other aspects of clients' identity such as SES, religion/spirituality, family structure, disability status, etc. Most research being conducted with "diverse" children is specific to racial and ethnic diversity. By documenting other aspects of identity, and targeting identities that lacks research findings, we can further support the effectiveness of play therapy to children from diverse backgrounds (not just racially and ethnically diverse).

f   Increase studies (both quantitative and qualitative) on play therapists' implicit racism in working with racially and ethnically diverse children. Given that the U.S. health service psychology workforce is 88% White, the historically White mental health field may have implicit norms on ways to conduct therapy that marginalizes people of color (e.g. Hook et al., 2017; Owen et al., 2016). Having more research on play therapists' implicit racism is therefore crucial in anti-racism effort.

g   Conduct more qualitative research studies on how racism/systemic bias/oppression is manifested in children's play. Various qualitative approaches to observing themes in session may provide valuable information on how children play out experiences and perceptions of racism and oppression.

h   Diversify the field of play therapy and increase the number of diverse play therapists. While reviewing both quantitative and qualitative research on this topic, we were surprised at the small number of play therapy studies specifically focusing on racially and ethnically diverse populations. We further noted that most of the researchers in these studies themselves are from diverse backgrounds. Aside from their passion in helping their communities, perhaps they had an "in" with the community, which facilitated the recruitment of participants. Therefore, the diversification of play therapists may facilitate the increase of research with diverse populations.

Positionality Statements

Yung-Wei Dennis

I am an Associate Professor in a public university in the northeast of the United States. I originally came from Taiwan and completed my play therapy and counselor education training at the University of North Texas (UNT). With my undergraduate degree in statistics, I have been mainly involved in quantitative research since my PhD training at UNT. I also conducted a meta-analytic study for CCPT, which was published in 2015. When I was at UNT providing play therapy to children either in the community counseling centers on campus or in the local pre- and elementary schools, I clearly experienced the therapeutic power of humanistic play therapy to my child clients. Even when I recognized the cultural differences between myself and my child clients (I still remember that my poor English pronunciation was corrected by my child clients so many times), I was still able to closely work with them in playrooms through the humanistic perspectives and observe their change and growth.

Since I started my career as a counselor educator, I have mainly focused on play therapy training and research and have not been doing clinical practice. Humanistic play therapy, especially CCPT, has a long research history and all the research findings have clearly demonstrated its treatment effectiveness. From my research experience, however, I am also fully aware of more and more needs in play therapy research. For example, research has demonstrated the general effectiveness, but researchers have not yet explored the specific therapeutic factors/components in humanistic play therapy; researchers have not yet empirically demonstrated the selection of toys in the playroom; researchers have not yet discovered the unique cultural meanings in child's play behaviors... etc. I can probably continue this list forever.

Terence

I am an Assistant Professor who completed my play therapy training at the University of North Texas. I am an international counselor educator from Malaysia. As an immigrant to the United States, I am acutely aware of the ways race and immigration status play a role in one's development. From a humanistic perspective, the being of the play therapist cannot be separated from the doing. As a counselor educator, I explore my students' beliefs and implicit attitudes because it affects their being.

For example, I recently discussed with my students how they would respond if a child asked them if they believed in Santa Claus. Most of them stated they would reflect the child's curiosity. Most, if not all, hesitated to answer honestly because there is an unspoken rule about who gets to break the Santa Claus bubble. The students' being is affected by their beliefs and implicit attitudes regarding who has the privilege of telling the truth to the child.

For play therapists to be a healing being, I reckon that we need to examine our implicit biases towards children of color. What are our beliefs about an Asian child, a Black child, a child who is an immigrant? How would we answer if our child clients ask us about our stance on Black Lives Matter? Or if we believe in Allah? How would we respond if parents were to ask us on our anti-racist practices in relation to therapy? Apart from our implicit biases and attitudes, we also need to question societal norms and ways of doing that are so ingrained, often accepted as a way of life. Why is it that most play therapists are White? What are some barriers for people of color to be trained as play therapists and to receive the Registered Play Therapist credential?

My musings lead me to one answer which can support change and advocacy: research. By doing more research, we can know more about how play therapists can mitigate the influence of racism on children, how to be better play therapists, and how to diversify the field of play therapy. Research holds the key to bettering us and the field.

References

American Counseling Association (2014). 2014 ACA Code of Ethics. Retrieved from www.counseling.org/resources/aca-code-of-ethics.pdf.

American Psychological Association (2017). Ethical Principles of Psychologists and Code of Conduct: Including 2010 and 2016 Amendments. Retrieved from www.apa.org/ethics/code.

Baggerly, J., & Parker, M. (2005). Child-centered group play therapy with African American boys at the elementary school level. *Journal of Counseling & Development*, 83(4), 387–396. doi:10.1002/j.1556-6678.2005.tb00360.x.

Barcenas Jaimez, G. (2017). *Child-Centered Play Therapy with Latina/o children exhibiting school behavior problems: Comparative effects of delivery by Spanish-speaking and*

English-speaking counselors [Unpublished doctoral dissertation]. University of North Texas.

Bratton, S., Ray, D., Rhine, T., & Jones, L. (2005). The efficacy of play therapy with children: A meta-analytic review of treatment outcomes. *Professional Psychology: Research and Practice*, 36(4), 367–390. doi:10.1037/0735-7028.36.4.376.

Ceballos, P., & Bratton, S. C. (2010). School-based child-parent relationship therapy (CPRT) with low-income first-generation immigrant Latino parents: Effects on children's behaviors and parent-child relationship stress. *Psychology in the Schools*, 47(8), 761–775.

Chau, I., & Landreth, G. (1997). Filial therapy with Chinese parents: Effects on parental empathic interactions, parental acceptance of child and parental stress. *International Journal of Play Therapy*, 6(2), 75–92. doi:10.1037/h0089409.

Cohen, J. (1988). *Statistical power analysis for the behavioral sciences* (2nd ed.). Lawrence Erlbaum.

Ebrahimi, E., Mirzaie, H., Borujeni, M. S., Zahed, G., Baghban, A. A., & Mirzakhani, N. (2019). The effect of filial therapy on depressive symptoms of children with cancer and their mother's depression, anxiety, and stress: A randomized controlled trial. *Asian Pacific Journal of Cancer Prevention*, 20(10), 2935–2941.

Edwards, N. A., Ladner, J., & White, J. (2007). Perceived effectiveness of filial therapy for a Jamaican mother: A qualitative case study. *International Journal of Play Therapy*, 16(1), 36–53. doi:10.1037/1555-6824.16.1.36.

Garza, Y., & Bratton, S. C. (2005). School-based child-centered play therapy with Hispanic children: Outcomes and cultural considerations. *International Journal of Play Therapy*, 14, 51–79. doi:10.1037/h0088896.

Garza, Y., Kinsworthy, S., & Watts, R.E. (2009). Child-parent relationship training as experienced by Hispanic parents: A phenomenological study. *International of Play Therapy*, 18, 217–228. doi:10.1037/a0017055.

Glass, G. (1976). Primary, secondary, and meta-analysis of research. *Educational Researcher*, 5(10), 3–8.

Glover, G., & Landreth, G. (2000). Filial therapy with Native Americans on the Flathead Reservation. *International Journal of Play Therapy*, 9(2), 57–80. doi:10.1037/h0089436.

Grskovic, J., & Goetze, H. (2008). Short-term filial therapy with German mothers: Findings from a controlled study. *International Journal of Play Therapy*, 17(1), 39–51. doi:10.1037/1555-6824.17.1.39.

Hassey, F., Garza, Y., Sullivan, J. M., & Serres, S. (2016). Affluent Mexican immigrant parents' perceptions of child–parent relationship training. *International Journal of Play Therapy*, 25(3), 114–122. doi:10.1037/pla0000028.

Hook, J. N., Davis, D., Owen, J., & DeBlaere, C. (2017). *Cultural humility: Engaging in diverse identities in therapy*. American Psychological Association.

Jang, M. (2000). Effectiveness of filial therapy for Korean parents. *International Journal of Play Therapy*, 9(2), 39–56. doi:10.1037/h0089435.

Kale, A. L., & Landreth, G. L. (1999). Filial therapy with parents of children experiencing learning difficulties. *International Journal of Play Therapy*, 8(2), 35–56. doi:10.1037/h0089430.

Kidron, M, & Landreth, G. (2010). Intensive child parent relationship therapy with Israeli parents in Israel. *International Journal of Play Therapy*, 19(2), 64–78. doi:10.1037/a0017516.

Kwon, Y. J., & Lee, K. (2018). Group child-centered play therapy for school-aged North Korean refugee children. *International Journal of Play Therapy*, 27(4), 256–271. doi:10.1037/pla0000077.

Landreth, G. (2012). *Play therapy: The art of the relationship* (3rd ed.). Routledge.

Landreth, G. L., & Bratton, S. C. (2020). *Child parent relationship therapy: (Cprt): a 10-session filial therapy model* (2nd ed.). Routledge.

LeBlanc, M., & Ritchie, M. (2001). A meta-analysis of play therapy outcomes. *Counseling Psychology Quarterly*, 14, 149–163. doi:10.1080/09515070110059142.

Lee, M., & Landreth, G. (2003). Filial therapy with immigrant Korean parents in the United States. *International Journal of Play Therapy*, 12(2), 67–85. doi:10.1037/h0088879.

Lim, S., & Ogawa, Y. (2014). "Once I had kids, now I am raising kids": Child-parent relationship therapy (CPRT) with a Sudanese refugee family – a case study. *International Journal of Play Therapy*, 23(2), 70–89. doi:10.1037/a0036362.

Lin, Y., & Bratton, S. C. (2015). A meta-analytic review of child-centered play therapy approaches. *Journal of Counseling and Development*, 93(1), 45–58. doi:10.1002/j.1556-6676.2015.00180.x.

Lipsey, M. W., & Wilson, D. B. (2001). *Practical meta-analysis*. Sage.

Lopez, H. T. (2000). *The effects of a therapeutic play intervention on Hispanic students' reading achievement, self-concept, and behavior* (Publication No. 3056916) [Doctoral dissertation, University of North Texas]. ProQuest Dissertations and Theses Global.

Manoharam, B. P. (2020). Effectiveness of play therapy in the behavioral response of children with burns during wound dressing. *Asian Journal of Nursing Education and Research*, 10(4), 517–520.

McGee, L. (2010). *The efficacy of Child-Centered Play Therapy with Hispanic Spanish-speaking children when conducted by a monolingual English-speaking counselor* (Publication No. 3430297) [Doctoral dissertation, Texas A&M University-Commerce]. ProQuest Dissertations and Theses Global.

McLeod, B. D., Islam, N. Y., & Wheat, E. (2013). Designing, conducting, and evaluating therapy process research. In J. S. Comer & P. C. Kendall (Eds.), *The Oxford handbook of research strategies for clinical psychology* (p. 459). Oxford University Press.

Naderi, F., Heidarie, A., Bouron, L., & Asgari, P. (2010). The efficacy of play therapy on ADHD, anxiety and social maturity in 8 to 12 years aged clientele children of Ahwaz metropolitan counseling clinics. *Journal of Applied Sciences*, 10(3) 189–195.

Nezu, A. M, & Nezu, C. M. (2008). Ensuring treatment integrity. In A. M. Nezu & C. M. Nezu (Eds.), *Evidence-based outcome research: A practical guide to conducting randomized controlled trials for psychosocial interventions* (pp. 263–281). Oxford University Press.

Ojiambo, D., Bratton, S. C. (2014). Effect of group activity play therapy on problem behaviors of preadolescent Ugandan orphans. *Journal of Counseling and Development*, 92(3), 355–365. doi:10.1002/j.1556-6676.2014.00163.x.

Olson, J. (2016). A trauma-informed approach to play therapy interventions with African American male children. In W. Ross (Ed.), *Counseling African American males: Effective therapeutic interventions and approaches* (pp. 237–251). Information Age Publishing.

Owen, J., Drinane, J. M., Davis, D. E., Tao, K. W., Hook, J., & Kune, N. F. (2016). Client perceptions of therapists' multicultural orientation: Cultural (missed) opportunities and cultural humility. *Professional Psychology: Research and Practice*, 47, 30–37. doi:10.1037/pro0000046.

Patterson, L., Stutey, D. M., & Dorsey, B. (2018). Play therapy with African American children exposed to adverse childhood experiences. *International Journal of Play Therapy*, 27(4), 215–226. doi:10.1037/pla0000080.

Prout, T. A., Bernstein, M., Gaines, E., Aizin, S., Sessler, D., Racine, E., Spigelman, A., Rice, T. R., Hoffman, L. (2020). Regulation focused psychotherapy for children in clinical practice: Case vignettes from psychotherapy outcome studies. *International Journal of Play Therapy*, 29(1), 43–53. doi:10.1037/pla0000111.

Ray, D. C., Armstrong, S. A., Balkin, R. S., & Jayne, K. M. (2015). Child-centered play therapy in the schools: Review and meta-analysis. *Psychology in the Schools*, 52 (2), 107–123. doi:10.1002/pits.21798.

Sangganjanavanich, V. F., Cook, K., & Rangel-Gomez, M. (2010). Filial therapy with monolingual Spanish-speaking mothers: A phenomenological study. *The Family Journal*, 18(2), 195–201. doi:10.1177/1066480710364320.

Schneider, C., & Jones, E. E. (2009). *Child Psychotherapy Q-Set coding manual*. University of California.

Shashi, K., Kapur, M., & Subbakrishna, D. K. (1999). Evaluation of play therapy in emotionally disturbed children. *NIMHANS Journal*, 17(2), 99–111.

Sheely-Moore, A., & Bratton, S. (2010). A strength-based parenting intervention with low-income African American families. *Professional School Counseling*, 13(3), 175–183 doi:10.1177/2156759X1001300305.

Sheely-Moore, A., & Ceballos, P. (2011). Empowering head start African American and Latino families: Promoting strengths-based parenting characteristics through Child Parent Relationship Training: An evidence-based group parenting program. *A Research-to-Practice Journal for the Early Childhood Field*, 14(1), 41–53. doi:10.1080/15240754.2010.541567.

Shen, Y. (2002). Short-term group play therapy with Chinese earthquake victims: Effects on anxiety, depression, and adjustment. *International Journal of Play Therapy*, 11(1), 43–63. doi:10.1037/h0088856.

Socarras, K., Smith-Adcock, S., & Shin, S. M. (2015). A qualitative study of an intensive filial intervention using child–parent relationship therapy (CPRT). *The Family Journal*, 23(4), 381–391. doi:10.1177/1066480715601681.

Solis, C. M., Meyers, J., & Varjas, K. M. (2004). A qualitative case study of the process and impact of filial therapy with an African American parent. *International Journal of Play Therapy*, 13(2), 99–118. doi:10.1037/h0088892.

Su, S., & Tsai, M. (2016). Group play therapy with children of new immigrants in Taiwan who are exhibiting relationship difficulties. *International Journal of Play Therapy*, 25(2), 91–101. doi:10.1037/pla0000014.

Taylor, L., & Ray, D. C. (2021). Child-centered play therapy and social-emotional competencies of African American children: A randomized controlled trial. *International Journal of Play Therapy*, 30(2), 74–85.

Trostle, S. (1988). The effects of child-centered group play sessions on social-emotional growth of three- to six-year-old bilingual Puerto Rican children. *Journal of Research in Childhood Education*, 3, 93–106.

Villarreal, C. E. (2008). *School-based Child Parent Relationship Therapy (CPRT) with Hispanic parents* (Publication No. 3302011) [Doctoral dissertation, University of North Texas]. ProQuest Dissertations and Theses Global.

Whiston, S. C., & Li, P. (2011). Meta-analysis: A systematic method for synthesizing counseling research. *Journal of Counseling and Development*, 89 (3), 273–281.

Yee, T., Ceballos, P., & Swan, A. (2019). Examining the trends of play therapy articles: A 10-year content analysis. *International Journal of Play Therapy*, 28(4), 250–260. doi:10.1037/pla0000103.

Yuen, T., Landreth, G., & Baggerly, J. (2002). Filial therapy with immigrant Chinese families. *International Journal of Play Therapy*, 11(2), 63–90. doi:10.1037/h0088865.

Appendix: Reflective Questions

This appendix consists of reflective questions proposed by the chapter authors with the intent to facilitate play therapists' self-awareness in moving forward on the journey of cultivating cultural humility and cultural comfort. We focus on the reflective questions from the chapters centering on group populations and special topics given that these questions have incorporated the concepts and ideas from those chapters discussing cultural humility, cultural opportunities and comfort, and social justice. The questions are organized by chapter and play therapists are encouraged to incorporate journaling, expressive arts, or other forms of creativity in their process of exploration.

Chapter 4: Cultural Opportunities with LGBTQIA Populations

1   Consider aspects and experiences of nature (biology) nurture (development and socialization), and culture and context that have informed and helped create your own understanding of gender and your gender identity. Draw, paint, write, or make a sandtray of your own gender web.
2   What are your current beliefs, attitudes, values, biases, about gender? Sexuality?
3   Consider the context and environment of your play therapy practice (building, playroom, toys/materials, etc.). What are specific actions you may take to make your play therapy practice affirming for LGBTQIA children and families?
4   Consider your play therapy relationships and interventions (language, nonverbal and verbal skills, attitudinal conditions, relational dynamics, etc.). What are specific actions you may take to make your play therapy practice more affirming for LGBTQIA children and families?
5   When in your play therapy practice have you experienced barriers in the relationship related to gender? Sexuality? When have you experienced opportunities and transformation?

Chapter 5: Cultural Opportunities with Religious Populations

1   Where would you assess your own level of religiosity? How much does it or does it not play into your day-to-day life?

2   What comes up for you when you hear about clients who are fundamentalist? Muslim? Jewish? Mormon? Christian?

3   When working with a client with a different religion or level of religious affiliation, what challenges have come up for you? How have you successfully navigated this relationship?

4   What system would be more challenging for you to work with? Why? Which might feel more accessible? Why?

5   Think about potential clients from various religions. What do you feel in your body as you imagine these parents/caregivers telling you about their religious beliefs or the child acting out a religious practice in session?

Chapter 6: Cultural Opportunities with Children with Disabilities

1   What training and supervision experiences have prepared you to work competently and ethically with children with impairments?

2   How has the medical model of disability impacted your understanding of working with children with variabilities?

3   As a result of what you have learned from reading this chapter, how can you enhance your scope of competence for working with children with impairments in play therapy?

Chapter 7: Cultural Opportunities with Indigenous Populations

1   How is child-centered play therapy compatible with Native People's values?

2   What is an Adverse Childhood Experiences (ACEs) score and how can it be used to inform services for Native children and their families?

3   Identify some of the historical factors that have negatively impacted Native families and discuss how this legacy continues to impact on children and families.

4   What specific interventions or recommendations might be effective when working with Native families?

Chapter 8: Cultural Opportunities with African American Populations

1   How has the Black Lives Matter movement shaped your experience and perceptions of the African American community?

2   In what ways can you advocate for this population in your local community? In your profession?

3   How has the media influenced your perceptions of the African American community?

4   After completing this chapter, what are some steps you can take to better engage with your African American client and their family that remains culturally empathic?

Chapter 9: Cultural Opportunities with Latinx Populations

1   How can you better support and advocate for the Latinx population in and out of the playroom?

2   How comfortable are you with the possibility of physical touch and increased self-disclosure within a cultural context? What are your thoughts and beliefs about physical touch and self-disclosure?

3   Are the toys you currently have an accurate cultural representation of the diverse children that will enter this room?

4   What Latinx leaders and community advocates can you build a relationship with to provide additional support for Latinx clients? To support advocacy for systemic change?

Chapter 10: Cultural Opportunities with Asian Populations

1   Given the variability among the Asian population, can you identify ethnic groups that you find yourself needing continuing learning and exploration in?

2   When thinking about working with child clients and their families from Asian cultural backgrounds, what are your initial thoughts, feelings, and body reactions? What might these reactions be telling you about your attitudes, beliefs, assumptions, and/or biases about this population?

3   Imagine when you hear an Asian parent say, "Our family is very traditional." What comes to your mind? What are some assumptions you hold about the expectations within this family? Reflect on how you would clarify whether your understanding of this parent is accurate.

4   When you are trying to put together a playroom that is culturally inclusive and sensitive to Asian cultures, what toys and/or play materials come to your mind? How can you refrain from being stereotypical about the toys you select?

5   (For non-Asian readers) What was your first exposure to an Asian? Was it your neighbor? Friend? Classmate? Movie? Literature? Or in any other context? Did it impact your perception of this population? If so, how?

6   (For Asian readers) What was your environment growing up? Was it a big Asian community or were you a minority surrounded Whites or by other minority groups? Did it impact your perception of Asians? If so, how?

Chapter 11: Cultural Opportunities with Middle Eastern Populations

1   What was your experience of the 9/11 terrorist attacks, and how have your perceptions of Middle Eastern Americans changed as a result?
2   How have portrayals of Middle Eastern individuals in the media impacted your understanding of this population?
3   What is your comfort level in working with parents whose parenting strategies may differ from yours in relation to level of strictness, role of education, and expectations?
4   As a result of reading this chapter, what are ways in which you can engage in advocacy for this population?

Chapter 12: Becoming a Culturally Inclusive White Play Therapist

1   Take a minute to reflect on the last webinar, conference session, or university class you attended. Who was in attendance? Who was presenting? What did they look like?
2   Take a minute to review Table 1 in Chapter 12 and identify where you were given unearned or earned privilege? Also identify your points of oppression.
3   What does being a White play therapist mean to you? What do you need to do to counteract your cultural norms that hold Whites to privilege and power?
4   From an epistemological perspective, consider: whose voices and knowledge are included in the planning, assessment, and play therapy sessions for a particular client or family?
5   Leaning into cultural humility, how might you embrace an opportunity to discuss race and culture in parent consultations?
6   Whom do you consult with related to your play therapy practice? What are the racial/ethnic identities of individuals of whom you are receiving direction and perspective?

Chapter 13: Play Therapy with Children in Poverty

1   What are your own experiences of class privilege and/or oppression? How have these influenced your values and worldview?
2   What challenges to accurate empathic understanding may emerge when working with children experiencing poverty? How can you work to address these?
3   Reflect on the societal messages you have received about those in poverty. How may these influence your perspectives of children in poverty? Parents?

4   What logistical barriers to access for families in poverty can you identify in your current (or ideal) counseling position? What steps can you take to advocate for the removal of these barriers?

Chapter 14: Inclusive Play Therapy Supervision

1   How would you rate your knowledge of and comfort with discussing cultural issues with supervisees?
2   Do you talk about race in supervision?
3   What was your earliest experience with racism? What impact did this experience have on you at that time? Does your earliest experience with racism still have an impact on you today?
4   Why is it important for us to be aware of our privilege? Why don't we (have to) attend to it on a regular basis?
5   What does it mean for us to have multiple, intersecting identities – where we experience some privileges (around some identities) and some oppression (around others)?
6   What insight can an awareness of our privilege give us in connecting with our supervisees or clients?

Chapter 15: The Multicultural Playroom: A Delphi Study

1   In what ways does your playroom environment remain consistent with results from this chapter? In what ways does it differ?
2   Considering your own cultural exploration, describe how this chapter may affect your cultural humility.
3   Considering the results of this chapter, how might you continue to add to the progression of cultural inclusion by the field of play therapy?
4   How have your experiences with your clientele shaped your cultural awareness? What have been some adaptations made to your playroom based off these experiences?
5   Cultural humility, particularly in the playroom, is an ongoing, ever evolving process. How might you continue to remain culturally empathetic as you practice/teach play therapy topics?
6   What are some collective ways the play therapy field as a whole can work together to move the field towards cultural inclusion?
7   After completing this chapter, how might you consider adapting your playroom, research topics, advocacy plan, or curriculum to be more culturally inclusive?
8   Can you think of additional materials not included in this chapter that you think may enhance the play experience that remains culturally inclusive?
9   How might this chapter challenge your ideas of a multiculturally inclusive playroom?

Index

Note: Page numbers in *italic* refer to author positionality statements; page numbers in **bold** refer to tables

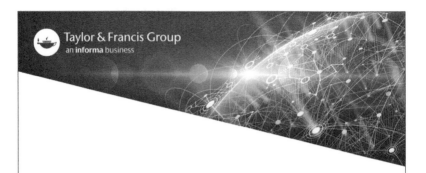

For Product Safety Concerns and Information please contact our
EU representative GPSR@taylorandfrancis.com Taylor & Francis
Verlag GmbH, Kaufingerstraße 24, 80331 München, Germany